INFORMAL NORMS IN GLOBAL GOVERNANCE

T0271998

Global Health

Series Editor: Professor Nana K. Poku,
John Ferguson Professor, University of Bradford, UK

The benefits of globalization are potentially enormous, as a result of the increased sharing of ideas, cultures, life-saving technologies and efficient production processes. Yet globalization is under trial, partly because these benefits are not yet reaching hundreds of millions of the world's poor and partly because globalization has introduced new kinds of international problems and conflicts. Turmoil in one part of the world now spreads rapidly to others, through terrorism, armed conflict, environmental degradation or disease.

This timely series provides a robust and multi-disciplinary assessment of the asymmetrical nature of globalization. Books in the series encompass a variety of areas, including global health and the politics of governance, poverty and insecurity, gender and health and the implications of global pandemics.

Also in the series

Ethics and Security Aspects of Infectious Disease Control
Interdisciplinary Perspectives
Edited by Christian Enemark and Michael J. Selgelid
ISBN 978 1 4094 2253 2

Migrants and Health
Political and Institutional Responses to
Cultural Diversity in Health Systems
Christiane Falge, Carlo Ruzza and Oliver Schmidtke
ISBN 978 0 7546 7915 8

The Political Economy of Pharmaceutical Patents
US Sectional Interests and the African Group at the WTO
Sherry S. Marcellin
ISBN 978 1 4094 1214 4

The Politics of AIDS Denialism
South Africa's Failure to Respond
Pieter Fourie and Melissa Meyer
ISBN 978 1 4094 0405 7

Informal Norms in Global Governance

Human Rights, Intellectual Property Rules and Access to Medicines

WOLFGANG HEIN
GIGA German Institute of Global and Area Studies, Germany

SUERIE MOON
Harvard University, USA

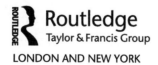

LONDON AND NEW YORK

First published 2013 by Ashgate Publishing

2 Park Square, Milton Park, Abingdon, Oxon OX14 4RN
711 Third Avenue, New York, NY 10017, USA

Routledge is an imprint of the Taylor & Francis Group, an informa business

First issued in paperback 2016

British Library Cataloguing in Publication Data
Hein, Wolfgang, 1949-
  Informal norms in global governance : human rights,
  intellectual property rules and access to medicines. --
  (Global health)
  1. Drug accessibility--International cooperation. 2. Right
  to health. 3. Agreement on Trade-Related Aspects of
  Intellectual Property Rights, (1994) 4. Intellectual
  property (International law) 5. Foreign trade regulation--
  Health aspects. 6. Non-state actors (International
  relations) 7. Drugs--Economic aspects. 8. Antiretroviral
  agents--Patents. 9. Drugs--Patents.
  I. Title II. Series III. Moon, Suerie.
  344'.04233-dc23

Library of Congress Cataloging-in-Publication Data
Hein, Wolfgang, 1949-
  Informal norms in global governance : human rights, intellectual property rules and access to medicines / by Wolfgang Hein and Suerie Moon.
    p. cm. -- (Global health)
  Includes bibliographical references and index.
  ISBN 978-1-4094-2633-2 (hbk) 1. Public health-- International cooperation.
  2. Right to health--Developing countries. 3. Drugs--Prices--Developing
countries. 4. Foreign trade regulation--Developing countries. 5. Patents (International law) I. Moon, Suerie. II. Title.
  RA441.H45 2012
  362.1--dc23

                                                                2012026010

ISBN 978-1-4094-2633-2 (hbk)
ISBN 978-1-138-26133-4 (pbk)

Contents

List of Figures and Tables

Figures

Tables

For my wife, Brigitte Mármora

For my parents, Ineon and Youjae Moon

Foreword

In 1994, when governments adopted the Agreement on Trade-related Aspects of Intellectual Property (TRIPs) in the World Trade Organization, no one anticipated the firestorm that would erupt just a few years later over the HIV/AIDS pandemic and access to medicines. HIV/AIDS activists, the Brazilian government, and South African activists rose up to protest the high costs of antiretroviral HIV/AIDS drugs. Faced with a devastating health care crisis, access campaigners linked drug patents to the unaffordable medicines that they desperately needed. In 1997 the new, post-apartheid, South African government sought to make legislative changes to facilitate more affordable access to medicines. In response, global pharmaceutical firms and powerful champions of the global intellectual property rules, including the United States, doubled down and sued the South African government for its efforts to make the drugs more accessible. In response the access to medicines campaigners pushed back and through a dedicated and nimble coalition of non-governmental organizations, developing country governments, experts, and civil society organizations achieved surprising and lasting victories in promoting key aspects of a global norm of the right to health. Against long odds, this coalition effectively re-framed the issues from trade and property rights, to access to essential medicines.

Words matter in global governance, and the discursive strategy of framing intellectual property rights as a public health issue helped to galvanize institutions such as the World Health Organization, the United Nations Development Program, the UN Committee on Economic, Social and Cultural Rights, and the UN Sub-Commission on Human Rights to support the informal norm of access to medicines. Hein and Moon trace the rise of the access to medicines movement, and explore the process by which an informal norm (not enshrined in formal international law) can come powerfully to shape results on the ground. Despite the fact that there have been minimal changes to formal international law (TRIPs), access to HIV/AIDS treatment has increased from about 400,000 people in 2003 to 6.6 million in 2011. Over 60 countries have made use of TRIPs flexibilities, and by 2008 over 95% of donor-funded ARVs used in developing countries were generic drugs.

Hein and Moon present a powerful case for an emerging form of global governance that facilitates rapid change, remains flexible, is open to influence from traditionally weaker actors, and establishes and reinforces informal norms that effect positive outcomes. Characterized by nodal governance and polylateral diplomacy, shifting and complex interfaces between civil society organizations, international organizations, governments, and transnational corporations have resulted in profound change even without being formally codified into international law. Hein and Moon are skeptical that informal norms and discursive strategies *alone* can effect lasting and irreversible change. At some point these must intersect with structural power and formal law. Only then will they become predictable, stronger, and more enforceable. Yet at this point the access norm seems sufficiently stable, and broadly accepted, that it would be very difficult for intellectual property rights-holders to secure stronger protection that would erode access to essential medicines. Too many people are watching too closely for them to get away with that. Forward movement continues to address the problem of neglected diseases, including work on a new global framework for financing and managing health R&D. The World Health Assembly's Global Strategy and Plan of Action on Public Health, Innovation and Access has kept the access norm on the agenda.

Hein and Moon's book highlights an important trend in global governance. Informal norms can play a crucial role, in a policy landscape of overlapping regimes, dense thickets of institutions, increasing legalization of policymaking, and the important role of non-state actors, that challenges conventional international relations wisdom about power and outcomes. As Hein and Moon state, "if the more powerful had always been able to protect the status quo, history would reveal no significant social changes." The rise of the access to medicines norm, and new policies to deliver it, is a significant change in the human right to health and is one well worth celebrating.

Susan K. Sell
George Washington University and
Woodrow Wilson International Center for Scholars
Washington, DC
September 25, 2012

Preface

Networking is not only an important topic in this book, but is also at the root of it. The two authors of this book met for the first time at the 2010 International Studies Association Convention in New Orleans, a gathering where projects are born that had not been imagined before. In New Orleans the authors each presented research papers on the panel "The Right to Health": Suerie Moon on "Re-Embedding Liberalism in the Global Public Domain: Reforming the Global Intellectual Property Regime for Health & Human Rights" and Wolfgang Hein on "Universal Access to Essential Medicines: The Emergence of a Precarious Norm in Global Health Governance."

Through the work on her dissertation "Embedding Neoliberalism: Global Health and the Evolution of the Global Intellectual Property Regime (1994–2009)" as well as her work as a staff member or adviser to civil society organizations and intergovernmental organizations involved in access to medicines issues, Suerie Moon had intimate knowledge of many details of the conflict on access to medicines. In addition, this book built on her ongoing work at the Harvard School of Public Health and Kennedy School of Government on the implications of global governance processes for health.

Wolfgang Hein has worked at the Hamburg-based German Institute of Global and Area Studies (GIGA) for more than 20 years on various aspects of global governance, and since 2002 with a special focus on global health governance. His ISA paper was based primarily on the results of a research project on "Global Health Governance and the Fight Against HIV/AIDS" in which the proliferation of actors in the conflicts around access to antiretroviral medicines played a significant role.

It was, however, the initiative by Ashgate Publishers and the editor of the Global Health series, Nana Poku, which played the final catalyzing role, when they proposed a book manuscript after having seen the ISA papers. We are grateful to Ashgate and to Professor Poku for the opportunity. We also thank the anonymous reviewer whose deep expertise, thoughtful critique and always very pertinent comments helped to give the manuscript its final shape.

We thank GIGA, which supported this project by integrating it into its research program and facilitating two work meetings of the authors through its financial support. The GIGA Information Centre readily assisted in the acquisition of the newest publications about our topic. Our colleagues at the global health research team at GIGA, Sonja Bartsch, Gilberto Calcagnotto, Lars Kohlmorgen, Christian von Soest, and Jan Peter Wogart, as well as the Research Team for "Global Governance and Norm-Building," in particular Cord Jakobeit, Robert Kappel, and

Ulrich Mückenberger, provided stimulating ideas on global health governance and a better understanding of global norm-building processes. Among the innumerable colleagues we spoke with at many conferences on global health and in various Geneva organizations, we want to highlight in particular the ideas and the background knowledge we owe to Ilona Kickbusch, Kent Buse and Nick Drager.

At Harvard we are grateful to John G. Ruggie, William C. Clark, and Sofia Gruskin, whose guidance, expertise and incisive comments shaped earlier versions of this work. We also thank Julio Frenk and Sue Goldie at the Harvard Global Health Institute, who provided the intellectual impetus, time and space to delve into the broader issues of global governance for health. We also thank Andrei Valan for his assistance with bibliographical inquiries and some of the more technical aspects of the production of the final manuscript, Johannes Schulz for help with the index, and Alyssa Yamamoto for excellent research assistance throughout.

Finally, we thank the many activists who fought long and hard to realize the human right to access to medicines, and continue to fight today. Among the many who have served as inspiration, mentors, teachers and supporters, special respect and admiration go to Daniel Berman, Yuanqiong Hu, Jamie Love, Chan Park, Bernard Pécoul, Ellen 't Hoen, and Tido von Schoen-Angerer.

Wolfgang Hein, Hamburg
and Suerie Moon, New York
June 2012

List of Abbreviations

AAI	Accelerating Access Initiative
access norm	the principle that access to essential medicines should be universal, and should take precedence over the protection of patents
ACTA	Anti-Counterfeiting Trade Agreement
ACT-UP	AIDS Coalition to Unleash Power
ACWL	Advisory Centre on WTO Law
AFP	Agence France-Press
AIDS	Acquired Immune Deficiency Syndrome
ART	Antiretroviral Therapy
ARV	Antiretroviral (antiretroviral drug)
AZT	Azidothymidine (zidovudine)
BHAP	Brazilian HIV/AIDS Programme
BIT	Bilateral Investment Treaty
BMGF	Bill & Melinda Gates Foundation
BMS	Bristol-Myers Squibb
BRICS	Brazil, Russia, India, China and South Africa
CDC	US Centers for Disease Control and Prevention
CESCR	Committee on Economic, Social and Cultural Rights
CEWG	Consultative Expert Working Group on Research and Development
CIEL	The Center for International Environmental Law
CIPIH	Commission on Intellectual Property Rights, Innovation and Public Health
CIPR	UK Commission on Intellectual Property Rights
CL	Compulsory License
CMH	Commission on Macroeconomics and Health
CML	Chronic Myeloid Leukemia
CPAA	Cancer Patients Aid Association (India)
CPF	Collaborative Partnership on Forests
CPTech	Consumer Project on Technology (United States)
CSIR	Council of Scientific and Industrial Research (India)
CSO	Civil Society Organization
CSR	Corporate Social Responsibility
DCGI	Drug Controller General of India
ddI	Didanosine (ARV)
DFID	United Kingdom Department for International Development

DG	Directorate General
DNP+	Delhi Network for Positive People
DRA	Drug Regulatory Authority
DRC	Democratic Republic of the Congo
DSB	Dispute Settlement Body
ECPR	European Consortium for Political Research
EDL	WHO Essential Drug List
EML	WHO Model List of Essential Medicines
EMR	Exclusive Marketing Rights
ESC(R)	Economic, Social and Cultural (Rights)
EU	European Union
EWG	Expert Working Group on Research and Development
FAO	Food and Agriculture Organization
FDA	United States Food and Drug Administration
FDC	Fixed-Dose Combination
FIND	Foundation for Innovative New Diagnostics
FTA	Free Trade Agreement
GATB	Global Alliance for TB Drug Development
GATS	General Agreement on Trade in Services
GATT	General Agreement on Tariffs and Trade
GAVI (Alliance)	Global Alliance for Vaccines and Immunization
GF (GFATM)	Global Fund to Fight AIDS, Tuberculosis and Malaria
GHG	Global Health Governance
GHP	Global Health Partnerships
GIGA	German Institute of Global and Area Studies
GIPAP	Glivec International Patient Assistance Program
GIST	Gastrointestinal Stromal Tumors
GHI	Global Health Initiative (US)
GNI	Gross National Income
GNP+	Global Network of Positive People
GPO	Government Pharmaceutical Organization (a Thai state-owned drug manufacturer)
GPPP	Global Public-Private Partnership
GSK	GlaxoSmithKline
GSPoA	Global Strategy and Plan of Action on Public Health, Innovation and Intellectual Property (WHA)
H1N1, H5N1	subtypes of influenza A virus
HAART	Highly Active Antiretroviral Therapy
HAI	Health Action International
HDI	Human Development Index
Health GAP	Health Global Access Project
HHS	US Department of Health and Human Services
HIV	Human Immunodeficiency Virus
IBFAN	International Baby Food Action Network

ICC	International Criminal Court
ICESCR	International Covenant on Economic, Social and Cultural Rights
ICMR	Indian Council for Medical Research
ICTSD	International Centre for Trade and Sustainable Development
IDA	International Dispensary Association
IFPMA	International Federation of Pharmaceutical Manufacturers & Associations
IGO	Intergovernmental Organization(s)
IGWG	Intergovernmental Working Group on Public Health, Innovation and Intellectual Property (WHA)
IIPA	International Intellectual Property Alliance
IISD	International Institute for Sustainable Development
ILC	UN International Law Commission
ILO	International Labour Organisation
IoWH	Institute for OneWorld Health
IP	Intellectual Property
IPAB	Intellectual Property Appellate Board
IPCC	Intergovernmental Panel on Climate Change
IPR	Intellectual Property Right
IUCN	International Union for the Conservation of Nature
IUFRO	International Union of Forest Research Organizations
KEI	Knowledge Ecology International
KETAM	Kenya Treatment Access Movement
LDCs	Least Developed Countries
LICs	Low Income Countries
LMIC	Lower middle-income country
MEP	Member of the European Parliament
MIC	Middle-Income Country
MoPH	Ministry of Public Health
MSF	Médecins Sans Frontières
NAFTA	North American Free Trade Agreement
NCD	Non-Communicable Disease
NGO	Non-Governmental Organization
NHSO	National Health Security Office (Thailand)
OECD	Organisation for Economic Cooperation and Development
OHCHR	Office of the High Commissioner for Human Rights
OXFAM	Oxford Committee for Famine Relief
PDP	Product Development Partnership
PEPFAR	US President's Emergency Plan for AIDS Relief
PhRMA	Pharmaceutical Research and Manufacturers of America
PLWHA/PLHIV	People Living With HIV/AIDS
PMA	Pharmaceutical Manufacturers Association
PPP	Public Private Partnership

PreMA	The Pharmaceutical Research and Manufacturers' Association (Thailand)
PRV	Priority review vouchers
R&D	Research & Development
S&T Plan	Medium to Long Term Plan for the Development of Science and Technology (China)
SPS	Agreement on Sanitary & Phytosanitary Measures (WTO)
TB	Tuberculosis
THB	Thai Baht (currency)
TNC	Transnational Corporation
TNP+	Thai Network of Positive People
TNPC	Transnational Pharmaceutical Corporation
TRIPS	Agreement on Trade-Related Aspects of Intellectual Property Rights
TRIPS+	measures that restrict the use of TRIPS flexibilities in signatory countries
UN	United Nations
UNAIDS	Joint United Nations Programme on HIV/AIDS
UNCTAD	United Nations Conference on Trade and Development
UNDP	United Nations Development Programme
UNEP	United Nations Environmental Program
UNESCO	United Nations Educational, Scientific and Cultural Organization
UNFPA	United Nations Population Fund
UNGASS	United Nations General Assembly
UNHCHR	United Nations High Commissioner for Human Rights
UNHCR	United Nations High Commissioner for Refugees
UNICEF	United Nations Children's Fund
UNITAID	An international facility for the purchase of drugs against HIV/AIDS, Malaria and Tuberculosis
UPOV	International Convention for the Protection of New Varieties of Plants
USAID	United States Agency for International Development
USD	United States Dollar
USTR	United States Trade Representative
WHA	World Health Assembly
WHO	World Health Organization
WIPO	World Intellectual Property Organization
WTO	World Trade Organization

Chapter 1

Introduction

(a) Formal and informal norms in the governance of a global society

Globalization entails a growing density of social relations that has made possible the emergence of a global society, albeit nascent and inchoate. Political actors in this global society include not only those widely-recognized to wield power on the global stage, such as major states and transnational firms, but also developing country governments, civil society networks, journalists, experts and the public at large. This society is governed not only by norms codified in formal international law, but also by informal norms that emerge through complex political processes.

Recent key developments in the field of global health give us reason to hope that the emergence of a global society may lead to a more inclusive vision of equity and interdependence beyond national borders, and that this may be conducive to the protection and promotion of human rights in general, and the progressive realization of the right to health[1] in particular. Informal norms may have an important role to play in this societal evolution. Such key developments include the following:

First, awareness of the dramatic disparities in health status between richer and poorer populations has increased, and created the normative groundwork for acts of solidarity such as resource transfers to improve health. Development assistance for global health increased dramatically, nearly quintupling from 1990 to 2010 from about $5.7 billion to $26.9 billion (Murray et al., 2011). The growing density of social relations suggests that systems analogous to national social safety nets may one day be constructed at the global level, and make more concrete the realization of economic, social and cultural rights.

Second, tighter relations of interdependence between populations, economies and states have increased the degree to which societies face common health threats, such as the spread of pandemic influenza or harmful effects of tobacco marketing. This increased interdependence has, arguably, strengthened the willingness to transfer resources but also exacerbated governance challenges at the global level.

---

1 As it is frequently done, we use this as a short form for "the highest attainable standard of physical and mental health," although it is not entirely correct. "Highest attainable" not only refers to limitations in health care due to the specific economic and social restrictions of a given society, but is also linked to innate disabilities and health problems.

Third, information on significant scientific advances, such as the development of new life-saving drugs or vaccines, travels more quickly and can create higher expectations and new political demands for access to healthcare. However, even with increased levels of aid, development spending for health amounts to an annual per capita "subsidy" of only about $4 for people living outside the developed world,[2] an amount that is far from sufficient for ensuring a minimum standard of healthcare to all people in need. Thus, increased political demands for health rapidly bump up against resource constraints.

Finally, the development of transnational networks has strengthened the political power of health advocates, who share information, devise joint strategies, and mobilize to put pressure on other powerful actors such as governments and multinational firms to be responsive to health concerns.

A remarkable illustration of the combined impact of these four developments is the case of the access to medicines movement and the emergence of a robust, albeit informal, "access norm." Starting in the 1990s, global trade rules required many developing countries to begin granting patents on medicines in their domestic laws for the first time. Patent monopolies enabled high drug prices that put them out of reach for the majority of the population. Most high-income countries have social protection systems such as public or private insurance to ensure the provision of even highly-priced medicines to their citizens, whether rich or poor. In many developing countries, however, low incomes and weak social safety nets mean that few will be able to access high-cost medicines.

Nevertheless, global trade rules allowed governments to apply certain flexibilities in patent rules to access lower-cost medicines for their populations. However, whether or not they would do so depended heavily on prevailing global norms on the proper balance between intellectual property protection and public health. At the heart of these debates lay the question of what priority would be given to health—particularly the health of some of the world's poorest people— and what priority to economic interests, particularly those of the most powerful nations and firms.

Against long odds, after a decade of heated political contestation and negotiation, a stable, widely-accepted and reliably-enforced informal norm had emerged that all people should have access to essential medicines—what we call the "access norm" for brevity. It is this informal norm that is the core focus and analytical puzzle of this book.

A "norm" is a basic concept in the social sciences. Finnemore and Sikkink (1998) define it as "a standard of appropriate behavior for actors with a given identity." The behavior could be appropriate within a small group of friends, an ethnic group, a nation or even a global society. There is a whole family of phenomena that can be categorized as "norms" (principles, standards, guidelines, and rules (Braithwaite and Drahos, 2000; see also Wiener, 2008) and that help to

---

2   In 2007 around 5.4 billion people lived in less developed regions (United Nations Population Fund (UNFPA), 2007).

create stable expectations with regard to behavior within the respective group, thereby simplifying human interactions.

Formal norms are generally such norms that have been accepted by a formally legitimized body (from a general meeting of an association to the General Assembly of the United Nations). If this body is a legislative body of a political unit, these norms are normally called "laws" and they are reinforced by the threat of sanctions.

Informal norms also play a role at all levels of social organization (from routines in everyday life to diplomatic conventions), but they are based on shared norms and beliefs[3] and not on formal institutional decisions. There is no formal (legal) obligation to comply with these norms, but social sanctions against non-compliance can be rather severe (e.g. exclusion from an important social group, loss of public support).

When it comes to international law, however, there is no global political authority or world government that can implement or enforce formal norms against the will of sovereign nation states.[4] For example, despite the dense web of international rules produced since the 1940s through the United Nations system and other international institutions, including a comprehensive human rights system, the right to health remains poorly implemented. Great disparities in the burden of disease persist between populations, as well as the resources to address them. Health spending per capita is about $7300 per year in the US, Norway, and Luxemburg, but just $9 in Eritrea, Ethiopia, and the Democratic Republic of the Congo (World Health Organization, 2010). Ensuring the protection and promotion of human rights basically remains the responsibility of sovereign nation states. Nevertheless, international human rights instruments obligate richer countries to assist poorer states, which face challenges in fulfilling economic, social and cultural human rights, including the right to health. However, there is no institution with the authority to implement the necessary measures to realize this right, such as mandating a level of resource transfers from high-income to lower-income countries. The persistence of extremely high levels of inequality in global health

---

3   This goes back to Emile Durkheim (1982 [1895]), who pointed out that informal norms embody shared social understandings. Such understandings frequently characterize multilateralism even when they do not coincide with expressed national interests (which may thus prevent any agreement on corresponding formal international norms) (Finnemore, 1996; Ruggie, 1992).

4   The comparatively reliable implementation of specific international regimes has mostly been discussed in the context of hegemonic power structures. Regimes based on international "hard" law (such as the World Trade Organization regime) have been contrasted with international "soft" law, in particular in the field of economic, social and cultural human rights (ESC rights). We distinguish between the concepts of formal vs. informal law, which refer both to codification and agreement by nation states, and the debates regarding hard and soft law, which refer mostly to questions of enforceability. (See further discussion of norms and law in chapters 2 and 3.)

seems to reflect the overall failure of global governance processes to implement the right to health.[5]

Nevertheless, in the access to medicines case, global governance processes have resulted in surprisingly widespread respect for and adherence to the access norm. Implementation of the access norm involved both greater flexibility in the application of patent rules and considerable resource transfers to improve access to medicines for HIV and other high-burden diseases.

This case, then, raises some provocative questions: Could informal norms also "work" in other sectors of global governance to produce a transnational web of implementable norms to strengthen the realization of economic and social human rights? Can we think of informal norms as a step towards the development of formal norms with a solid institutional foundation for their implementation? Or does the emergence of a global society against a backdrop of rigid state-based governance structures imply an increasing dependence on informal norms? If so, how stable, inclusive and effective are informal norms?

(b) The emergence of the "access to medicines" norm

Access to essential[6] medicines is now recognized as an integral part of fulfilling the human right to health. However, the lack of resources in some countries makes the fulfillment of this right a major challenge. At the same time, the development of new medicines requires significant investments into research and development (R&D). The knowledge component of a medicine can be considered a global public good (Moon, 2009). That is, the knowledge that 200mg of compound X can safely and effectively treat disease Y is the end result of a long process of drug development, and is potentially non-excludable and non-rival—all people can benefit from this new knowledge, and sharing this knowledge with others does not diminish the amount that is left for others. However, somebody must bear the high costs and risks of developing this knowledge. How can universal access to medicines be ensured in a world of vastly unequal resources, growing political demands for health, and an ongoing need for investment into the development of

---

5   The situation of health contrasts against the success story of global trade expansion, based on the WTO Agreements and the dispute settlement process, which includes the most extended mechanism of legal sanctions ever accepted in an international agreement.

6   We use the term "essential medicines" throughout this book to refer broadly to the WHO concept of essential medicines, not only to the specific medicines included on the WHO Model List of Essential Medicines at any given point in time. WHO has defined essential medicines as "those that satisfy the priority health care needs of the population. They are selected with due regard to public health relevance, evidence on efficacy and safety, and comparative cost-effectiveness. Essential medicines are intended to be available within the context of functioning health systems at all times in adequate amounts, in the appropriate dosage forms, with assured quality and adequate information, and at a price the individual and the community can afford" (World Health Organization, 2011).

new drugs? Who should pay for the development of new medicines, how much, and who decides?

The patent system, with its roots going back for centuries, pre-dates the emergence of the modern pharmaceutical industry in the mid twentieth century. The industry came to rely on patent-based monopolies as the primary legal tool that enabled them to recover investments into research and development. Patents are state-granted time-limited monopolies that allow patent-holders to sell the patented product at the highest price the market will bear without being exposed to competition. However, high prices can make medicines unaffordable to many of those who may need them.

The problem of ensuring universal access to medicines can be seen as essentially a problem of global public goods provision—how can the global community ensure that medicines are affordable to all while maintaining continued investment into R&D? This is not merely an economic problem, but a political one that goes to the heart of global governance challenges. Complicating these challenges is the 1994 World Trade Organization (WTO) Agreement on Trade-Related Aspects of Intellectual Property Rights (TRIPS), which required all WTO Members to adopt minimum standards of intellectual property protection. In many countries, TRIPS required the introduction of patents on medicines into domestic law for the first time. The TRIPS Agreement came into force just as the HIV pandemic was decimating populations, particularly in the developing world. For HIV/AIDS, the challenge of how to allocate payment for medicines R&D at the global level was resolved with an implicit political compromise:

High-income countries accepted to pay the R&D costs for the antiretroviral (ARV) drugs used to treat HIV/AIDS by paying the high monopoly prices enabled by the patent system, while many developing countries paid roughly the costs of production by procuring competitively-produced generic ARVs.[7] This solution did not come easily, but rather, was reached after a decade of intense political struggles and hard-fought concessions over the degree of flexibility developing countries would be allowed to apply in the way they implemented TRIPS in their domestic legal systems. A normative landmark was the 2001 WTO Doha Declaration on TRIPS and Public Health, in which all WTO Members agreed that TRIPS should not block the protection of public health, and should be implemented in a manner that would ensure access to medicines for all.

In the case of HIV drugs, the norm of universal access to medicines has been at least partially implemented through a limited and informal (from a legal point of view), but strong consensus among concerned state and non-state actors, supported by civil society organizations (CSOs) and important sections of the global public. The consensus is most explicit and visible in the UN General Assembly commitment in 2005 to achieve universal access to treatment and care for HIV/AIDS by 2010

---

7   In most high-income countries, relatively well-resourced public or private insurance systems made it possible for individuals to get access to high-cost medicines.

(United Nations General Assembly, 2005). With only one-third of people in need getting access to HIV/AIDS treatment by 2010, the universal access goal was not achieved by the deadline (WHO, UNICEF, UNAIDS 2010). Nevertheless, the progress in increasing access to HIV medicines in developing countries was extraordinary: access to treatment increased over 16-fold from about 400,000 people in 2003 to 6.6 million in 2011 (UNAIDS, 2011; WHO, UNICEF, UNAIDS 2010). Over 60 countries made use of flexibilities in TRIPS rules, including but not limited to those enumerated in the Doha Declaration, to get access to lower-cost generic versions of widely-patented medicines ('t Hoen, 2009). This widespread government authorization of the use of generic HIV medicines resulted in over 95% of donor-funded ARVs used in developing countries coming from generic sources by 2008 (Waning, Diedrichsen and Moon, 2010).

This process of norm-implementation was accompanied by a continuing push to broaden and clarify understandings of the "access norm" beyond the implicit meaning of the early days of the global access to medicines movement, which focused almost exclusively on ARVs—that is, there was an effort to expand the norm to include not only HIV drugs but medicines for all diseases. With respect to the so-called "neglected diseases," which almost exclusively affect poor populations and therefore do not constitute a sufficient incentive for private sector R&D investment, a consensual arrangement was reached in which public and philanthropic money was invested into R&D through public-private product development partnerships, which decreased costs and investment risks for pharmaceutical companies participating in neglected disease research collaborations. On the other hand, transnational pharmaceutical companies (TNPCs) and the industrialized countries in which they were based continued to contest the expansion of the access norm beyond the narrow confines of HIV/AIDS or neglected diseases.

However, populations in developing countries need access to a range of newer, widely-patented medicines, particularly as they are facing a growing burden of disease from both communicable and non-communicable diseases. In particular, TNPCs and their home countries continued to use their political and economic power to discourage IP-related measures to reduce drug prices, such as compulsory licensing and other patent law flexibilities, as was demonstrated clearly in the negotiations leading up to the UN High-Level Meeting on Non-Communicable Diseases held in September 2011 at the UN General Assembly. Industrialized countries strongly—and successfully—opposed any mention of the Doha Declaration in the meeting's final declaration, arguing that Doha only applied to infectious diseases such as HIV/AIDS; in contrast, many developing countries had pushed to include the Doha Declaration in the text, arguing that patents on cancer drugs, among others, were increasing prices to unaffordable levels (Fink and Rabinowitz, 2011). CSOs and some developing country governments had consistently advocated for the right to make use of TRIPS flexibilities across a broad range of medicines, with some success. We discuss further the expansion of the access norm in chapters 5 and 6.

Overall, by 2011, there was widespread acceptance, both formally and informally, of the norm that access to essential medicines should be universal, and should not be blocked arbitrarily by patent protection—what we call the "access norm," for brevity. This norm was driven forward and implemented most legibly in the area of HIV/AIDS. However, it rests largely on *informal* political understandings between the actors involved (governments, CSOs, TNPCs) that developing countries will enjoy some degree of flexibility in how they implement international intellectual property obligations—that is, no major changes were made to the TRIPS Agreement itself.

These major steps towards implementing at least one aspect of the human right "to the highest attainable standard of physical and mental health" (International Covenant on Economic, Social and Cultural Rights, ICESCR, Art. 12) are encouraging, but they raise at least three key questions:

(1) How stable is the access norm? In a global system with few enforceable rules and no binding system for resource transfers, how stable is the access norm likely to be? For example, there is no institution that can guarantee through the authoritative control of financial means and the potential use of coercive means that HIV medicines will be delivered continuously to people in need of them. Can the current levels of access to antiretroviral therapy (ART) and the commitments to expand access be upheld? In particular, can TNPCs be continuously put under sufficient pressure to adhere to the range of "access policies" that have been put in place to facilitate access to HIV drugs, including for newly developed medicines? Can the policy space for developing country governments to use flexibilities in the TRIPS Agreement to access generic medicines be preserved? And how can the necessary level of financial transfers to pay for access to treatment in poor countries be guaranteed?

(2) How inclusive is the access norm? The scope of the access norm remains contested along two dimensions—which diseases it will cover, and which countries will be allowed greater flexibility in managing patents. Universal access to essential medicines concerning all diseases has been accepted in principle, but not in practice. Beyond HIV and clearly-defined emergencies such as pandemic flu, the degree to which drugs for other diseases are included in the access norm remains highly contested. The issue has become particularly heated over drugs for cancer, for which mortality rates are far higher in poorer regions of the world (Ferlay et al., 2010).[8] In addition, while the Doha Declaration clearly applied to all WTO Members—and *de facto*, to all countries—the issue of which countries would be afforded greater flexibility remains politically contested. While the poorest countries (UN-defined Least-Developed Countries [LDCs] or World Bank-defined Low Income Countries [LICs]) are given relatively greater policy space, middle-income countries—particularly the emerging economies—come under immense

---

8   See also (Coleman et al., 2008; Merletti, Galassi and Spadea, 2011).

political and economic pressure to observe stringent patent standards and to pay higher prices for medicines.

(3) What are the relative strengths and weaknesses of formal vs. informal norms for implementing the human right to health? Despite its appearance in a number of political documents and consensus texts, the access norm remains largely informal and somewhat precarious. The central normative language of the Doha Declaration (Paragraph 4), for example, has not been incorporated into the TRIPS Agreement. Nevertheless, as noted above, it has been possible to achieve major concrete progress since the turn of the millennium in access to HIV medicines. This progress was enabled by the widespread use of TRIPS flexibilities to procure lower-cost generic versions of patented ARVs and the widespread practice of TNPCs to sell originator drugs at discounted prices in lower-income countries. The process also included a large number of financing initiatives (including the Global Fund to Fight AIDS, Tuberculosis and Malaria (GFATM), internationally-operating foundations, and various NGO and church initiatives), which was necessary to finance ART in many poor countries, even with reduced drug prices.

However incomplete the implementation of the human right to access to essential medicines might be, this dramatic increase in funding and the major shift in IP norms is not easily explained by dominant theories of international relations and international law. We suggest that the intensive discourse on the characteristics and the threat of HIV/AIDS made the access norm nearly impossible to reject; at the same time, the informal character of the norm reduced the costs for TNPCs and industrialized countries to adhere to it. The pharmaceutical industry could accept special treatment for ARVs and sell them at lower prices in poorer countries or allow them to be sold as generics, based on the political agreement that TRIPS remained intact and they could still recover their R&D costs by selling the same drugs at high prices in high-income countries. In other words, the TRIPS flexibilities served as a political pressure-release valve that allowed the TRIPS Agreement—and by extension, the political legitimacy of the WTO—to be preserved without any major formal changes. In some ways, the Doha Declaration may have precluded more dramatic formal changes to TRIPS (such as a provision allowing countries to exclude certain medicines from patentability), which may have proven a more reliable way to ensure the right to health in the long run. This line of reasoning leads us to ask, what are the relative merits of informal and formal norms for protecting and promoting the right to health?

(c) Informal norms and human rights

The aim of this book is to analyze in detail the meaning and the significance of our claim that "universal access to essential medicines" has been established as an informal, but nevertheless effectively implemented norm in global politics. "Effectively implemented" means that breaking the norm produces important costs (e.g. in terms of public image and political support),[9] and that the pressure to adhere to the norm will be upheld without great fluctuation, though there may be flexibility to adapt the norm to changing circumstances. Thus, we will look into the conditions that make the *acceptance of norms without legally-defined obligations* possible. Can we assume that a tendency in the process of global socialization towards certain forms of global solidarity will continue to operate in the future? A framework for implementing informal, but rather clearly defined norms can be observed—can we expect such a framework to operate more broadly to strengthen ethical convictions and global social norms based on human rights and to produce strong human rights informed compromises when there are normative conflicts between different international regimes (e.g. such as the regimes governing trade and health)?

To pursue these questions, we take a closer look at the transformative character of globalization, which includes the challenges it poses for a policy field like health as well as the opportunities it offers to address them. Globalization has arguably increased the need for international and transnational coordination to "govern" the many global forces that can impact human health. Yet, in the absence of a central political authority, it is unclear how the multiple sets of often conflicting rules and norms will interact, and what their collective impact on health will be. Health rules and norms act at different levels (from the global to the local) as well as cover a very broad range of health issues (from disease prevention to medicines approval to health worker certification). Some rules are primarily normative, such as the human right to "the highest attainable standard of mental and physical health", and are mostly seen as international soft law as there are apparently few "hard" sanctions to ensure their implementation. Other rules have more binding force, such as the International Health Regulations, national laws that regulate health systems, the rules for the approval of new medicines, and finally (in particular in federal systems) specific rules set by sub-national entities. Last but not least, rules developed outside of traditional health circles, such as trade or migration laws, can have significant impacts on health. The regulation of intellectual property rights at the national and international level is, perhaps, the highest-profile example of such a set of rules.

While human rights norms should, in theory, take precedence over other sets of rules, there is no clear formal mechanism to ensure that in practice such norms

---

9   Costs are basically incurred through the loss of public support. Industry had fought hard to get US government support for negotiating the TRIPS agreement (Sell, 2003; Sell and Prakash, 2004) and needed continuous government cooperation to make use of the agreement (as only states can bring complaints to the WTO's Dispute Settlement Body). The access norm had broad public support (see Chapter 9) and thus governments could no longer unconditionally back the positions of TNPCs. (See, for example, the US stepping back in the TRIPS dispute with Brazil in 2001, in Chapter 5.)

prevail over other (e.g. economic) rules. In fact, however, the implementation of norms not only depends on what normally is considered to be "hard (international) law." Human action can also be driven by the "logic of appropriateness" (March and Olson, 1989). If a specific norm is accepted by a broad transnational public as highly appropriate, sufficient public pressure might build up to determine a course of action, even if no "hard sanctions" (economic or directly coercive) are threatened by law. We discuss this in more detail in chapters 2 and 3.

This book concentrates on one specific conflict between two sets of international rules: those providing for stringent intellectual property rights protection, which pharmaceutical companies rely upon to generate profits and finance R&D for new medicines (encapsulated in the TRIPS Agreement and backed by hard trade sanctions), and the emergent norm regarding universal access to medicines based on the "human right to health." This right is entrenched in formal international law, but its implementation can be impeded by high prices of patented medicines in contexts where most patients and/or health systems are unable to pay. However, there are no *legally defined sanctions* for not complying with this norm.

Another aspect of this conflict is that between patents as a market-based system of setting R&D priorities according to potential market-size, and the need to invest sufficient resources into medicines for diseases that only affect the poor or the few (neglected or orphan diseases), and who therefore do not comprise a sufficient market to incentivize private investment. Frequently this is characterized as the 10/90 gap: only 10% of financial resources are invested in research on diseases that affect 90% of the world population.[10]

Global civil society played a central role in the emergence, consolidation, and expansion of the access norm. It remains an open question whether this will end up in the codification of new legal norms, as was the case in global norm-building processes discussed in the dominant discourse on the role of civil society (Keck and Sikkink, 1998). In addition, CSOs are broadly seen as significant actors in supporting the implementation of international "soft law" (in particular, the human rights obligations of states). On the access to medicines issue, CSOs have played both roles—pushing simultaneously for a human-rights-compatible interpretation and limited revision of TRIPS, and for access to treatment in all countries and the necessary financial support for those who cannot afford it.

---

10   The 10/90 gap was introduced by the Global Forum on Health Research, which explained: "In 1990, the Commission on Health Research for Development estimated that only about 5% of the world's resources for health research (which totaled US$ 30 billion in 1986) were being applied to the health problems of low- and middle-income countries, where 93% of the world's preventable deaths occurred ... Some years later, the Global Forum coined the term '10/90 gap' to capture this major imbalance between the magnitude of the problem and the resources devoted to addressing it. Since its foundation in 1998, the Global Forum advocated effectively around the '10/90 gap' and gave a voice to people who would otherwise not have had one" (see http://www.globalforumhealth.org/about/1090-gap/, accessed October 11, 2011).

A careful analysis of the evolution of the access conflict suggests that, at least with respect to access to ARVs, an effective informal norm demanding universal access to essential medicines has developed on the basis of subsidiary rules giving priority to human rights norms when conflicts arise with norms in other sectors. This development has allowed for authoritative legal comments on specific human rights issues, and the mobilization of civil society as a very reliable actor to protest against norm-breakers. Though the Doha Declaration has strengthened the acceptance of public health norms within TRIPS, it still appears improbable that the actors involved will agree on major changes to the formal TRIPS rules. Rather, the informal norm of universal access to medicines allows TNPCs to comply without having to make further formal concessions in the field of IPRs.

At the level of formal international negotiations, an agreement on changing TRIPS on a relatively peripheral point (the so-called "Paragraph 6 negotiations") was reached in 2003, and a "Global Strategy and Plan of Action on Public Health, Innovation and Intellectual Property" was endorsed by WHO Member States at the 2008 World Health Assembly. However, both of these formal texts exclude any major amendments to the global rules for intellectual property rights protection and did little to resolve the question of how to finance a program of support to boost R&D on diseases that primarily affect developing countries. The complexities of achieving these agreements, the many compromises required, as well as the difficulties of fully implementing them has made the relevant processes difficult and long. Nevertheless, it was possible to achieve significant strengthening and expansion of the access objective, largely through *informal* norm-building processes.

We posit that the growing discrepancy between the progressing density of social relations within a global society on the one hand, and the lack of a unified political authority on the other hand, leads to a situation in which some human rights norms can be effectively implemented through informal networks of state and non-state actors, but with important limitations. We then assess where these limits may lie, and when changes to formal international agreements may appear necessary. The book elaborates on this thesis, analyzes the changes in global social relations and global governance that underlie changing processes of global norm-building and presents evidence from the analysis of political conflicts around the access norm.

(d) Overview of the book

The book begins with an introduction of the global context in which the access conflict arose and led to a consolidated informal norm, positing universal access to essential medicines as a subsidiary norm to the right to health (with some remaining conflicts about the meaning of "universal"). In Chapter 2 we discuss the impact of globalization on international relations. In the attempts to deal with inter- and transnational problems, global governance has increasingly substituted for conventional intergovernmental relations. The emergence of a new set of transnational non-state actors in a global society produced a much more flexible field of alliances and conflicts as compared to the classical "Westphalian"[11] system of international relations. This development also provides the framework for the growing number and complexity of actors constituting the newly emerging field referred to as "global health governance" (GHG). The specific challenge of HIV/ AIDS and the issue of access to treatment gave rise to the "access norm," which was closely linked to the emergence of new forms of coordination in the complex field of GHG, as characterized by the concept of *nodal governance* (see Burris, Drahos and Shearing, 2005; Hein et al., 2009).

Chapters 3 and 4 bring us closer to our main field of empirical analysis. In Chapter 3 we discuss in more detail the relationship between the access to medicines norm and the human rights system in general. The UN human rights system is generally based on the two international covenants on Civil and Political Rights and on Economic, Social and Cultural Rights and a number of human rights conventions on specific aspects. Human rights as defined in these international treaties are *formal international law*, but most of these rules are generally seen as *soft law* (with some exceptions, such as with respect to genocide, and possibly, over the past two decades with respect to some basic democratic rights, which are increasingly backed by international sanctions). A system of formal subsidiary rules, which could offer clear criteria for adjudication, does not exist, as there would in any case be no way to enforce them. This is where informal norms based on shared beliefs in an emerging global society come in.

The specific problem with "access to medicines" is, as we have already highlighted in this introduction, that it is *not* a field without any effective international law, but, on the contrary, it is covered by the most effectively implemented corpus of international law—the WTO Agreements, of which TRIPS is one. In Chapter 4 we deal in more detail with the basic characteristics of intellectual property rights (IPRs) in general and with access to medicines in particular, and explain the relationship between IP and medicines R&D. We will also refer to the concept of knowledge as a global public good, and its relationship with the access problem as well as with the problem of financing research and development (R&D) for medicines.

Chapters 5 to 8 constitute the empirical heart of this book; we use a process tracing methodology in order to provide evidence for the effectiveness of the informal norm in contributing to the (partial) implementation of the human right to health. Chapter 5 deals with the history of the emergence and consolidation of the "access norm" embedded in a series of conflicts particularly with respect to access to ARVs. Our analysis shows that the implementation of this norm has been largely

---

11   The term "Westphalian" system of international relations refers to the Westphalian Peace of 1648, which accepted the sovereignty of the territorial state as the main principle of international relations after the demise of the claims of the Pope and the Emperors as "universal powers."

dependent upon its broad acceptance by the actors involved (CSOs, TNPCs and states) without clearly defined obligations in the framework of international law. The informality of the norm made it possible to accept very inclusive declarations ("all essential medicines") but to leave some important questions effectively open to successive steps by developing countries, such as "testing" the reactions of TNPCs to issuing compulsory licenses first on ARVs, and then on an expanding range of drugs on non-communicable diseases.

Already in Section (b) above we referred to the most important problems produced by the informality of the norm. These problems are dealt with in the subsequent chapters: Chapter 6 discusses the aspect of the inclusiveness of the norm (concerning the range of medicines and countries included). Though—with reference to the human rights discourse—in more general statements, high-income countries as well as TNPCs accepted that access must be provided to essential medicines irrespective of the disease concerned and (in principle also) irrespective of the average income of a country. We discuss in more detail specific conflicts in India and Ecuador, and also look at the positions of different actors concerning the provision of medicines in the cases of pandemic flu and non-communicable diseases. This analysis includes several accounts of national-level political contests over domestic IP rules—with middle-income countries as a new battlefield—and discusses how the practices and discourse of state and non-state actors interacted at the international level to produce global normative change.

Chapter 7 deals with the second principle weakness of informal norms, the question of the stability of the norm. While a formal legal rule remains in force even when public attention to a particular problem decreases, an informal norm that depends on the discursive power of a mobilized public could weaken due to changing power relations between the actors involved. For example, immediately after the adoption of the Doha Declaration, in most statements the pharmaceutical industry spoke of an important achievement, but in the years to follow, there were other occasions where TNPCs insisted on maintaining stringent international IP norms and pushed for agreements that restricted the use of TRIPS flexibilities: these included free trade agreements, the negotiation of WTO accession agreements (e.g. in the accession of China) and other channels of IP rulemaking (such as bilateral investment treaties, and the Anti-Counterfeiting Trade Agreement (ACTA)).

Chapter 8 then turns to another arena: There are still no formal international rules that link the (hard law) rules of the TRIPS Agreement with the (soft law) rules of ESC human rights. However, health advocates have promoted for a number of years—starting with the (expert) WHO Commission on Intellectual Property Rights, Innovation and Public Health in 2004—a discourse and then negotiations on a formal agreement on "Public Health, Innovation and Intellectual Property" (note the changed sequence of the terms) concerning research on neglected diseases as well as access to essential medicines. In these negotiations the access norm has been re-framed as an "access and innovation norm," linking the issue of affordability of medicines to the challenge of designing optimal incentives for pharmaceutical innovation that are driven by public health needs and do not trade away access.

Whatever the success of formal negotiations on access and innovation will be, it is certain that non-state actors will continue to play an important role. Without a strong global political authority, only strong pressure from a global public might be able to produce a new formal agreement with real normative force. Though in the access case, public demands can be said to be legitimized by the close link to human rights, the question of the legitimacy and authority of informal norms remains important. In Chapter 9 we look back at the access to medicines case to draw out broader propositions regarding the nature of informal norms and nodal governance in processes of global governance. We address the question of the foundations of legitimacy and accountability in global governance, and the implications for the appraisal of global democracy.

Finally, in the conclusion, we summarize our findings about the limits of global change through informal norms, and the arguments for turning back to the possibility of changes in formal international law. We discuss the conditions for a strengthening of human rights norms through both informal and formal processes as well as the continuous interaction between them, and link this discussion back to the broader context of politics in a global society.

Chapter 2
Towards a Global Society

(a) Globalization

Globalization can be briefly defined as the intensification and acceleration of cross-border flows of people, goods, services, and ideas.[1] This process has been accompanied by innovation in many fields and new opportunities for economic and social development, but also growing inequalities and risks, in particular, due to the decreasing capacity of national governments to control globally-networked economic, social and political forces. These processes have affected countries in different degrees depending on their size and power (Keohane and Nye, 1997). This trend has led to increasing attempts at more effective collective action by governments, business and civil society to better manage these risks and opportunities. Globalization has also opened up new fields of political conflicts in an emerging arena of global politics that can be characterized as a global public domain (Ruggie, 2004), in which various actors assert their claims, defend their interests, debate rules and policies, contest truths, and construct norms. In short, the globalization process has intensified the density of social and political interactions on a global scale.

Globalization has been facilitated by new technologies and by changes in institutions and regimes at the international and national levels, such as the promotion of trade and investment liberalization (Held, McGrew, Goldblatt and Perraton, 1999) and rules- and norm-building processes in transport and communication. It extends far beyond the economy to political, cultural, environmental, and security issues and implies an increasing transnational interconnectivity between people and communities. Such connectivity leads to a growing density of transnational social relations and the creation of common identities based on characteristics other than nationality—for example among people in civil society networks fighting for more equity in global health.

Globalization entails processes that contribute to the constitution of a *global society*. So far we have used the term "global society" in a somewhat pre-theoretical way. For the full development of our argument, however, it is necessary to point to a few essential aspects of our understanding of this concept. Our starting-point is a critique of methodological nationalism, i.e. "the assumption that the nation/state/society is the natural social and political form of the modern world" (Wimmer and Glick Schiller, 2002). Historically, social and political institution

---

1 This definition summarizes the basic features of contemporary globalization as characterized by (Held, McGrew, Goldblatt and Perraton, 1999, 15–16).

building proceeded as a co-evolutionary process with nation-building.[2] Similarly, the development of transnational health policies can be seen as co-evolving with other institutions demanded by a global society.

Max Weber called "societal" (or "associative") relations (*Vergesellschaftung*) those where "the orientation of social action rests on a rationally motivated adjustment of interests or a similarly motivated agreement" (Weber, 1978). Thus, the (rationally motivated) building of social and political institutions historically focused on limited territories, which then for one or the other reason expanded (through integration, conquest or colonization) or remained small (Monaco, San Marino etc.). Based on this understanding of the building of societies, we can see why social relations might become denser transnationally when conditions change—and when there is then a rational motivation for "an adjustment of interests" that transcends existing institutions. As summarized above, the recent phase of globalization has led to such a re-structuring of economic and political interests taking into account the narrowed potential of states to pursue national interests due to international regimes, particularly in the field of trade.

Seen in an abstract way, the formation of a "society" does not imply the constitution of a "national community." Weber speaks of communal relationships, "if and so far as the orientation of social action is based on a subjective feeling of the parties, whether affectual or traditional, that they belong together" (Weber, 1978: 40). Weber continued, "Every social relationship that goes beyond the pursuit of immediate common ends, which hence lasts for long periods, involves relatively permanent social relationships between the same persons and these cannot be exclusively confined to the technically necessary activities" (Weber, 1978: 41).

Strictly speaking, the idea of community implies direct personal interactions. However, when focusing on the symbolic dimension of communal relations, the term comprises much larger social entities such as nations. It is well-documented that nation-building processes went far beyond the consolidation of sovereignty within a clearly-defined territory and a "rationally motivated adjustment of interests"; rather, strategies of nation-building systematically supported the rise of "nations" as "imagined communities" (Anderson, 1983; Djelic and Quack, 2010). The centrality of the "nation" (in terms of identification) and the "nation state" (in terms of an institution for the adjustment of interests) in social development help explain the role of methodological nationalism in the social sciences in most of the nineteenth and twentieth centuries. However, it is important to note that empirically during the same period there were no insurmountable barriers to the formation of transnational communities e.g. in the fields of literature, science, and in various civil society activities (such as the fight for the abolition of slavery), and also via significant flows of migrants.

---

2   It is beyond the scope of this book to take up in detail the complex discussion on the definitions of "society" and "community" (see, as a good summary, Djelic and Quack, 2010).

In recent decades, the growth of transnational interdependence has led to the formation of many transnational communities of shared norms and political goals. This has produced changing constellations between (globalizing) non-state actors, nation states and international organizations. So far, it is still very rare to find empirical research that approaches the analysis of global social relations from a sociological perspective and effectively overcomes methodological nationalism (Holton, 2005; Mau, 2010); other publications in this field either concentrate on the idea of cosmopolitanism (Held, 1995) or take an actor-oriented perspective on transnational political cooperation and conflicts between different groups of non-state actors (see Section b below). Yet such research is increasingly necessary to understand and explain the implications of increasingly dense transborder social interactions.

Due to a growing global interdependence and the greater role of transnational communities in politics, globalization has brought an increasing awareness of conflicts and social problems linked to the inequality of global development. People in richer countries are more and more exposed to information regarding social problems in other parts of the globe, which serves as a reminder that such problems may be, to some extent, also their problems. Such is the case with HIV/AIDS or other infectious diseases that threaten the economic and political stability of some countries and regions, which might in turn threaten international peace and security (Hein and Kohlmorgen, 2008). Individuals as well as activist and epistemic communities in wealthier countries may feel greater solidarity with those in poorer countries, after being exposed on a more regular basis to the needs and inequalities between them. As the global risks of infectious disease and the importance of health to social and political stability are acknowledged, health is increasingly perceived as a global public good that requires strengthened global efforts (Chen et al., 1999).

In part due to the inadequate responses of nation states and IGOs to many global problems, civil society and private sector actors play a prominent role in global governance—particularly in social and health policy. Their involvement has a twofold effect. On the one hand, corporations and business associations maneuver in this political space to pursue their interests and to foster market liberalization that can undermine social rights. On the other hand, actors like CSOs, advocacy groups and foundations that strengthen social rights put pressure on large enterprises to behave in a more socially responsible manner and push governments to refrain from undermining the realization of social rights in other countries and/or demand that they fulfill their regulatory functions. These actors target not only governments and corporations based in the industrialized countries, but those in developing countries as well. These dynamics, which include partnerships between various types of non-state actors (CSOs, TNCs, international foundations, transnational media) as well as state actors (IGOs and governments), have been characterized in the growing literature on GHG as a proliferation of actors, producing a number of benefits but also a serious problem of coordination (see below, Section (d)).

Still, the global health system is not merely a hodge-podge of undifferentiated organizations and actors. The difference between private for-profit actors, civil society actors and public institutions remains important. The role of national public institutions as the primary setters of binding rules and authoritative decision-making might weaken over time, and the implementation of norms in the transnational space might depend for a longer period on voluntary, legally unenforceable forms of cooperation between business and civil society actors; nevertheless, it is important to trace the changing, but still distinguishable functions of these basic types of actors in modern society during globalization. We will take a closer look at the transformation of the system of "International Relations" into a system of "Global Governance," then look at the character of and the relations between transnational actors in global politics and in global health governance. We then return to the basic question of this book concerning the potential force of informal norms to implement human rights.

(b) From international relations to global governance

In traditional international relations theory, international agreements were conceived in a rather simple way: the system of international relations was based on *an aggregation of interests at the national level* (see Figure 2.1: A1, A2 and A3 represent the various interest groups—business, unions, CSO—in nation A, and so on). Thus, negotiations at the international level were led by governments on the basis of these nationally aggregated positions, which, in the first instance, reflected power relations within nation states. The outcome of these negotiations was a result of power relations between nation states, partially mediated by decision-making procedures within intergovernmental organizations (IGOs).

Meanwhile, globalization has established new transnational political spaces that prevent the full aggregation of interests at the national level. Rather, the transnational interaction of state and non-state actors produces dynamics and opportunities that increasingly limit the political options of nation states. We have arrived at quite a complex structure of interaction and relations between the different actors (see Figure 2.2). Whereas in the ideal Westphalian system[3] there are basically two alternatives—cooperation or conflict within an IGO or bilateral cooperation or conflict between states—in the post-Westphalian structure there are many possibilities for cooperation and conflict among nation states, IGOs, CSOs, and transnational corporations. The "old" actors of the Westphalian system remain relevant, but their roles are transformed by the challenges to their political monopoly brought on by the emergence of new, genuinely transnational actors. New nodes appear in the transnational political space $(N_1; N_2)$ (see below, and also Hein et al. (2009), for the concept of nodal governance), which coordinate

---

3   On the specific background of the use of the terms "Westphalian" and "post-Westphalian era" in international relations theory see Linklater (1998).

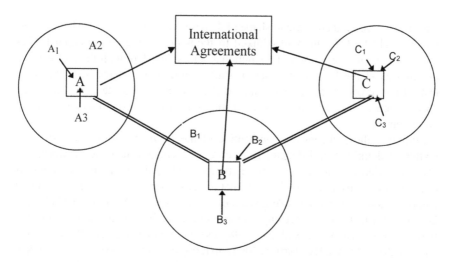

Figure 2.1   International agreements in traditional IR theory

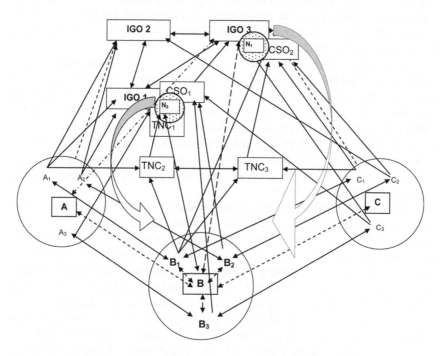

Figure 2.2   Global politics in a post-Westphalian system

power resources and compete to shape global governance processes. These nodes, which might be CSO networks linked to IGOs or specific coordinating bodies within IGOs integrating other transnational actors, interfere with the aggregation of interests at the level of the nation state. While nation-states were the main institutions involved in norm-setting in the Westphalian system, we can now observe new modes, spatial levels and institutions that are also influential in global norm-setting.

Whether these changes are indicative of the *birth of a global society*, is a matter of definition and debate. But certainly there is a tendency towards the decomposition of interaction at the national level, and the creation of patterns of interaction across national borders that are at least partially based on common identities and interests between groups of actors (see also Scholte, 2011; Sklair, 2001). Empirical studies focusing on these processes include those on CSOs and norm-building (Keck and Sikkink, 1998) and sociological analyses (Gaventa and Tandon, 2010; Mau, 2010; Tarrow, 2005). In terms of political system building, key developments include incipient processes of the development of a *global demos*, in particular, the acceptance by a growing number of actors that global democracy implies more direct involvement of people in global governance than merely being represented by their respective *governments* in international institutions; and that human rights are not rights *granted* to people, but entitlements that must be fought for by people as "global citizens."

The greater the density of global social relations, the more important become result-oriented policies that improve effectiveness, and the more dysfunctional seems an international system focusing on national power and struggles for hegemony. Max Weber might have seen it as one effect of globalization that a "rationally motivated adjustment of interests" is increasingly orienting social action towards people affected by a specific problem in any part of the world. In such a process of "global socialization", national governments might be seen as important allies by specific actors, but not necessarily as representing the "interests" of a specific country.

Whereas nation-building can be interpreted as a process in which the nation developed into the center of norm-building, economics (including labor relations), culture and politics, globalization can be seen as a process of "decentration"—that is, norms and economic, cultural and political relations beyond the nation have gained in importance. Increasingly, transnational relations between individuals, as well as collective actors from the sub-national level, challenge the central role of the nation. If we take Modelski's conceptualization of globalization as an evolutionary process, one would expect continuously growing pressure to adapt existing—or create new—institutions to cope with problems (Modelski, 2008).

Yet, the construction of a world based on territorial states and "nations" has been a process of very *longue durée* (Braudel, 1958)—as will be its deconstruction by a proliferation of transnational actors and the rise of genuinely global institutions. The basic institutions of the "age of nations" are highly resilient to fundamental change, trying to adapt to new developments and to incorporate new types of actors. Indeed, in spite of the decentration process, *larger nation states remain centers of power.* Although their regulatory capacities tend to be challenged and their tax bases suffer from transnational competition and relocation, they continue to command important financial resources. They are still, in many ways, at the center of societal organization, and social expectations continue to be focused on services and benefits to be delivered by nation states.

Due to the uneven and non-simultaneous character of modern world development, *decentration affects different regions and countries in these regions in different forms and degree.* Many poor countries are still in the process of the development of effective state structures while the *emerging powers* are trying to use their rapidly rising economic and financial power to challenge and change the post-World War II structures in the world system, which are biased towards Western institutions and values.

In the absence of a world state, *nation states still play a central role in the creation of binding legal norms;* the implementation of international agreements basically depends on their effective integration into national legal systems and even most norms created by non-state networks depend in some way on the *shadow of state authority.*[4]

The engagement of nation states in new institutional forms, including the acceptance of non-state actors as their near-equals in some decision-making processes, is part of these developments and has become a quite common feature in the case of global environmental organizations (see the International Union for the Conservation of Nature (IUCN), founded in 1948 as an early example[5]) and in global health (see below).

These developments also imply a changing role for foreign policy with respect to health. When "national interests" are increasingly linked to the results of global governance processes driven by cooperation and competition between and within transnational communities, foreign policy may no longer primarily focus

---

4   This concept is used in the recent discussion on the regulatory state to underline that "the state creates conditions in which civil society and market economies can operate" (Hutter, 2006).

5   The IUCN was founded in 1948 by delegates of 18 governments, seven international organizations and 107 national organizations concerned with nature protection in cooperation with UNESCO. The central objective is to "encourage and facilitate co-operation between governments and national and international organizations concerned with, and persons interested in, the "Protection of Nature" (Constitution of IUCN; http://data.iucn.org/dbtw-wpd/edocs/1948-001.pdf). The IUCN developed a complex system of voting in their highest body, the World Conservation Congress: each state member has three votes, each national non-governmental organization has one, each international non-governmental organization two votes (http://cmsdata.iucn.org/downloads/statutes_en.pdf, Annex: Rules of Procedure of the World Conservation Congress). Another example is the Collaborative Partnership on Forests (CPF) which consists of 14 international organizations, among intergovernmental organizations also the IUCN and the International Union of Forest Research Organizations (IUFRO) a non-governmental international network.

on promoting national interests vis-à-vis those of other nations, but may have to assume increased responsibility for advancing efforts at cooperation and the provision of global public goods (e.g. related to health or security) in global policy domains.

What does this mean for the characterization of our concept of global governance? If "governance" means the "management of the course of events in a social system," global governance sets out to manage the most complex social system conceivable, more complex than any system of inter-governmental organizations, such as the UN system. In the introduction we noted that there is no hierarchical global political authority, and from the perspective of the implementation of international law this could be seen as problematic. On the other hand, these processes of self-organization of specific groups of actors in the global system could be a way to deal with this institutional complexity.

Considering that the aim of this book is to deal with a specific facet of "global governance," we will not review the discourse of global governance here, but use a general, open definition that links very well with our definition of governance. We define "global governance as the totality of collective regulations to deal with international and transnational interdependence problems," following Bartsch and Kohlmorgen (2007b), who refer to the definitions of global governance by Mayntz (2005) and by Rosenau (1995): "... global governance is conceived to include systems of rule at all levels of human activity—from the family to the international organization—in which the pursuit of goals through the exercise of control has transnational repercussions." Going a step further, global governance might be seen as a totality of complex processes of self-organization in a global society (characterized by Fidler (2007) as "open-source anarchy"; see Section d), which produce manifold interfaces between various sets of rules, and between state and non-state actors and intergovernmental organizations. This perspective, however, raises the question of how such a process of self-organization relates to aspects of legitimacy, accountability and democratic control of power which are basic elements of democratic political systems and are generally seen as challenges in global norm-building.

Global governance has taken its most differentiated forms at the sectoral level as can be observed in the case of global health governance (GHG). The relationship between health and intellectual property rights, however, points to the fact that sectoral global governance includes important interactions with other sectors. International and transnational interdependence problems exist not only in various aspects of global health activities, but also between different sectors in global affairs. Conventional IGOs—like WHO—tend to be overstrained by the growing complexity of actors and issues in many policy fields, which has led to the rise of new forms of coordination, cooperation, and networked governance in dealing with many kinds of problems. Following the observation regarding the importance of network structures involving many actors of different types— as indicated in Figure 2.2—we apply the concept of nodal governance (Burris,

Drahos and Shearing, 2005; Hein et al., 2009) to such new forms of interaction, which also have played an important role in the conflicts on IPRs and access to medicines.

(c) Transnational actors in global governance

The conflict over intellectual property rights (IPRs) and access to medicines mobilizes two groups of transnational actors that are at the core of the transformation towards a global society: private for-profit enterprises aiming at opening-up (and shaping) international markets for maximizing profits, and welfare-oriented actors aiming at strengthening human welfare (and securing human rights) in a situation where social inequalities within and between countries have been growing. Within national territories, if conflicts cannot be resolved among the actors involved, in theory, it is the task of the modern nation state to find compromises between conflicting interests, to set rules and to interpret and implement them, and to transfer financial resources for social and environmental policies. At the international level, institutions to carry out these functions are weak or non-existent. In the international arena, the UN system developed a large number of agencies to deal with specific issues, but in many cases the preponderance of "national interests" has prevented issue-specific solutions.[6] While post-Westphalian global politics have opened up policy arenas for participation by transnational social actors, they have not (yet) succeeded in creating transnational institutions that can take authoritative decisions that will then be reliably implemented.

As indicated in Section (a) private economic actors are generally seen as the main drivers of the liberalization of international trade rules that greatly facilitated globalization since the early 1980s. At the center is the global trade regime building on the General Agreement on Tariffs and Trade (GATT) of 1947. Until the 1970s, the grand compromise of "embedded liberalism" (Ruggie, 1982) limited trade liberalization to those sectors that were politically acceptable to the domestic societies of major trading partners. For various reasons, lengthy discussion of which is beyond the scope of this book, the post-1945 growth model reached its limits during the 1970s. The main causes for the "exhaustion of Fordism" (i.e. the standardized mass production of durable consumer goods supported by a sustained rise in the real wages of industrial workers due to collective bargaining) are

---

6 This has been a notorious problem for the UN Security Council; another example is the major difficulty UN organizations were facing in particular during the 1990s as some of the larger financial contributors to UNESCO, FAO, WHO and other specialized UN Agencies withheld their dues because they considered the organizations "inefficient" – among other reasons, due to the rather consistent bloc-voting of most developing countries against the neoliberal turn on many issues (see also below Chapter 5, Section (i) concerning WHO).

usually seen as the growing scarcity of fossil fuels (oil price rises) on the one hand and the scarcity of labor in the industrialized countries (and thus a strengthening of labor unions) on the other hand (see e.g. (Marglin and Schor, 1990) and various contributions in (Amin, 1994)). Glyn and Sutcliffe (1972) pointed to a "profit squeeze" in Britain. The transnationalization of industrial production was increasingly seen as a chance to overcome this crisis by optimizing the choice of production locations and avoiding the pressure of labor unions.

Neoliberalism and its insistence on the removal of barriers to international trade and capital movements provided the theoretical and ideological framework for policies that would allow large firms to use technological innovations (communication and transport, computer-aided manufacturing, just-in-time concepts) to open up new global spaces for generating and maximizing profits. In international negotiations to this end, firms used the strong position of their home states to push for the desired results. Thus, business became an actor of both "worlds," using the tension between the "Westphalian" world of states (e.g. through lobbying powerful governments to defend business interests) and their own role in constructing the economic infrastructure of a world society to pursue their own interests.

The transformation of GATT into a much more encompassing World Trade Organization—fortified by a strong regime of sanctions—was a decisive step towards creating the political framework for a global market. Given the growing importance of high-tech industries in international trade and investment, research-intensive sectors like information technologies and pharmaceuticals pushed for an Agreement on Trade-related Aspects of Intellectual Property Rights (TRIPS) to become an essential part of the WTO (Sell, 1998) (see also Chapter 4 for more details).

The accelerating mobility of capital could be interpreted as a factor favoring an underlying tendency towards a "race to the bottom", i.e. investors trying to avoid locations where costs of higher social (including health) and environmental standards cannot be compensated through increases in productivity, thus exerting pressure to keep standards low if there is no direct linkage between higher social and/or environmental standards and productivity growth.[7] Adam Smith had already warned: "The proprietor of stock is a citizen of the world, and is not necessarily attached to any particular country. He would be apt to abandon the country in which he was … assessed to a burdensome tax, and would remove his stock to some other country where he could either carry on his business or enjoy his fortune more at his ease" (Smith, 1937(1776)).

---

7 On the "race to the bottom" through the evasion of regulations etc., see Tonelson (2000); for competition related to working conditions, see Vogel and Kagan (2004); for pressure on regulatory policies see Drezner (2006) (also for a critical review).

Though many authors agree that there is no general "race to the bottom,"[8] there is wide-spread agreement that the regulatory capacities of individual nation states have been reduced and that social inequalities have grown.

While business has played a central role in driving forward economic globalization, the development of transnational civil society networks has also played a key role in the gradual emergence of a global society. Social inequalities have not only mobilized opposition in many countries, but we can also observe improved conditions for transnational communication and cooperation among CSOs, and between them and other actors in global affairs. We referred above to the important social and political dimensions leading to fundamental changes in transnational politics, of which the rapidly rising importance of transnational CSOs constitutes one of the central elements. We subsume under the term "CSO" all non-state, non-profit and basically voluntary organizations, that is, the large variety of collective actors that are neither part of the state apparatus (responsible for the authoritative handling of a society's affairs) nor a private for-profit enterprise. They include the "classical" non-governmental organizations (NGOs),[9] more precisely called advocacy organizations, social membership organizations (organizing internal affairs and lobbying for members' interests in their political environment), national and ethnic organizations, and philanthropic foundations. We define social movements as part of civil society, but not as organizations (though most of them are supported by a number of CSOs), and faith-based organizations as a special case in the landscape of civil society activities (since, on the one hand, they are taking part in public life like other CSOs, but on the other hand, they are based in religious organizations, nearly all with a long history of shaping social life and orienting the identity of peoples (Bartsch and Kohlmorgen, 2007a)).

According to various studies (for example (Anheier, Glasius and Kaldor, 2004; Union of International Associations, 2004), at the turn of the millennium there were approximately 51,000–59,000 international CSOs; of these, approximately 3000 international CSOs were in the health sector. Due to their professionalization, many CSOs are important advisors to governments and intergovernmental organizations.[10] Some of them, in particular the large foundations, are important funders of international activities. In addition, by organizing transnational support

---

8   See Drezner (2006) for a clear statement on this and a large amount of literature in support of his critical view (see ibid., footnotes 58–61).

9   This is an unfortunate term, as—taken literally—it encompasses every organization not part of any government (thus including for-profit enterprises), but has been customarily used to refer just to a very specific group of advocacy organizations.

10   See e.g. Martens (2005); concerning public relations, see Waisbord (2011). There have also been panels on this topic in various international conferences, e.g. ECPR General Conferences 2011 in Reykjavik (Panel: The Professionalisation of Organised Civil Society), International Political Science Convention, July 2009, Santiago de Chile, Panel MT01.256 (Nongovernmental Organizations: Professionalisation and Democratization).

for specific global campaigns, advocacy CSOs are becoming influential players on many issues. Mostly organized along specific topics and sectoral issues, and generally less restrained by bureaucratic and hierarchical structures than governmental actors, CSO networking is playing an increasingly important role in global problem-solving and norm-building (Khagram, Riker and Sikkink, 2002; Tarrow, 2005).

Transnational business has been primarily interested in securing general framework conditions for their economic operations,[11] but these firms are increasingly vulnerable to public complaints against the environmental or social impacts of their activities, and a possible backlash of such conditions on the firm itself. In former times, the ability of the local state to guarantee the general conditions of production was not the most significant factor in choosing new locations for conducting business outside the industrialized world. Investments in the extraction of raw materials, plantations of tropical agricultural products or the establishment of trade posts either took place in colonial areas or in enclaves of (in some cases only formally) independent states. Under both circumstances, to a large degree foreign investors took care of the establishment of the necessary infrastructure and frequently also the security of the region concerned.[12] The more important transnational activities and investments became for the day-to-day business of big companies, however, the more risky it appeared for them to keep out of local affairs and to ignore the external effects of their activities in areas where they were economically involved. If they chose a location for long-term investment, they were affected by the environmental impact of their activities, had an interest in supporting a "healthy" political environment and contributing to the health of workers in whom they had invested (see e.g. Thauer, 2011).

Increasingly, however, political pressure on TNCs to take on social and environmental responsibilities beyond their own rather narrowly-defined interests has grown—a phenomenon broadly known as "corporate social responsibility" (CSR). Since the 1990s a number of international efforts have been made to develop a general understanding of the relevant respective norms (see: OECD Guidelines for Multinational Enterprises, UN Global Compact; ISO 26000; and most recently, the Guiding Principles on Business and Human Rights, elaborated under the auspices of the UN Secretary General's Special Representative for Business and Human Rights), which has required a closer comprehension of the requirements of economic, social and cultural human rights, including in particular labor standards and core values in the fields of environmental protection and anti-

---

11   There is an enormous literature on multinational or transnational enterprises; though the relative importance of specific factors depends on the characteristics of the firm, basically two dimensions have been stressed in recent work: The external economies of regional linkages and clustering of firms, and systemic government support of business for economic development (see the standard work: Porter, 1990, see also: Dunning, 1999).

12   The concept of "enclave production" has been frequently used in critical development theory, see e.g. Leonard and Straus, 2003 and Furtado, 1970.

corruption measures.[13] Michael Porter and Mark Kramer speak of a "corporate social agenda": "A corporate social agenda looks beyond community expectations to opportunities to achieve social and economic benefits simultaneously. It moves from mitigating harm to finding ways to reinforce corporate strategy by advancing social conditions" (Porter and Kramer, 2006).

Over the past two decades, the idea of CSR has gained considerable weight in the relationships between TNCs and CSOs. Many large corporations have a director responsible for CSR on their board or board committees responsible for overseeing CSR activities.[14] Socially-motivated concessions regarding medicines prices or licensing patents to third parties such as generic firms can be marketed to the public as a gesture of social responsibility. We show in the following chapters that this has played a significant role in the implementation of the "access norm." The global activities of CSOs, their reference to core human rights norms, and the successful framing of global disparities in access to medicines as ethically unacceptable in major industrialized societies—as reflected in public opinion and the reaction of politicians—exerted strong pressure on TNPCs. Pharmaceutical companies could not deny that the industry as a whole was highly profitable, and that space existed to take measures to improve access to lifesaving medicines in the poorest countries. As we will see later on, offering to cooperate to improve access, at least to ARVs, and working on neglected diseases, were indispensable elements in a strategy to defend (or better re-establish) the image of the industry and to uphold the TRIPS system (see, for example, the UK government's guide to "good practice in the pharmaceutical industry" (DFID, 2005)).

In the context of global governance CSR played a different role than in the "old" nation states: While within high income countries, state regulations and transfer payments could counteract the social impacts of IPRs (or of other economic activities), this could not be taken for granted in poor countries or in cases where international rules produced effects for which no single nation state was ready to take responsibility. Where state control and public stewardship met with difficulties—because of weak states or isolated "race to the bottom" effects (e.g. threats to relocate production)—CSR could to a certain degree substitute for the implementation of political regulation. Indeed, oftentimes, business may seek to avert regulation and other more compulsory measures by engaging in CSR.[15]

---

13 See, for example, the UN Global Compact, "The Ten Principles" (www. unglobalcompact.org/AboutTheGC/TheTenPrinciples/). On the Global Compact and the social legitimacy of business, see Kell and Ruggie (1999).

14 Information based on Google results on "Boards of Directors," CSR; see also, Strandberg (2008).

15 "Voluntary Commitments," which constitute one expression of CSR, are particularly popular with private companies as substitutes for environmental regulation (see e.g. Böhringer and Frondel (2002) and Kinderman (2010)). The engagement of TNCs in GPPPs can play a similar role (see fn. 25).

In many cases, corporate social responsibility constitutes an important motivation for TNPCs to cooperate as part of a rather new group of transnational actors: the so-called global public-private partnerships (GPPP).[16] These are *hybrid actors*[17] in the sense that they give formal governance roles to both state and non-state actors. While in intergovernmental organizations non-state actors have been admitted as "observers" and therefore as actors on the margins of political processes (at least formally), in hybrid organizations state and private actors (including for-profit as well as not-for-profit actors) cooperate at eye-level. These hybrid organizations are neither public, nor private. GPPPs can be seen as another mechanism to respond to a situation where states are not in a position to provide the necessary services and business does not consider it economically attractive to do it alone (e.g. to invest into research on neglected diseases). In global health this has led to the development of public-private partnerships (also called "Global Health Partnerships") not only as limited projects, but as stable hybrid organizations. A number of scholars consider Global Health Partnerships to be the core institutions of global health governance and therefore we will characterize this rather new institutional form in more detail in the following sections.

(d) Post-Westphalian global health governance

Transformation from a Westphalian system of international relations to a post-Westphalian system of global governance has had a fundamental impact on the institutional structure of global health; several authors attest that the change has been more radical than in other sectors (Dodd et al., 2007; Florini and Sovacool, 2009). Many actors, especially but not only civil society organizations, started to build transborder networks and coalitions focusing on global issues. The growing strength of a global demos and of human rights norms can be seen as basic to the many activities of CSOs in global health, not least among those involved in campaigning for access to medicines. Globalization has impacted health not only through the increased spread of infectious disease or the discourse of human rights, but also in other important ways. Many of the health effects of globalization are closely related to "society building": for example, the bio-medical model of Western health-care that focuses on the pathology, biochemistry and physiology of diseases; disease-focused vertical programs of treatment (see Lee, 2009) and the spread of specific lifestyles and consumption habits. As outlined above, the many new problems, but also possibilities related to globalization are at the root of understanding (a) the complexity of interrelations between global health and

---

16   See Buse and Walt (2002), Huckel Schneider (2009a), International Federation of Pharmaceutical Manufacturers and Associations (IFPMA) (2007).

17   Though hybrid organizations play a rapidly growing role in public politics, political scientists have been rather reluctant to use this concept (Boyd, Henning, Reyna, Wang and Welch, 2009; see Koppell, 2001).

many other aspects of social and economic development and (b) the proliferation of actors aiming at improving human health in one way or another.

Until the late 1980s the institutional architecture of international health was still comparatively simple, firmly based in intergovernmental institutions founded at the end of World War II. The World Health Organization (WHO) was created in 1948 to "act as the directing and co-coordinating authority on international health work" (WHO Constitution, Article 2). Its role was based on the general acceptance of the norms that governed the understanding of universality and multilateralism as embodied in the United Nations. For the first decades after its founding in 1948, this position of the WHO was not challenged by any other organization; only UNICEF played a rather significant role in issues concerning children's health. In the 1970s the World Bank's entry into health financing created some competition concerning approaches to supporting health care in developing countries.[18] But it is only during the 1990s that a fundamental change can be observed, which has been characterized as a transformation from "*international health*" to "*global health*" and from "*international health governance*" to "*global health governance*" (Berridge, Loughlin and Herring, 2009; Brown, Cueto and Fee, 2006).

GHG as a complex multi-actor system

Today, a large number of different health activists, experts, and organizations interact with each other at various levels, including national governments, IGOs, bilateral agencies, and hybrid players such as public-private partnerships (PPP).[19] All of these actors have their own agendas, are guided by specific interests, and operate from disparate power bases. Their ability to influence politics at the global level varies depending on the actors' properties and the specific interfaces in which they interact. The flexibility of organization and cooperation characterizing this evolving system of global governance may offer multiple ways to overcome perceived barriers and rigidities within UN organizations. This development has contributed to a dynamic of a proliferation of actors and variation of institutional forms in global health. The establishment of the Global Fund to Fight AIDS, Tuberculosis, and Malaria (GFATM) illustrates this trend. The G8 proposed to make large-scale funding available for the fight against HIV/AIDS and was supported by then-UN General Secretary, Kofi Annan. Since some G8 members refused to allocate funds via a UN organization (which was seen as not sufficiently "results-oriented"), an independent fund was established, based on the PPP model with a Board comprising nation-state governments, representatives of private enterprise, and civil society organizations as decision makers (IGOs were only involved as non-voting members).

---

18 On the role of international governmental organizations in GHG see, for example, Kohlmorgen (2007).

19 For an interesting attempt to map the "global health architecture" see Walt, Spicer and Buse (2009).

The implementation of the human rights norm of "universal access to essential medicines" can be seen as another example of the emergence and role of organizational flexibility in GHG. The intellectual property system, which encourages R&D-intensive industries to finance product development, is a factor obstructing universal access to essential medicines in an unequal global society. The emerging norm to assure universal access to essential medicines has gained strength during the last decade. It has necessarily demanded changes in policies by pharmaceutical companies (supported by some form of financial subsidy) towards *voluntarily* selling medicines in specific places and/or to specific populations at greatly reduced prices. As noted above, it has also strengthened the political position of developing country governments to take compulsory measures when voluntary measures by the industry fall short.

In this post-Westphalian system of global governance, traditional forms of state regulation through nation states and IGOs are both complemented by and competing with new forms of trans-national activities through non-state actors and the hybrid organizations referred to above. Furthermore, global health has become an issue in quite a number of other policy fields such as foreign policy, geopolitics, security, trade and migration.

Global health partnerships

Beyond the fight against HIV/AIDS, PPPs or "global health partnerships" (GHPs) have contributed significantly to the changing approach to global health. By integrating a number of different actors (government health departments, multi- and bilateral organizations, pharmaceutical enterprises, private foundations and civil society organizations) in different combinations as required by the specific tasks and social and political environments, flexible forms of cooperation have become possible. These partnerships combine specific needs identified by governments, IGOs, or CSOs with the scientific and technological capacities of private corporations and the financial resources of donor countries, public funds, or private foundations.

A number of such partnerships have attempted to address the absence of research and development on neglected diseases and products (for instance, the Drugs for Neglected Diseases Initiative, Medicines for Malaria Venture, the Global Alliance for TB Drug Development, the International AIDS Vaccine Initiative, and the Foundation for Improved Diagnostics). A different group of partnerships has been established to address the lack of access to existing medicines. These initiatives include drug donation programs by drug manufacturers (e.g. ivermectin (Mectizan) for river blindness, fluconazole (Diflucan) for the treatment of AIDS-related opportunistic fungal infections, and atovaquone/proguanil (Malarone) for malaria in Africa), as well as those aiming to reduce the costs of medicines (e.g., the Green Light Committee for TB medicines, the Accelerating Access Initiative for ARVs[20]). Other alliances catalyze action and try to improve coordination on a range of issues, from TB (the Stop TB Partnership) and malaria (the Roll Back Malaria Partnership) to health measurement (the Health Metrics Network), and the crisis in human resources for health (the Global Health Workforce Alliance).

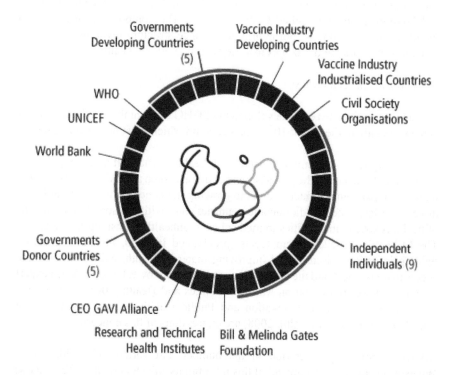

Figure 2.3   Composition of the GAVI Board
Source: GAVI Alliance website:http://www.gavialliance.org/about/in_partnership/index.php.

UNITAID constitutes another, in many ways even more groundbreaking international organization in the field of coordinating finance, acquisition of medicines and the provision of access—it is an international facility for the purchase of drugs against HIV/AIDS, malaria and tuberculosis, financed primarily

---

20   The Accelerating Access Initiative (AAI) is a cooperative endeavor of UNAIDS, the World Health Organization, UNICEF, the UN Population Fund, the World Bank, and seven research-based pharmaceutical companies (Abbott Laboratories, Boehringer Ingelheim, Bristol-Myers Squibb, GlaxoSmithKline, Gilead Sciences, Merck & Co., Inc. and F. Hoffmann–La Roche) (http://www.ifpma.org/health/hiv/health_aai_hiv.aspx, accessed July 18, 2010).

through a solidarity levy on airline tickets, and founded in September 2006 on the initiative of Brazil, Chile, France, Norway, and the United Kingdom. (see more details in Chapter 5)

Some of these partnerships have taken over a broad field of activities, either concerning the fight against a specific disease (like Roll Back Malaria, Stop TB) or concerning a specific area of health services like the Global Alliance for Vaccines and Immunization (now called GAVI Alliance). The composition of the GAVI Board (Figure 2.3) points to a hybrid governance structure involving both state and non-state actors and linkages to varied actors in global health.

GHG: Basic characteristics

We can summarize the recent development of GHG by a number of characteristics that are specific to the recent 10–15 years and on which most observers agree:[21]

(i) GHG implies a substantive concern with health threats that affect populations worldwide (for example the global spread of disease, such as HIV/AIDS, the much-feared new pandemic influenza and the growing incidence of non-communicable diseases in low- and middle-income countries) and with the social determinants of health (extreme inequalities in medical care, unhealthy consumption patterns). The Millennium Development Goals (proclaimed in 2000, including goals on fighting infectious diseases and improving maternal health, child mortality and access to medicines) and the themes discussed in depth by WHO-sponsored expert commissions (Commission on Macroeconomics and Health, 2001; Commission on Intellectual Property, Innovation and Public Health 2006; Commission on Social Determinants of Health, 2008) are expressions of this concern.

(ii) An important proliferation in the number and variety of health actors. Whatsoever might be the impact of this multiplicity of actors on the effectiveness of global action on health (see below), there is no doubt that it has contributed to a rapid rise of financial resources available in the form of "development assistance for health" (from about 5 billion USD in 1990 to close to 27 billion in 2010 (Murray et al., 2011).

(iii) A growing impact of civil society organizations (CSOs).

21   See only the most recent books which summarize and give critical assessments of the origins and development of GHG: Buse, Hein and Drager, 2009; Cooper and Kirton, 2009; Kay and Williams, 2009; MacLean, Fourie and Brown, 2009; Rosenberg, Hayes, McIntyre and Neil, 2010. For a conceptual overview of the "Global Health System," see: Frenk, 2010; Keusch, Kilama, Moon, Szlezak and Michaud, 2010; Moon et al., 2010; Szlezak et al., 2010.

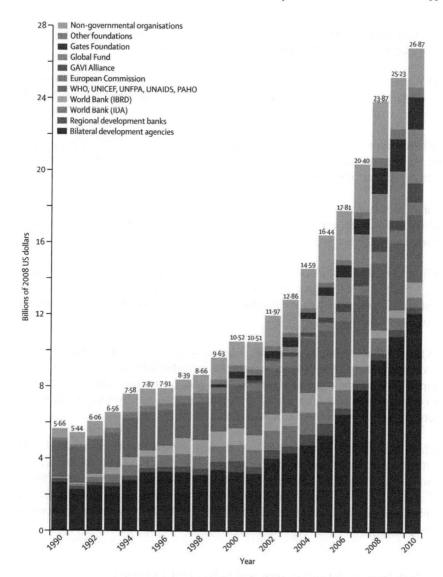

Figure 2.4   Development assistance for health from 1990 to 2010 by channel of assistance

Note: The bar graph represents the contributions of specific (groups of) donors in the same sequence as the legend.

Source: Reprinted from Murray, C., Anderson, B., Burstein, R., et al. (2011). Development Assistance for Health: Trends and Prospects. *The Lancet*, *378*, 8–11, with permission from Elsevier.

(iv) A growing involvement of private corporations, including the acknowledgment in principle of social responsibility by corporate actors.

(v) A growing importance of private funders (e.g. foundations), while national governments do not hesitate to sideline intergovernmental organizations through alliances with non-state actors.

(vi) New types of hybrid actors and global initiatives (e.g. foundations, public-private partnerships, the GFATM) interacting with national governments and intergovernmental organizations.

(vii) The dominance of state actors (WHO, etc.) in international/global health affairs is no longer accepted without question, but states and intergovernmental arenas are still extremely relevant.

(viii) Increasing interlinkages between health and other areas of global governance (e.g. trade and intellectual property rights; environment; agriculture), among which the conflict between intellectual property rules and access to medicines is a prominent example.

(ix) More than before, poor health is not only seen as a consequence of poor development but also as a cause; investments in health "pay" through their positive impact on development. The Commission on Macroeconomics and Health played a central role in changing global understandings on the two-way relationship between health and economic development.

While until the turn of the millennium the term "global health governance" was virtually unknown, since then research in GHG has produced a considerable number of publications linking this new field of research to analyses in the fields of globalization and international relations. More than many other sectors of global governance, GHG allows deeper insights into the relationship between an emerging global society and actors in global politics.

(e) Interfaces, nodal governance, and polylateral diplomacy: Elements of the social construction of global health governance (GHG)

In one way or the other, many analyses have turned to the impact of the growing institutional complexity on the "architecture", or the construction principles, of GHG. Depending on the vantage point, one can see GHG as an anarchy of actors that constitutes a "creative, unstructured plurality"[22] in managing global health

---

22   The term "unstructured plurality" has been first used to characterize global health in Bartlett, Kickbusch and Coulombier (2006) based on Beck and Lau (2004).

(at every moment raising new health issues and proposing new ways of solving them), or as a waste of material and political resources through an uncoordinated fragmentation of actors and activities in dire need of coordination. In the real world, simple models do not prevail, a third model appears to be much closer to capturing the complex interactions between anarchical developments and forms of binding coordination and decision-making, which can be characterized by the concepts of nodal governance and polylateral diplomacy.

David Fidler (2007) characterized governance of the global health system as a form of "open-source anarchy," which is broadening and deepening the normative basis for global health action. In this conceptualization, global health governance is comparable to open-source software, in which "anybody can access, use, modify and improve" upon components of the system (Fidler, 2007). This concept suggests that the interactive space of relations between national societies is no longer dominated by inter-state relations. Transnational relations are not squeezed into diplomatic rules and traditional means of exerting pressure on other states in the field of power politics or through complicated mechanisms of international organizations. Actors can use their specific strengths—such as financial and expert resources, or discourse and its power to mobilize support—to reach their goals, such as influencing international law-making processes. Transnational networks between health-oriented actors have been formed that focus on specific issues (such as access to medicines, neglected diseases, and tobacco control, among others), constituting a complex web of global social relations whose net result is to influence the social response to global health challenges.

Severino and Ray (2010) discuss a similar change in the field of development aid (which partially overlap with global health): the surge of an "institutional jungle" and a tendency towards the privatization of international cooperation. They propose the term "hypercollective action" to characterize this "new mode of production of global policies" (Severino and Ray, 2010). The authors acknowledge the mobilizing and creative dimension of these dynamics, but also the "considerable costs in terms of efficiency, time, coherence and ... credibility" (Severino and Ray, 2010). Severino and Ray's critique calls into question the potential for effective self-organization through "open-source anarchy."

When the need for "effective coordination" is expressed in the political debate, people frequently continue searching for a central institution of coordination. The interactive processes of global health governance, however, have created new forms of coordination in this field. Multiple forms of transnational links in fact coordinate all kinds of activities: research, production, marketing campaigns, political strategies, CSO campaigns, and whatever might be of interest for a transnational group of actors. In these networking processes important actors or institutions emerge as nodes of information and coordination (in the pursuits of specific goals such as improving access to medicines, improving support systems for primary health care, etc.), which frequently link various fields of activities and types of actors. This creates forms of coordination, cooperation and networked power that have been characterized by the concept of *nodal governance* (Burris et al., 2005; Hein et al., 2009). Informal and formal networking in Geneva and at other regular global health events (e.g. international AIDS conferences, meetings of the Global Forum for Health Research) plays an important role in creating flexible links between global health actors, who are often pursuing common goals related to the solution of specific health challenges.

As we have seen, these construction principles of GHG were even more complicated by the fact that the achievement of health goals substantially depended on norms and rules set in other sectors following quite different aims. Compromises mean stepping back on the basic aims of one's own group of actors to accept some basic rights in other social domains. While it is obvious that the pharmaceutical industry is closely related to health, the health of a population also depends on other economic sectors where this link is not as obvious, such as the food industry and the creation of unhealthy consumption habits, and the automobile industry and the potential neglect of the health impact of emissions (in particular in LMICs where a majority of the population do not own vehicles[23]). The concept of "health in all policies" (Kickbusch and Buckett, 2010; Stahl, Wismar, Ollila, Lahtinen and Leppo, 2006) refers to this need for a holistic perspective on these interrelationships between social activities that are seemingly far apart.

While it is already difficult to establish a "health in all policies"-perspective within nation states, in global politics such a perspective is only assumed by a limited group of observers (including commissions set up for such purposes), which might have a certain type of impact on decision-making at one or the other policy node. Nodal governance offers a useful way of thinking about the "power map" in a governance system, and the key characteristics of effective governing nodes. The concept of interfaces can then be used to refine the study and analysis of the power relations between different nodes and/or networks. Although there has been some research on interactions within particular categories of nodes—for example non-state actors (Arts, Noortmann and Reinalda, 2001; Baker and Chandler, 2005) and international organizations (Rittberger and Zangl, 2006)—the linkages between these actors have, to date, not been well examined. Moreover, there are only a few theoretical approaches explicitly dealing with interactions in governance and global governance. Oran R. Young scrutinized the "institutional interplay" of regimes and their relations to their institutional environment[24]—with regimes seen as sets of "principles, norms, rules, and decision-making procedures around which actors' expectations converge in a given area of international relations" (Krasner, 1982). Our approach refers more to Jan Kooiman, who defines interactions as "mutually influencing relations between two or more actors or entities" (Kooiman, 2003), and differentiates between a structural and an intentional level of interaction. The intentional level is comprised of actors and their objectives and interests,

---

23 Automobile-centered transportation systems in poor countries furthermore encourage the continued use of cars, buses and trucks that produce both emissions and pollutants.

24 See among others: Oberthür and Gehring (2006); Stokke (2001); Young (1996).

whereas the structural level refers to the "material, social and cultural context" (i.e., institutions, social constructs, forms of communication, technological development, power relations) in which interactions take place.

In an attempt to develop a concept that allows us to integrate Kooiman's structural and intentional levels and at the same time open up the term 'institutional interplay' for more actor-oriented analysis, we propose to take up Norman Long's concept of "interfaces" (1989) and to discuss its value in analyzing the interactive process of institutional change in global health governance. Long's work follows an essentially constructivist perspective, and in our work on informal norm-building, we demonstrate that discursive power plays an important role in making people understand the importance of access to medicines as an essential element of the human right to health, and thus in promoting and implementing the norm. This finding sheds some light on the importance of the "social construction of reality" for transnational norm-building processes, but we are far away from a position of radical constructivism which is based on philosophical idealism (reality as we can know it, is basically mentally constructed). Basically, we accept the idea that constructivist approaches can be well linked to the more classical approaches in international relations theory, such as realism and idealism. The interface-concept and the identification of different types of power are consistent with a more eclectic approach to constructivism. While discursive power might support a different understanding of important global political issues, the impact on the distribution of resources and on the interpretation and on possible changes of international law are not simply a matter of changes in the perception of specific issues, but will only be effective and sustainable if accompanied by a transformation of institutions and of power relations.

While the term "interfaces" is used loosely and can be found to describe meetings in coffee houses as well as interactions in governing bodies of international organizations, Norman Long's concept of "social interface" provides the first detailed conceptualization of this term. Long defines a social interface "as a critical point of interaction or linkage between different social systems, fields or levels of social order where structural discontinuities based upon differences of normative value and social interest, are most likely to be found" (Long, 1989).

Long explains that "studies of social interfaces should aim to bring out the dynamic and emergent character of the interactions taking place and to show how the goals, perceptions, interests, and relationships of the various parties may be reshaped as a result of their interaction" (Long, 1989). Thus, interfacing might have an influence and might even radically change the actors' original strategies (as described later in the chapter in relation to the pharmaceutical corporations in South Africa through their interactions with civil society over two court cases). Often, experiences at the interfaces have a mutual influence on the actors' behavior even if they are in an antagonistic relationship and/or if there are great disparities in power. This reciprocity may lead to a harmonization of conflicting strategies. If interactions continue, the development of boundaries and shared expectations is likely, which shape the interaction and may constitute "an organised entity of interlocking relationships and intentionalities" (Long, 1989). Interfaces frequently entail complex processes particularly when a variety of actors with different interests, relationships and modes of rationality are clashing. Moreover, Long stresses that it is important to focus not only on one single interface and the related actors and institutions, in a kind of micro perspective, but also to include the actors and institutions beyond this concrete interface in a macro perspective. Interface analysis should be based on broader institutional frameworks and fields of power (Long, 1989) and should not be understood as a mechanical point where two actors, programs or similar meet. In nodal terms, governance operates in a landscape of multifarious social interactions and conflicting or merging cultural and political habits and behaviors, meeting in related sets of specific interfaces—the complex web of institutions and informal networks linked to GHG in Geneva serves as a good example. In Chapter 9 we discuss in some detail the role of Geneva as a supra-node in GHG (the "Geneva connection").

Long applies the social interface approach mostly to interfaces between the global and the national/local level in the field of "development," that is, to vertical interfaces. Most of the elements of Long's approach, however, can also be used for our approach to the analysis of global governance, including the analysis of horizontal interfaces between different types of actors at the global level. We will modify Long's approach by concentrating less on cultural practices and sociological aspects (though not denying their importance), but focusing instead on the political processes and dynamics of power (i.e. adapting it to institutionalist approaches in international relations theory).

Due to their specific social and institutional environment, specific types of interfaces will provide quite different ways for individuals or groups to achieve "a position to carry out his own will despite resistance" (Weber, 1947). We distinguish four major types of interfaces that are closely related to the use of various forms of power:[25]

1. Discursive interfaces are interactions aiming at changing perceptions, concepts and norms held by different nodes of governance (e.g. mass media, campaigns, or expert commissions). *Discursive power* is linked to the central role of communication in the very production of social relations and thus related to the acceptance of basic beliefs on specific issues, and also to broad values like human rights. Discursive power shapes the demands and perceptions of actors' interests. Based on normative claims, advocacy and the impact of mass media, normative power plays an important role in discursive interfaces. Also influential in discursive interfaces is expert

---

25   For a more detailed discussion of forms of power in international politics, see Barnett and Duvall (2005). We leave out what might be called violent interfaces, closely related to the use of compulsory power, which certainly plays an important role in international relations theory, but not in the issue of access to medicines and intellectual property rights.

knowledge, which depends on the acceptance of a scientific foundation of political positions on disputed issues (expert power).

2. Resource-transfer interfaces involve various kinds of economic relations such as investments, loans and aid. At these interfaces the resources required to support economic development, to finance innovation and to tackle problems are identified, mobilized and disbursed; they are frequently closely linked to organizational interfaces, where decisions on using resources are made or conditions to attract investments are made. Although political institutions (with the backing of discursive power) might try to intervene, economic power is essential where resource transfers are needed. We will see that e.g. in relation to the insistence of the US not to confer responsibility for a global health fund to the WHO (see Chapter 5, Section (i)) or the conflicts on financing the Global Strategy and Plan of Action on Public Health, Innovation and Intellectual Property (see Chapter 8, Section (a)).

3. Organizational interfaces refer to decision-making structures linking different actors within relevant organizations and institutions. The "institutional power" of each actor depends on the rules of representation in the decision-making bodies including their potential to forge alliances around their positions. Actors with significant resources, but who do not see a chance within existing institutions to have them used in a way which serves their interests, might try to establish new institutions to pursue their goals (consider the foundation of the Global Fund to Fight AIDS, Tuberculosis and Malaria (GFATM)).

4. Finally, the level of legal interfaces (as a specific outcome of processes at state-based organizational interfaces), relates to the most formalized norms for regulating human relations and "civilizing" social and political conflicts—that is, for solving them without recourse to violence—due to the monopoly of the state on the legitimized use of force. We call this "structural power" as it is based on the structural position of the state in modern, territorially defined societies. As, however, there is no enforceable legal system at the global level, the implementation of international law depends to a large extent upon conflicts at other types of interfaces (consider the role of popular mobilization—discursive interfaces—in the outcome of conflicts linked to TRIPS regulations later in this book).

From this characterization of interfaces and forms of power, it is clear that different actors are more or less powerful at different types of interfaces. For example, CSOs typically have been at their most powerful in discursive interfaces, while corporations are dominant at resource-based ones. In some states, though rarely at the international level, legal interfaces provide an opportunity for CSOs to exercise power against better-resourced entities and government itself. Thus, the outcome of conflicts depends to a large degree on the types of interfaces at which conflicts are fought (see already with reference to characteristics of institutions,

Schattschneider (1960), and players will be successful in nodal governance if they are able to move a conflict to a field where they dispose of an optimum "portfolio" of different power resources (e.g. through forum shifting).

The "simple" form of nodal governance refers to the role of nodes in networks.[26] It characterizes many issue-oriented activities like the Campaign for Access to Essential Medicines, where MSF in Geneva acts as the central node linking the activities of many NGOs, the Peoples' Health Movement as a large network of grassroots organizations, or Knowledge Ecology International (KEI) as a communication platform on the internet. KEI provides an information exchange on the impact of intellectual property rights on medical research and access to medicines (through its website keionline.org and its widely-followed ip-health listserve). In this form "nodal" is more or less a synonym for "networked" governance.

The real strength of the nodal governance concept, however, lies in its approach to understanding the workings of interconnected governance networks, which operate in a landscape of mixed social interactions and of conflicting or merging cultural and political habits and behaviors. Nodal governance encompasses "a plurality of mechanisms that enable or constrain the exercise of power and rapid adaptive change" (Hein et al., 2009), which allows for a high degree of flexibility as characterized by Shearing and Wood (2003).

"Within a nodal conception of governance, no set of nodes is given conceptual priority. Rather, the exact nature of governance and the contribution of the various nodes to it are regarded as empirically open questions. It is assumed that the specific way in which governmental nodes relate to one another will vary across time and space. While these arrangements might very well become entrenched for considerable periods in many places, this should be regarded as an empirical state of affairs rather than an analytical constant" (Shearing and Wood, 2003).

Thus a system of nodal governance in a sector of global governance like health consists of interfaces between a considerable number of individual nodes. Some of these interfaces might arise just for the purpose of specific negotiations; others might be stable but are related to the management of very closely defined issues. On the other hand, some institutions might develop into clearing-points for discussions and informal negotiations on a more continuous basis. They have been called by some authors *superstructural nodes* (Burris, 2004). These complex interactions between various types of nodes of very different positions of authority (furthermore varying according to issues) has led to "landscapes of nodal governance" with flexible interfaces and changing hierarchies of power.

The World Health Assembly is the central superstructural node in GHG (beyond WHO's role as an intergovernmental organization). The WHA ensures the interface between the delegates of its members (nation-states) as well as the interface of these delegates with the representatives of many other global health

---

26   "A node is any formal or informal institution that participates to any degree in a governance network" (Hein, Burris and Shearing, 2009).

actors. Quite independent from what is being discussed on the assembly's formal agenda, the new "polylateral diplomacy" (Wiseman, 1999) is conducted throughout the WHA: Formal and informal meetings take place, agreements are reached, deals are struck, NGOs exert influence, the private sector lobbies, receptions are organized. In short, key global health players participate in the Assembly even if they are not part of the formal meetings.[27]

Concerning the establishment of an institutionalized link between the dynamics of GHG, basically shaped by a creative plurality of non-state actors and the role of WHO in authoritative and legitimate decision-making in global health, we can conclude:

> In the present complex global environment no single actor can or should set the agenda for action. ... Broad-based, participatory processes for agenda setting, anchored by WHO's global political legitimacy, will be required to define priorities, avoid unnecessary duplication, and share knowledge. (Moon et al., 2010)

In spite of a certain reconfirmation of the importance of WHO in GHG, it should be taken into account that in post-Westphalian global politics, non-state actors and hybrid global health initiatives are in a fundamentally different position than in the "old" international system:

a. they have acquired their own legitimacy drawn directly from the voice of people supporting them in pursuing transnational issues;
b. power in global politics is increasingly used in networks and coalitions independent from governments, including governmental actors themselves, which cooperate in global affairs with non-state actors;
c. in the medium and long run, the emergence of a global society might lead to further questioning of the legitimacy of national governments as representing the interests of their citizens, while at the same time independent links between people and transnational actors organized around specific goals will grow—as it does e.g. in human rights affairs.

---

27   Based on these observations, the proposal has been made to establish a Committee C of the WHA, which would involve the active participation of international agencies, philanthropic organizations, multinational health initiatives, and representatives from major civil society groups, particularly those who legitimately represent the most vulnerable populations. Some participants at the World Health Assembly 2011 took up this idea indirectly in the context of the WHO reform debate by proposing the introduction of a World Health Forum, but as of late 2011, despite widespread recognition of the need to engage non-state actors in decision-making processes, the WHA had not yet taken any decisions on the establishment of any permanent institutional arrangement for doing so (Hein and Kickbusch, 2010; Kickbusch, Hein and Silberschmidt, 2010).

To predict whether in the very long-run, a new re-centering of the nexus between voice (participation, representation) and entitlement (rights and obligations) in the form of a global state might develop, is out of reach for contemporary social science. We presume that in the coming decades *a new structure of multiple, interdependent, but not hierarchically organized forms of global governance* will prevail and increasingly shape norm-building processes at all levels of the global polity—linked among each other through a complex system of nodal governance. Flexible constellations of interfaces adapting to the solution of specific problems (like access to patented medicines) can react rather promptly to newly emerging issues and can also focus decision-making processes much more closely on the stakeholders affected, as compared to IGOs and inter-state relations bound by law and fixed institutional arrangements. Nation-states negotiating on the basis of highly aggregated interests tend to tie non-related goals into political deals and thus to make it more difficult and time-consuming to reach agreements. Sometimes specific issues which might be seen as relatively less important by national negotiators are also given up in exchange for other goals (see Chapter 4, Section (e), on IPR provisions in Free Trade Agreements). Initially, nodal governance processes do not aim at reaching binding and generalizable solutions but will allow for results-oriented interventions at short notice, which—if it proves to be effective in the long-run—might serve as a foundation for institutionally accepted formal rules and/or regimes.

Thus, increasingly norms—in particular in the field of human rights—might be implemented through social pressure based on a common understanding of their fundamental content arrived at in discursive processes rather than through diplomatic negotiations. On the other hand, we should not forget that formal international agreements—whenever they can be achieved—create legal interfaces where actors can refer to the structural power of the state. In this situation, the implementation of norms will become less dependent on the mobilization of discursive power. Universal access to essential medicines is such a case: Discursive power played a decisive role in the acceptance and the implementation of the norm, but certainly the norm would gain further stability if it were included in formal agreements.

(f) Global society, global politics and human rights

Human rights norms—especially economic, social and cultural (ESC) norms— have frequently been called "soft norms," as there are no "hard" sanctions against violators of these norms. In fact, however, in a world of nation states another problem has to be solved before the question of sanctions can be seriously approached: the material capacity of the respective states to implement these rights. Article 2(1) of the International Covenant on Economic, Social and Cultural Rights (ICESCR) declares that a state ought to implement these rights "to the maximum of its available resources." Theoretically, there are two possibilities to support effectively the implementation of ESC rights, i.e. either to clearly define obligations (including obligations to assist poor states) and to agree on sanctions (see discourse about introducing social and environmental standards into WTO agreements[28]) or to rely on the power of global society (CSOs, including alliances with state actors, media) to put pressure on the stakeholders involved to take responsibility in the implementation of human rights. The first path towards formal rules is complicated and difficult to negotiate since states are likely to resist agreeing to new norms that expose them to new sanctions and imply new responsibilities in fields where ESC rights did not prevail in the aggregation of national interests.

Post-Westphalian global politics, however, open up chances for the second path. Implementation then takes a formally voluntary character. Systems of *nodal governance* create links between actors demanding the fulfillment of rights and those with the resources to to meet the commitments—not only states, which according to international law are responsible for implementation, but also pharmaceutical companies, which could exercise flexibility in the use of their patents, other private producers of medical implements and services, philanthropic organizations, new global health initiatives and other providers of aid. Discursive power may convince actors to change their strategies, and may also be converted into institutional power through changes in voting behavior in IGOs or by creating new organizations focusing on specific tasks related to the implementation of human rights. Finally, when a specific norm is well established, a revision of international law might be accepted. In such a process of informal norm building, legal adaptations might occur at the end of the chain of norm implementation, after the flexibility of norm compliance had been, possibly for decades, a condition for its acceptance.[29]

Earlier publications on the role of CSOs in transnational norm-building mostly focused on forms of blaming and shaming (Finnemore and Sikkink, 1998; Keck and Sikkink, 1998; Price, 1998; Sikkink, 1986). More recently, however, the capacity to frame an issue in a specific way—for example, high prices of essential medicines as a human rights violation—has been stressed in the literature (Tarrow, 2005). Stakeholders in the norm-building and implementation process engage in increasingly dense communications. They are represented in numerous conferences on access to medicines in particular, or on GHG in general, within

---

28   This is a complex discourse reaching back to times of GATT. On the one hand, WTO power to sanction norm-breaking behavior is sought to be used to support the implementation of labor and environmental norms in traded goods and services, on the other hand, this is seen as beyond the objectives of WTO and/or as forms of hidden protectionism. See e.g. Nankivell (2002); United Nations Environmental Program (UNEP) and International Institute for Sustainable Development (IISD) (2005).

29   These hypothetical arguments on nodal governance and informal norm-building illuminate the link between the transformation of international relations and informal global norm-building, which will be dealt with in substance in the central part of this book.

and beyond WHO; they have an impact on public opinion and thus potentially also on the public image of political parties. International expert commissions like the Commission on Intellectual Property Rights, Innovation, and Public Health (CIPIH) offered broadly observed fora for discussion. What has transformed these events into a system of nodal governance is the density of communication, which has created a sole, albeit multi-faceted, discursive network. As discussed in the following chapters, the ensuing impact of discursive power (in the form of framing issues as well as in the form of public opinion) has influenced processes of decision-making (including the mobilization of resources) and the management of formal agreements. Even if it remains difficult to change formal international law or to agree on new formal regulations, discursive processes might lead to different attitudes of state actors (including different interpretations) towards formal regulations. *The 2001 Doha Declaration on TRIPS and Public Health* constitutes a prominent example in GHG, which in itself did not change international law but had an important impact by insisting on interpretations of the TRIPS Agreement favorable to access-oriented politics. Still, as we discuss in this book, the inclusiveness and stability of the access norm remained hotly contested, and were shaped by processes of nodal governance. The extent to which there will be future legal clarifications of such human rights norms still remains an open question, which we discuss in the final part of this book.

Chapter 3

Access to Medicines:
A Matter of Human Rights

Attention to health as a human right is a relatively recent phenomenon. Although, health is recognized as a right in the 1948 Universal Declaration of Human Rights (Art. 25) and in the 1966 International Covenant on Economic, Social and Cultural Rights (ICESCR, Art. 12), during much of the 1990s, health was not at the forefront of the human rights discourse nor of the global discourse on poverty. Health was basically seen as one aspect of global inequalities. The situation began to change in the late 1990s, when the lack of access to life-saving medicines particularly for people living with HIV/AIDS in developing countries became a global scandal and succeeded in mobilizing extended networks of CSOs and, quite rapidly, wider public opinion around the issue of the "human right to health" (Fischer-Lescano and Liste, 2005). The prominent role of health in the Millennium Development Goals was another factor strengthening public attention to health as a basic human right.

Civil and political rights have long been treated as the core of human rights, particularly in the Western world. In effect, the inclusion of economic, social and cultural (ESC) rights in the Universal Declaration of Human Rights and the negotiation of an international covenant on ESC rights were largely pushed by developing and socialist countries. Though the 1995 World Conference on Human Rights in Vienna declared that both are "universal, indivisible and interdependent," there is a fundamental difference between them. While civil and political rights refer to specific rights of individuals against the state and their protection against the illegitimate use of force (which does not directly depend on the level of economic development of a country), ESC rights generally refer to the duty of states to deliver specific goods. Frequently, one finds these distinguished as "negative rights" and "positive rights", respectively. In the case of ESC rights, a state may simply choose not to make available the necessary resources to deliver these goods.[1] As we observed in the last chapter, Article 2(1) of the ICESCR requires a state to implement these rights "to the maximum of its available resources" and "with a view to achieving (them) progressively." In addition, Article 11 stresses the importance of international cooperation for the realization of such rights.

There is a significant difference between the extra-territorial obligations implied for the realization of civil and political versus economic, social and cultural rights.

---

1   On the relationship between civil and political rights and ESC rights see Steiner and Alston (2000).

In the case of civil and political rights, extraterritorial obligations refer basically to the conditions under which military force might be used to force compliance upon a state, encapsulated in contemporary times in the "Responsibility to Protect" doctrine (International Commission on Intervention and State Sovereignty, 2001). In the case of ESC rights, however, many low-income countries, some of which have annual per capita public health expenditures of less than \$10 (CMH 2001, p56), are economically not in a position to fulfill ESC rights. Therefore, states also have the obligation to assist other states in fully realizing the right to health and to "ensure that the right to health is given due attention in international agreements" (General Comment 14, §39). General Comment 14 (§64), which provided the Committee on Economic Social and Cultural Rights' (CESCR) authoritative interpretation of the right to health, explicitly calls on a number of IGOs to "cooperate effectively with States parties, building on their respective expertise, in relation to the implementation of the right to health at the national level." This cooperation implies a net transfer of resources between countries—which could be realized through a large number of mechanisms, bi- and multilateral aid, international funds, private foundations, but also through restrictions on the transfer of resources from poor countries to rich by private actors.

However, there are no global institutions with the power to make binding decisions on the level and character of such resource transfers. Furthermore, as has been argued in the human rights discourse (Windfuhr, 2005), respect for ESC rights obliges States Parties not to take on international obligations (for example, through trade agreements) that might have adverse effects on the realization of these rights.

In practice, however, the past decades have witnessed the conclusion of many new trade and investment agreements that may very well undermine the right to health by enabling increases in the price of medicines beyond affordable levels through stringent IP policies (Correa, 2006; Drahos, 2003; Shaffer and Brenner, 2009). The tension between international human rights law and the rapidly developing set of international IP laws illustrates well the problem of regime complexity. "Regime complexity" (Alter and Meunier, 2009) refers to the emergence of nested, overlapping or parallel global regimes without any clear hierarchy, which has resulted from a proliferation of trans-border rulemaking activities (Koskenniemi, 2007). While, in principle, human rights norms should take precedence over other bodies of international law, the absence of any institution able to enforce such a hierarchy leads to conflict, confusion and ambiguity in practice. Such ambiguity can be used strategically by both relatively strong and weak actors, including not only states but also non-state actors such as firms, CSOs, and experts. The following chapters illustrate how access to medicines advocates both added to and took advantage of regime complexity, a theme to which we return in the Conclusion.

(a) The right to health and to access to essential medicines

Article 25 of the Universal Declaration of Human Rights states: "Everyone has the right to a standard of living adequate for the health and well-being of himself and of his family, including food, clothing, housing and medical care and necessary social services ..." This right was reinforced by Art. 12 of the ICESCR, a legally binding instrument—and thus formal international law for all those countries that ratified it—concluded in 1966 and ratified by all OECD countries with the exception of the US: "States Parties recognize the right of everyone to the enjoyment of the highest attainable standard of physical and mental health" (Art. 12.1), which includes "the prevention, treatment and control of epidemic, endemic, occupational and other diseases" and "the creation of conditions which would assure to all medical service and medical attention in the event of sickness" (Art. 12.2). These documents, however, are rather inconclusive with respect to the "standard of health" that is supposed to be "attainable."

Moreover, the "right to health" is codified in slightly different formulations in a number of other international agreements.[2] As such, it constitutes binding international law, but is widely seen as a typical example of "soft law," which corresponds to principles of basic human rights but is far from being enforceable at the international level. (In contrast, once codified into national constitutions or other national laws, both the right to health and to access to medicines have been found to be enforceable—at least in some cases (Hogerzeil, Samson, Casanovas and Rahmani-Ocora, 2006; Kinney and Clark, 2004).)

The global implementation of the "right to health" (or reformulated at the 1978 Alma Ata conference into the political goal "health for all") has been a difficult task not only because of its huge dimensions but also because of a lack of political determination; to some degree the dimensions of the challenge were in fact used as a legitimization of the second point. As briefly noted in the introduction, there is an important distinction between primary norms and secondary (or subsidiary) norms. Primary norms are those norms that are founded on general values or ideas shared by a community and upheld through diffuse social pressure. Such norms basically do not change even when they are laid down in binding international legal instruments. Secondary norms are designed to make sure that primary norms are in fact observed. In a world of sovereign nation states this is not an

---

2 In addition to the International Covenant on Economic, Social and Cultural Rights, see the Convention on the Elimination of All Forms of Discrimination against Women (Articles 10, 12 and 14), the Convention on the Elimination of All Forms of Racial Discrimination (Art. 5) and the Convention on the Rights of the Child (Art. 24). In addition, Art. 35 of the Charter of Fundamental Rights of the European Union refers to the rights established by "national laws and practices." Furthermore, we find commitments by governments to improve human health in a number of declarations and Programmes of Action (Agenda 21, chapter 6, §§1 and 12; Cairo Programme of Action, Principle 8 and §8.6; Copenhagen Declaration, Commitment 6, Beijing Declaration, §§17 and 30, Habitat Agenda §§36 and 128) and, of course, in the Millennium Declaration.

easy task—it took the UN International Law Commission (ILC) about 45 years to produce in 2001 "Draft articles on the Responsibility of States for internationally wrongful acts." In many cases, the determination of "wrongfulness" demands an authoritative interpretation of the international law concerned, which is a central part of the somewhat broader concept of secondary norms (see Hart, 1973).[3]

Hubert L.A. Hart, one of the foremost theorists of legal positivism, asserted that in developed legal systems the indeterminacy of primary rules was supplemented by secondary norms, which allow for clear decisions about their contents, changes and compliance with them (i.e. rules of recognition, change and adjudication (Hart, 1961[1997]). In international law, however, there are only rudimentary secondary rules, since "the formal structure of international law lack[ing] a legislature, courts with compulsory jurisdiction and officially organized sanctions" (Hart, 1961[1997]). Typical secondary norms are rules regulating the creation of norms within the subsystem (such as ESC rights), rules governing the consequences of a breach of primary rules (delineating responsibility and counter-measures), and rules of dispute settlement (Wellens, 1995 as quoted in Marschik 1998, 215). That does not mean that the extended realm of international law just consists of a huge patchwork of largely ineffective primary rules. Since the 1990s a growing process of *legalization* in world politics has been observed. This is characterized by three criteria: "the degree to which rules are obligatory, the precision of those rules, and the delegation of some functions of interpretation, monitoring, and implementation to a third party" (Goldstein, Kahler, Keohane and Slaughter, 2001). We have to take into consideration, however, that more precision, monitoring, and control of implementation does not necessarily overcome some of the most serious challenges to the implementation of human rights norms identified in the first chapters: the lack of flexibility to agree upon formal rules in a reasonable time frame when urgent problems have to be solved, and conflicts between norms in different sectors exist.[4] Notwithstanding these problems, within the UN system, important efforts have been directed towards "the progressive development of international law and its codification" (UN Charter, Art. 13 (1)), in particular through the International Law Commission (ILC) and the UN human rights system. Reports by these commissions, in particular the ILC, in most cases touch upon questions of secondary norms in international law—though, of course, they do not have the authority to take binding decisions in this respect.

Concerning ESC rights, such determination has been carried out by the Committee on Economic, Social and Cultural Rights (CESCR), (an independent body of experts charged with monitoring States Parties implementation of the ICESCR), in the form of various "General Comments". In 2000, the CESCR

---

3   See also footnote 46 in Bodansky and Crook (2002).

4   For example, while the relationship between the human right to health and the global trade regime are still being discussed, even more stringent IPR norms may be established through new agreements such as the Anti-Counterfeiting Trade Agreement (ACTA), creating further ambiguities between these two bodies of law.

issued General Comment 14, a 20-page document entitled "The right to the highest attainable standard of health."[5] General Comment 14 stated clearly for the first time in Paragraph 43 that State parties are obliged "to provide essential drugs, as from time to time defined under the WHO Action Programme on Essential Drugs" (ARVs have been included in this list since April 2002) and "to ensure equitable distribution of all health facilities, goods and services." The Committee continued that "A State party cannot, under any circumstances whatsoever, justify its non-compliance with the core obligations set out in paragraph 43 above, which are non-derogable" (§47). States also have the obligation to assist other states in fully realizing the right to health.[6] Violations of a State's obligation to respect the right to health included, inter alia, "the failure of the State to take into account its legal obligations regarding the right to health when entering into bilateral or multilateral agreements with other States, international organizations and other entities, such as multinational corporations" (Committee on Economic, Social and Cultural Rights, 2000).

But, what if states do not accept this obligation? The Draft Articles of the ILC in principle also apply to human rights but they do not refer explicitly to problems in this context. Certainly, the description of "countermeasures" which could be taken by an "injured state" (Draft Articles, Art. 49) are difficult to apply in the case of an infringement of human rights provisions, in particular ESC rights. Thus, there remains the "traditional" means of "blaming and shaming," which is playing an increasing role within the various bodies making up the UN human rights system. This is a consequence of a tendency towards dealing more openly with country reports and complaints against non-complying countries, underlined in particular by the creation of the UN Human Rights Council in 2006. Furthermore, it can be assumed that the effectiveness of "blaming and shaming" has been considerably strengthened by the growth of a global civil society and linked to the greatly increased importance of mass media in international communications. This is the starting point of the following analysis looking at the implementation of the right to universal access to essential medicines as a secondary norm to the right to health.

---

5   This document is part of a series of comments by the CESCR called 'Substantive issues arising in the implementation of the International Covenant on Economic, Social and Cultural Rights' adopted since 1989, here "General Comment No. 14" (document E/C.12/2000/4): http://www.unhchr.ch/tbs/doc.nsf/(symbol)/E.C.12.2000.4.En?OpenDocument.

6   Stephen Marks (2009) talks of a "derivative right," arguing that "When the main human rights instruments were drafted, the idea that lack of access to medicines was not considered, except that access to medicines was one of a number of reasonable measures constituting healthcare." Indeed, Art. 12 d demands "The creation of conditions which would assure to all medical service and medical attention in the event of sickness." Whether, in fact, "lack of access to medicines was not considered," or whether that was seen as a (possible) secondary norm determining the concrete content of this article, must be seen as an open question, but the content of that book (Clapham, Robinson, Mahon and Jerbi, 2009) rather points to the latter interpretation (one of a number of specifications of that right).

There are a large number of publications on the advocacy role of civil society organizations (CSOs) in the fight for universal access to medicines (mostly related to access to antiretrovirals for people living with HIV/AIDS) and also in a number of other issue areas. For example, many publications exist on the case of breastfeeding and the International Baby Food Action Network (IBFAN) (Adler and Haas, 1992; Keck and Sikkink, 1998; Meier and Labbok, 2010; Sikkink, 1986); other relevant cases include labor rights, in particular the anti-child labor and anti-sweatshop movements (Betz, 2002), indigenous peoples' rights, the conflicts on farmers' rights and access to (and the conservation of) seed varieties, and on agricultural trade liberalization and the conflicts around large dams relating to environmental impacts and displacement of people (Khagram, 2004). In these cases, the degree to which firms have accepted the asserted human rights norms has varied greatly, ranging from a basic acceptance in the cases of breastfeeding and child labor to hardly any significant changes in the cases of seeds, agricultural trade and large dams for the generation of hydroelectricity. So far, however, there has been little systematic research on the potential role of CSOs and non-state actors in general in *implementing* secondary norms in ESC rights.

Can civil society mobilization and normative pressure—that is normative and expert power at discursive interfaces—substitute for the lack of an enforceable system of rules for the implementation of human rights?

These considerations point to another aspect of the discussion of secondary norms: They could be either legally binding norms within international law (which is the case in a so-called self-contained regime like the WTO international trade regime, or with respect to supplementary norms negotiated in an international organization in a specific political field),[7] or "authoritative interpretations" that are not legally binding (as in the case of the "General Comments"), or they could be simply informal political norms broadly respected by responsible global actors. Whether it is advisable to consider the latter norms "as law under construction" (Coomans, 2005) or whether in specific cases—the conditions of which ought to be clarified and will be taken up again in the conclusion of this book— informal norms might be more effective than formal international law, will be discussed further. We should not forget that there is a close relationship between the social acceptance of norms and an effective (and basically non-coercive) implementation of law.[8]

---

7 See the following comment by Axel Marschik (1998): "The last decades have ... witnessed an increase in the number of subsystems in nearly all fields of international law. While this development has undeniably contributed to a better application of primary norms, the ensuing multitude and variety of subsystems has also resulted in a new structural disarray as each set of secondary norms can only assist in the operation of the specific primary norm within its own subsystem. Conflicts between subsystems have subsequently emerged, creating unprecedented difficulties for practitioners and scholars."

8 This is a central element of many legal theories and in particular of the sociology of law (see, for example, Licht, 2008).

(b) Sources of formal and informal norms on access to medicines

In addition to the CESCR's General Comment 14, a number of actors exercising considerable normative (or discursive) power began to promote the right to access to medicines in the late 1990s, and by extension, critiqued the expected impacts of TRIPS. Human rights norms could impact the interpretation of intellectual property laws in at least four ways: through the normative force of a human rights discourse; through binding human rights obligations codified in national law; by providing alternate international arenas for debating IP rules, and thereby helping to reframe an economic issue as a human rights issue; and finally, through the authority of opinions exerted by human rights experts and expert bodies. By 1999–2000, such critiques were emerging from UN bodies, experts, developing country governments and civil society groups. Each of these actors put forward normative claims that IP rules should not undermine social concerns such as public health, development, and human rights.

For example, the 1999, 2000 and 2001 UNDP *Human Development Reports* each carried substantive sections on TRIPS and its potential negative effects on developing countries in the areas of health, agriculture and traditional knowledge (UNDP, 1999; UNDP, 2000; UNDP, 2001). On the eve of the 1999 WTO Ministerial in Seattle, the CESCR issued a statement to the WTO highlighting its concerns regarding the negative consequences of TRIPS "particularly on food security, indigenous knowledge, biosafety and access to health care—major concerns of the Committee as reflected in articles 11 to 15 of the Covenant" (UN Committee on Economic, Social and Cultural Rights, 1999).

The following year, the UN Sub-Commission on Human Rights issued Resolution 2000/7, "Intellectual property rights and human rights," expressing concern regarding "restrictions on access to patented pharmaceuticals," among a range of other issues (United Nations High Commissioner for Human Rights, 2000). While noting that "the right to protection of the moral and material interests resulting from any scientific, literary or artistic production of which one is the author" is included among the rights delineated in the Universal Declaration of Human Rights and International Covenant on Economic, Social and Cultural Rights, the resolution also clearly stated that it was a right "subject to limitations in the public interest." In relatively strong language, the Resolution concluded that "the implementation of the TRIPS Agreement does not adequately reflect the fundamental nature and indivisibility of all human rights, including the right of everyone to enjoy the benefits of scientific progress and its applications, the right to health, the right to food and the right to self-determination, there are apparent conflicts between the intellectual property rights regime embodied in the TRIPS Agreement, on the one hand, and international human rights law, on the other" (United Nations High Commissioner for Human Rights, 2000).

Notably, each of these UN bodies (the UN Committee on Economic, Social and Cultural Rights, the UN Sub-Commission on Human Rights, and the Human Development Report office) was comprised of individual experts, not representatives of Member States. These experts played an important role in calling attention to the potentially negative social effect of IP rules, bolstered by the political legitimacy of the UN. The first significant statement from an *intergovernmental* human rights body followed in 2001, when Brazil put forward a resolution that was then adopted by the UN Commission on Human Rights on access to medicines for HIV/AIDS.

Less formally, advocates and civil society groups were making strong public claims regarding the right to access to medicines, though their claims were not often framed in the language of human rights. For example, on the eve of the WTO Ministerial in Seattle, the CSOs Médecins Sans Frontières (MSF), Consumer Project on Technology (which later became Knowledge Ecology International), and Health Action International (HAI) convened 350 participants from 50 countries at the Conference on Increasing Access to Essential Drugs in a Globalised Economy, which issued the Amsterdam Declaration. The Declaration outlined the shared agenda of the civil society groups, and included a range of goals including ways to ensure that TRIPS would be interpreted and applied in a manner sensitive to public health (including the use of compulsory licensing) and taking alternate approaches to ensure sufficient R&D into the diseases that affected the world's poor (the so-called "neglected diseases") ('t Hoen, 2009). These activities are described in further detail in Chapter 5, but it is important to note here the key role that CSOs played in asserting and strengthening the access to medicines norm.

These events, some orchestrated by individual experts, others by developing country governments, and others by CSOs, took place simultaneously and together began to create an emerging normative consensus at the turn of the millennium around the right to access to medicines within the new global IP regime.

(c) The UN Special Rapporteur on the Right to Health

Further elaboration of the secondary norm of access to medicines has been carried out through the work of authoritative independent experts. In 2002, the UN Human Rights Commission created for the first time a mandate for a Special Rapporteur on the right of everyone to the enjoyment of the highest attainable standard of physical and mental health (or, more concisely, the "right to health"). The Special Rapporteur is "an independent expert appointed by the Human Rights Council to examine and report back on a country situation or a specific human rights theme. He/she expresses his/her view in an independent capacity and does not represent his/her Government" (Office of the United Nations High Commissioner for Human Rights). From 2002–2008, human rights law professor Paul Hunt served as the first Special Rapporteur on the right to health. In this capacity, Hunt strongly re-affirmed the position of the CESCR's General Comment 14 that access to medicines was a core component of realizing the right to health, and that the obligation of states to make essential medicines available was immediate and not subject to progressive realization (Hunt, 2006). Furthermore, he endorsed the use of TRIPS flexibilities and argued that "no rich State should encourage a developing country to accept intellectual property standards that do not take into account the safeguards and flexibilities included under the TRIPS Agreement. In other words, developed States should not encourage a developing country to accept "TRIPS-plus" standards in any bilateral or multilateral trade agreement" (Hunt, 2006). (Industrialized countries have not abided by these recommendations, as reflected in negotiations over new trade agreements that contain stringent IP provisions, a topic to which we return in later chapters.)

As such, Hunt asserted that both states and non-state actors—particularly pharmaceutical companies—were subject to a set of obligations to support the progressive realization of this right. Hunt released a set of draft *Human Rights Guidelines for Pharmaceutical Companies in Relation to Access to Medicines* in September 2007 for public comment, and received input from states, investors, pharmaceutical companies, academics and CSOs. In August 2008, the Guidelines were circulated as a UN General Assembly document (A/63/263). Hunt also undertook a "mission" to GSK headquarters, and presented his findings to the UN Human Rights Council in June 2009 (Hunt, 2009). While the precise human rights obligations of non-state actors, and private businesses in particular, remain an area of considerable debate (Clapham 2006; GlaxoSmithKline, 2009b; Khosla and Hunt, 2009; Ruggie, 2008), Hunt argued that ensuring access to medicines was a "shared responsibility" between public and private actors, and that pharmaceutical companies had an "indispensable role to play" (Hunt, 2006).

While he included both patent-holding and generic pharmaceutical companies in his review, Hunt argued that patent-holders had a special set of obligations:

> Society has legitimate expectations of a company holding the patent on a life-saving medicine. In relation to such a patent, the right-to-health framework helps to clarify what these terms, and expectations, are. Because of its critical social function, a patent on a life-saving medicine places important right-to-health responsibilities on the patent holder. These responsibilities are reinforced when the patented life-saving medicine benefited from research and development undertaken in publicly funded laboratories. (Hunt, 2009)

The Guidelines are exhortatory rather than obligatory, but make clear normative assertions regarding the responsibilities of pharmaceutical companies with regard to access to medicines. It is difficult to measure their impact at this point, but they exemplify the normative pressure put on the industry and the consolidation of the "access norm."

The potential effect of the normative and expert power of the Special Rapporteur is indicated in the vehemence of the companies' responses. Some companies were not enthusiastic about the concept of obligations: in response to Hunt's report on his visit to GSK, the company issued a statement that

> The 'right to health' is an important issue, though not well defined, especially as it relates to non-state actors. Therefore we do not accept the suggestion—implicit in the development of this Report—that GSK's programme and ongoing commitment is in any way required by international legal norms, whether in human rights or other areas. (GlaxoSmithKline, 2009b)

In a similar vein, Merck's representative remarked, "we feel the approach to define guidelines specific to the pharmaceutical industry is misguided and will not result in meaningful improvements" (Sturchio, 2008). Nevertheless, it is notable that a number of companies had adopted some of the recommended practices in their access policies, as is discussed in the following chapters.

In 2008, Anand Grover, the director of the Indian NGO Lawyers Collective, was appointed the next Special Rapporteur. As an influential voice on Indian patent policies and a key strategist and legal counsel on a number of precedent-setting IP cases in India, Grover was well-versed in the relationship between TRIPS and access to medicines. In his annual reports to the UN Human Rights Council and the General Assembly, Grover has consistently raised concerns regarding the realization of the right to access to medicines and the impact of TRIPS and other IP provisions in trade agreements (Grover, 2009; Grover, 2011). In December 2010, he also publicly raised concerns regarding IP-related elements of the draft free trade agreement being negotiated between India and the European Union and its potentially negative impacts on access to medicines (Office of the High Commissioner for Human Rights (OHCHR), 2010).

By the first decade of the twenty-first century, the notion that access to medicines comprised a core component of realizing the right to health had gained relatively wide acceptance through the above-mentioned processes. The following chapters describe how this human rights norm rapidly came up against conflicting norms on intellectual property protection, and the global political contest that ensued.

Chapter 4
Access to Medicines and Intellectual Property

This chapter focuses on the driving forces behind the creation of global markets, the institutional structures of WTO and TRIPS, and the legal and organizational interfaces created by them. In this context, we explain the importance of intellectual property rights for pharmaceutical companies and summarize the process of the internationalization of intellectual property protection. We discuss the implications of TRIPS for the interests of the industry as well as for realizing the human right to health, in order to provide context for the conflicts and the building of the informal access norm that we analyze in detail in Chapter 5.

(a) Medicines and the global public goods problem

Classically, public goods have been characterized by two traits: non-rivalry in consumption (meaning that consumption by one person does not reduce the amount of good available for consumption by others) and non-excludability in access (no one can be excluded from consuming the good). Information and knowledge are classic pure public goods, and in an era of globalization and information technology, these have also become global public goods. A major element of the price of many patented medicines is attributed to the R&D costs of developing the knowledge encapsulated in a particular pill; arguably, the most valuable element of a new medicine is the knowledge that a certain dose of substance X can safely produce a certain therapeutic effect on the body. This knowledge can be considered a potential global public good. Once it has been produced—that is, once a stringent regulatory authority such as the US FDA has approved a new medicine—others can produce the drug at relatively low cost without having to bear the costs of developing this knowledge.

In some ways, the heart of the conflict over access to medicines can be seen as a problem of global public goods provision. While everyone can benefit from the development of new knowledge in the form of new medicines, the question of who should pay for the production of this knowledge is difficult to resolve.

There is a strong link between goods seen to be critical for the realization of human rights and the concept of global public goods as those that *should* be non-excludable—that is, goods to which all people should have access. Indeed, an important conceptual and normative evolution has taken place over the past several decades, such that it is accepted that the knowledge encapsulated in certain types of medicines (i.e. those deemed essential) should be made available as global public goods (Moon, 2009). This conceptualization is reflected in a number of claims, assertions, and consensus texts, not least of which is the recognition that access to essential medicines comprises a key component of realizing the human right to health (Committee on Economic, Social and Cultural Rights, 2000) (see a fuller discussion of this normative evolution in the previous chapter).

Yet, even if there is wide acceptance of the idea that certain medicines should be available as global public goods, some very practical questions remain: when certain goods are essential to the health of a potentially global population of end-users, how should access to those goods be ensured? Who should pay for the significant R&D costs involved, how should those costs be allocated on a globally equitable basis, and how should such decisions get made?

TNPCs are important contributors to the production of health-related knowledge. As private enterprises they do not directly produce global public goods, but are primarily oriented towards maximizing profits. However, some of the goods they produce are supposed to be made available publicly to those in need of them, either through the state or through some other form of publicly-regulated collective scheme such as insurance.

The conflicts that arise around access to medicines and intellectual property have their basis, in part, in the different modes of governance that play a role in the interface between institutions politically responsible for public health (e.g. national health ministries, WHO) and private for-profit organizations, which has often created tension regarding how to ensure that certain goods are available to all. The former must ensure the availability and affordability of needed inputs and/ or prevent public harm from the marketing of unhealthy products or concepts. For example, in the past, conflicts arose upon the introduction of the Essential Medicines concept in the 1970s, which the industry perceived as interfering with their ability to market their products (Laing, Waning, Gray, Ford and 't Hoen, 2003), and, quite prominently, with Nestlé on the issue of the marketing of baby milk to substitute for breastfeeding (the conflict over which CSOs marked their first major worldwide success on a health issue (Sikkink, 1986)).

The creation of global markets, enabled by the interaction of technical developments and international negotiations to reduce barriers to trade in goods and services, widened the transnational space for both TNCs and the development of international law to regulate them; this development is changing the legal interfaces between institutions responsible for access to public goods and the private producers of these goods. The effective international implementation of intellectual property rights constitutes one area of international law where two modes of governance—the state for guaranteeing the delivery of public goods and the market for using the incentive to maximize private benefits from offering these goods—have clashed concerning health issues. In short, this problem can be characterized as a problem of the global organization of private activities that produce global public goods for health.[1]

(b) Introducing the WTO

The WTO is the central public institution charged with creating and structuring markets at the global level. It has thus far developed an extended corpus of international law regulating the development of world trade. In 1994, member states of the General Agreement on Tariffs and Trade (GATT) transformed the post-World War II institution into the WTO with the signing of the Marrakesh Agreements. In contrast to the GATT, the newly-created WTO covered a broader set of subject matter (notably, expansion beyond trade in goods to trade in services and intellectual property), and included for the first time an enforcement mechanism adjudicated by the Dispute Settlement Body (DSB). Many of the WTO Agreements had the potential to impact public health in both industrialized and developing countries.[2] In recent years the Agreement on Trade-Related Aspects of Intellectual Property Rights (TRIPS) has been at the center of conflicts, but the General Agreement on Trade in Services (GATS) and the Agreement on Sanitary and Phytosanitary Measures (SPS) also have potentially important impacts on global health.

All of the Agreements are managed by WTO bodies, in most of which all WTO Members are represented. The Ministerial Conference is the highest-level governing body and is scheduled to meet at least every two years to decide on important issues and on the course of negotiations on new agreements. The General Council handles the day-to-day work of the WTO between the Ministerial Conferences, alongside the Dispute Settlement Body, the Trade Policy Review Body, the three councils for each broad area of trade (Goods, Services and TRIPS Council) and their subsidiary bodies ("Committees"). This broad representation of Members can mislead the observer with regard to existing inequalities, as many poor Members are not in a position to send delegates to all meetings. Critics have also raised concerns regarding informal meetings of a smaller number of "interested" delegations and the so-called Green Room[3] meetings, called by a committee chairperson or the Director General. Green Room meetings are intended to facilitate package deals that allow for complex compromises and tradeoffs across different areas. The WTO stresses that these negotiations are nevertheless

---

1   For further discussion of global public goods and health, see Chen, Evans and Cash (1999); Kaul (2003); Smith, Beaglehole, Woodward and Drager (2003).

2   For different perspectives, see Bermann and Mavroidis (2006); Blouin, Drager and Smith (2006); Blouin, Chopra and van der Hoeven (2009); Fink and Maskus (2005); Koivusalo (2003).

3   These types of meetings are named after the Director General's conference room even if they take place elsewhere.

"transparent," as every member is kept informed about what is going on and has an opportunity to provide inputs (The World Trade Organization (WTO)). This assumption, however, has been questioned by critics who contend that in practice the Green Rooms are small negotiating clubs where key decisions are made, and offered to the wider membership for endorsement thereafter (Hoekman and Kostecki, 2001; Jones, 2009).

The existence of a strong dispute settlement process is a powerful instrument to implement WTO rules.[4] If consultation and mediation processes do not lead to settlement of a dispute, the DSB establishes a panel[5] that produces a final report after half a year of examination of facts and arguments, as well as meetings with the parties and other interested states. Each party has the right to appeal the panel findings. Appeals are dealt with by the Appellate Body composed of seven persons broadly representative of WTO membership. Within 90 days a definite report is produced, which either rejects the complaint or allows the imposition of trade sanctions against the Member that has violated trade rules. The creation of an Advisory Centre on WTO Law (ACWL) in 2001 helped to compensate for inequalities in legal expertise, particularly between richer and poorer Members.[6] The uneven potential and effects of trade sanctions, however, constitute a problem: In fact, a developing country suspending tariff concessions to an industrialized country might create more problems to its own economy, it being dependent on particular imports, than doing harm to big industrialized countries, which do not depend on markets in those countries (Hoekman and Kostecki, 2001).

The Secretariat (including the Director General) plays a facilitating role—for example by trying to propose compromise solutions in the case of deadlocks. In addition, as part of their official mission, Secretariat staff play an important role in the delivery of technical assistance to developing countries (helping them to actively participate in WTO affairs); staff also participate in informal networks of communication in Geneva about issues important to other IGOs, CSOs, and governments present in Geneva (the "Geneva connection," see Chapter 9).

The central objective of the WTO is to regulate and facilitate world trade; it is not a welfare-oriented (or multipurpose) organization. Nevertheless, free trade has always been promoted on the premise that it will create a win-win situation for all participants. Thus, in a number of ways, it is normatively related to global welfare: the legitimacy of the WTO is based, at least in part, on the assumption that expanding trade has a generally positive impact on welfare. The preamble to the Agreement Establishing the World Trade Organization includes

---

4 For more details see Hoekman and Kostecki (2001) and Chapter 3 (see also the explanation given on the WTO website at www.wto.org/english/thewto_e/whatis_e/tif_e/disp1_e.htm.

5 Chosen from a list of potential panelists nominated by WTO members; Parties can reject proposed panelists.

6 For more information on the ACWL's mission, see http://www.acwl.ch (accessed November 29, 2011).

goals supporting "development" and improving standards of living. Furthermore, safeguard mechanisms can be used in situations of social and economic crisis, and specific WTO committees deal with welfare-related problems.

(c) Introduction to TRIPS—basic issues

Internationalizing and institutionalizing intellectual property protection has a long tradition, dating back into the nineteenth century (see David (1993); Drahos and Braithwaite (2002); Penrose (1951)).[7] In the area of patents, the form of IP most relevant for medicines, a push to internationalize patent protection culminated in the first major international IP agreement, the 1883 Paris Convention on the Protection of Industrial Property,[8] which is still in force today with 173 members (World Intellectual Property Organization, 2009).[9] In 1967, the Stockholm Convention Establishing the World Intellectual Property Organization (WIPO) was signed and the international protection of intellectual property rights reached a new level of institutionalization. Even then, many of the industrialized countries were not members, and it took another twenty to thirty years before advanced economies such as Canada, Austria, Spain, Switzerland and Norway adopted strong patent protection, which reflected the rules and regulations elaborated by WIPO in an international setting.

However, WIPO's one-country-one-vote rule led to stalemates. Furthermore, WIPO did not have any strong mechanism to enforce compliance. Industrialized countries faced the same situation as in other UN bodies such as the UN Conference on Trade and Development (UNCTAD) or the UN Educational, Scientific and Cultural Organization (UNESCO): developing country blocs could defeat Northern proposals and push their own preferred alternatives forward (Drahos and Braithwaite, 2002). Reacting to pressures from various IP-intensive industries (Drahos, 2002; Drahos and Braithwaite, 2002; Sell and Prakash, 2004), the US and other developed countries with strong interests in protecting IPRs insisted on negotiating an agreement on intellectual property rights in the context

---

7 After the Paris Convention for the Protection of Industrial Property (1883), and the Berne Convention for the Protection of Literary and Artistic Works (1887), a common international secretariat was established in 1893. During the first half of the twentieth century, the political and economic upheavals of the two World Wars and the economic problems associated with them did not allow any further institutionalization until 1967, when the Stockholm Convention Establishing the World Intellectual Property Organization (WIPO) was signed.

8 The 1886 Berne Convention for the Protection of Literary and Artistic Works was a landmark treaty for copyright, but is not discussed here because of its marginal relevance to the issue of access to medicines.

9 The 11 original signatories were: Belgium, Brazil, France, Guatemala, Italy, the Netherlands, Portugal, El Salvador, Serbia, Spain and Switzerland.

of the WTO[10] negotiations. The enforcement and dispute settlement system of the WTO agreements would make it possible to put pressure on advanced developing countries (at the time, the rising tigers such as South Korea, Taiwan, Hong Kong and Singapore) which were known not only to copy and re-engineer innovations, but also had been successful in exporting those more sophisticated products all over the world. In the field of medicines the increasing competition from international generic producers, which did not face the same strict patent laws domestically as in the US and other OECD countries, were increasingly perceived to hurt the sales of patented drugs, both at home and abroad (Gereffi, 1983).

Though IPRs and their internationalization are definitely not a market-based solution and therefore somehow contradictory to the general logic of the creation of a global market, they are the most well-established mechanism to address the innovation problem. It is not surprising that, in particular with respect to health and the global public goods character of pharmaceutical innovation, serious doubts have grown regarding whether IPRs are the optimal solution. These concerns are addressed in greater detail in Chapter 8. Nevertheless the private research-intensive industries, most orthodox economists as well as trade officials in the industrialized countries and many developing countries, have all defended IPRs as the accepted approach to promoting innovation.

Throughout the 1980s, industrialized countries and IP-intensive industries worked to construct a new set of global IP rules. Embodied in TRIPS, this treaty is a set of formal rules on intellectual property that have profoundly impacted the field of pharmaceuticals. TRIPS was one of the core treaties that came into force with the creation of the WTO in 1994. By requiring all WTO Members to provide a minimum level of IP protection domestically, TRIPS was intended to harmonize IP policies across industrialized and developing[11] countries against the backdrop of economic globalization. The final goal of the TRIPS Agreement[12] was to achieve a global harmonization of IPR rules with rather high minimum standards with which all WTO Members had to comply. All Members had to implement these standards into their national laws (for example minimum 20-year patent terms; rules on copyrights, trademarks, geographical indications and industrial design; and rules on IP enforcement).

However, as discussed in the introduction, TRIPS sparked a major public health controversy. According to its critics, TRIPS imposed a global intellectual property

---

10   The label "trade-related" was introduced after the Uruguay Round negotiations over TRIPS began, which appears primarily as a move to legitimize the introduction of intellectual property rights as a negotiating issue in the WTO framework.

11   We define "developing countries" as low- and middle-income countries, as classified by the World Bank (without drawing upon any theoretical considerations concerning the term "development").

12   See the summaries on TRIPS in Hoekman and Kostecki (2001); UNCTAD-ICTSD (2005); World Health Organization & World Trade Organization (2002).

regime on developing countries that was unsuited to meet their development needs in general, and threatened access to medicines in particular.

However, TRIPS contained a number of so-called "flexibilities" intended to address the concerns of some developing countries. These included transition periods, compulsory licenses, exceptions to patent rights, flexibility on patentability criteria, and other measures. In the case of TRIPS, the following clauses can be seen as "entry points" for social concerns:

The preamble recognizes the "developmental and technological objectives" of national IPR systems and the "special needs of the least-developed country Members in respect of maximum flexibility in the domestic implementation of laws and regulations in order to enable them to create a sound and viable technological base."

Art. 7 stresses that TRIPS "should contribute to the promotion of technological innovation [...] in a manner conducive to social and economic welfare"; Art. 8.1 highlights that: "Members may [...] adopt measures necessary to protect public health and nutrition, and to promote the public interest in sectors of vital importance to their socio-economic and technological development."

Furthermore, there are safeguard mechanisms. Art. 30 allows "limited exceptions to the exclusive rights conferred by a patent, provided that such exceptions do not unreasonably conflict with a normal exploitation of the patent."[13] Art. 31 deals with the authorization of compulsory licensing, which "in the case of a national emergency or other circumstances of extreme urgency" allows for use of a patent without the authorization of the right holder. Parallel importing, that is, imports of products supplied by the patent owner or a licensee at a lower price in another country, is also permitted, if not excluded by national patent law.[14]

The inclusion of variable transition periods can be seen as an important concession to developing countries, and was, in particular, a move to get India on board during the negotiations. In general, the TRIPS Agreement granted a one-year period to adjust national legislation to comply with TRIPS provisions, but developing countries were entitled to delay the date of application for a further period of four years (until January 1, 2000). In cases where a developing country already had a system of patent protection in place, but was obliged "to extend

---

13 Art. 30 allows the so-called Bolar provision. Countries may allow manufacturers of generic drugs to use the patented invention to obtain marketing approval without the patent owner's permission and before the patent protection expires. Generic products can then be marketed as soon as the patent expires (http://www.wto.org/english/tratop_e/ trips_e/factsheet_pharm02_e.htm, accessed June 19, 2006).

14 This refers to the issue of the exhaustion of patent rights, which means that the IPR embodied in a product or service is exhausted "when a good or service is first sold or marketed in a country". If a national patent law recognizes a doctrine of "international exhaustion", the IPR holder's right is extinguished whenever a good is sold or marketed anywhere in the world (UNCTAD-ICTSD, 2005). TRIPS Art. 6 allows a country full freedom with respect to the doctrine of exhaustion it uses in its patent law.

product patent protection to areas of technology not so protectable in its territory on the general date of application of this Agreement for that Member" (TRIPS Art. 65.4), there would be an additional transitional period of five years until 2005. This was the case in India, which had introduced a Patents Act in 1972 protecting only pharmaceutical production *processes* but not pharmaceutical products as such. LDCs were granted a transitional period of ten years originally set to expire in 2006, but since extended to 2013 with a request filed in 2011 for a further extension; a special exception was agreed in the 2001 Doha Declaration in the area of pharmaceuticals, granting LDCs an extension until at least 2016 to implement or enforce pharmaceutical-related patents.

While the *formal* provisions of TRIPS provided developing countries with some degree of flexibility to bring their national patent policies into compliance with the treaty, the exact shape and scope of this policy space was undefined and a subject of heated political contestation (Deere, 2008). The subject of greatest controversy was compulsory licensing. This measure could be used, for example, to authorize a generic version of an essential medicine if the patent-holder refused to supply it or to make it available at a price affordable to the local population. Compulsory licensing is intended to counteract the potential abuse of monopoly power by patent-holders, and is a standard feature of industrialized country patent systems.

In the case of an international agreement with "teeth" like the WTO, however, making broad use of these "flexibilities" was not without risks. Interpretations could be challenged by opposing parties, and in the case of a negative DSB panel decision there would be the threat of sanctions. The TRIPS Council is the first addressee for taking up new issues, such as those arising in the context of access to medicines, and for monitoring implementation. From 1994–2010, the DSB had received 29 TRIPS-related disputes, several of them directly relevant to pharmaceuticals and access to medicines in developing countries, as will be discussed below.

Even without resorting to the DSB, certain members use bilateral pressure to discourage the use of TRIPS flexibilities in developing countries. Most notably, the US Trade Representative has issued an annual report since the 1980s, known as the Special 301 report, assessing the IP protection measures implemented by its trade partners. Inclusion in the report, at the rank of Priority List, Priority Watch List, or Priority Foreign Country (rankings of progressive severity), is widely understood as a precursor to trade sanctions. The elaborate trade observation system of the USTR is a strong node within the US trade governance network (integrating a large number of trade lobbyists with informants on trade-related policies all over the world) and is linked to a narrow circle of IPR and trade advisors that constitute a superstructural node in global IPR governance.[15] The difficulties faced in making effective use of the existing options in a complex legal and political framework

---

15   Drahos points to the overlapping membership of the International Intellectual Property Alliance (IIPA), the Biotechnology Industry Organization, the Business Software

constitutes one of the central challenges for many developing countries in this system, as demonstrated by the experience of many countries (see sections on South Africa, Brazil, and Thailand in chapters 5 and 6).

In addition to state-to-state disputes at the WTO level, TRIPS-related disputes and legal challenges have also arisen at the national level. Actors, including both pharmaceutical companies and CSOs, can use national judicial systems to challenge national laws and decisions. Such cases, albeit national in nature, can impact the further development of TRIPS law and the way it is implemented in other countries (see sections on India and South Africa in chapters 5 and 6). These cases reflect the fact that there is room for alternate interpretations of many TRIPS provisions and legal interpretations and battles play an important role in defining the rights and obligations of states and firms (UNCTAD-ICTSD, 2005).

Thus, while most of the WTO Agreements sought to liberalize global trade by reducing state intervention in the transnational flow of goods and services, TRIPS required the opposite—it required governments to grant, protect and enforce a certain type of property right, generally for the benefit of IP rights holders. Several accounts of the negotiations behind the creation of TRIPS have pointed out that the industrialized countries sought expanded global IP rights to protect their competitive advantage in IP-intensive industries, such as entertainment, pharmaceuticals, information technology, and chemicals (Drahos and Braithwaite, 2002; Sell, 2003). Respected free-trade advocates such as economist Jagdish Bhagwati described the WTO's intellectual property protection as a tax that most poor countries pay on their use of knowledge, "constituting an unrequited transfer to the rich producing countries" as quoted in Sexton (2001). In other words, TRIPS created global trade rules that would increase rent transfers from IP rights users to IP rights holders.

However, an alternate rationale behind TRIPS has also been put forward: to increase innovation and to distribute globally the burden of financing research and development, such that one country could not "free-ride" on the investments made in another by refusing to recognize the intellectual property rights over a given invention. This rationale was particularly relevant in the field of pharmaceuticals, for several reasons. First, while there is heated debate over the average cost of R&D for a new medicine, there is consensus that the process is costly, risky and capital intensive. One analysis arrived at an estimate of $802 million for the average development costs for a new medicine, though this figure has been contested (DiMasi et al., 2003; Light and Warburton, 2011).[16] Second, the vast majority of R&D investment in pharmaceuticals is carried out in just a few highly-

---

Alliance and the Industry Functional Advisory Committee on IPRs for Trade Policy Matters, which advises the US Congress and President (Drahos, 2004).

16   These data are heavily debated (cf. the cost estimates for R&D in public-private partnerships which are much lower, e.g. between US$ 115 and 240 in the TB Alliance (Commission on Intellectual Property Rights, Innovation and Public Health (CIPIH), 2006), a number in line with those provided by the CSO Public Citizen in 2001 (Public

industrialized countries (namely, the US, Japan, Switzerland, Germany, France, and UK, along with several other members of the EU); if other countries did not grant patents on the medicines developed in these countries, firms would earn lower profits and national R&D investments (through grants, subsidies, tax breaks, or other R&D policies) would effectively go towards creating public goods for the global community. Third, medicines developed in one country were often found to be useful and/or needed, in all other countries. The development in the late 1970s of the WHO Essential Medicines List, which prioritized a list of medicines of particular public health importance, helped to sharpen this idea further (Laing et al., 2003). A consequence of this "universalization" of (primarily Western) medicines was a growing political demand for such medicines across a broad range of countries with highly variable ability to pay. How could medicines R&D be recovered on a global basis, across such diverse legal, economic, political and health contexts?

(d) TRIPS, TRIPS+ and the fight for social issues

Moving the focus of implementing international IPR rules from WIPO to the WTO represented the first round of "forum shifting" in this field, a strategy by which actors attempt to shift the main arena for international rulemaking to a different international organization or forum that is more favorable to their interests (Drahos and Braithwaite, 2002; Helfer, 2004; Sell, 2003; Sell and Prakash, 2004). That strategy was also used by the pharmaceutical industry and the US negotiators in bilateral trade agreements. The early ones, such as the North American Free Trade Agreement (NAFTA), were negotiated either before or at the same time as the TRIPS Agreement. Most of the others were signed in the late 1990s and the move has continued during the first decade of the twenty-first century. All of them contained so-called "TRIPS-plus" measures that restricted the use of TRIPS flexibilities in signatory countries and can be seen, at least in part, as a swift reaction by industrialized countries to the strengthening of TRIPS flexibilities in the Doha Declaration (see Chapter 5). These agreements, again, became rallying points of opposition to the trade agreements in their respective countries, as discussed in more detail in Chapter 7, which resulted in some trade negotiations being abandoned, while others continued to move forward.

It was certainly not in the interest of *developing countries* to create a strong international system of IPRs that would hamper technological learning through processes of product copying and reengineering. In the TRIPS Negotiating Group, India's demands that "[a]ny principle or standard relating to IPRs should be carefully tested against the needs of developing countries" (UNCTAD-ICTSD, 2005), did not achieve much more than a reference in the preamble of the Agreement (see

Citizen, 2001), see also the response by DiMasi et al. to the Public Citizen figures (DiMasi, Hansen and Grabowski, 2003).

above). One should assume that developing countries tried to defend and make use of the flexibilities TRIPS had left to them, as was the case concerning the Doha Declaration and the ensuing TRIPS amendment (the Paragraph 6 decision). In the process of interest aggregation at the national level, however, in many developing countries health considerations did not play a central role, and flexibilities in the field of IPRs were frequently sacrificed in favor of short term economic interests such as improving access to Northern markets, as has been demonstrated in negotiations on bilateral and multilateral free trade agreements (FTAs).[17]

In general, a situation of competing national systems striving for economic growth and economic development, where the most competitive economic actors and other elites have a better opportunity to influence the strategies of national governments than the poor, tends to relegate social issues to the second tier of priorities. If economic growth is accompanied by increasing inequalities (as is the case in many countries), the hopes for trickle-down effects seem to be rather empty promises. The actors that might throw their weight behind improving the situation of the poor appear to have more power in the context of global politics: these are: (a) a technocratic elite contemplating the costs and benefits in the long run and organizing reactions to threats on a global scale; and (b) a host of advocacy movements and organizations thinking in terms of a global society.

Thus, issues of social development constitute normative points of reference to interpret and readjust provisions of trade agreements—depending, of course, on relations of interests and power in global politics. In general, however, in the current world order, the problem of systematically relating trade order to social order is unresolved. The global governance system consists of a multiplicity of structures, as nation states still constitute barriers to the development of a unified legal system to organize politics and resource transfers. Nevertheless, in the ongoing process of globalization, the need for coordination and conflict resolution is increasing. This can explain the rise of new forms of interfaces that link organizations of global economic and global social governance. Social forces that are not locked into the "old" system of state-oriented institutions seem to be best situated to propel these links. As IGOs are by definition tied to nation states, their existing organizational interfaces are much less flexible than civil society organizations to deal with global social problems. We will discuss these developments in detail after having looked at the relationships between CSOs, TNPCs, nation states, and IGOs (see Chapter 9).

In the late 1990s, then, the odds were low that advocates for public health and IP flexibilities would gain the upper hand. The following chapter describes and

---

17   There are a large number of critical texts on Free Trade Agreements with TRIPS+ provisions. The UNCTAD-ICTSD Project on IPRs and Sustainable Development has presented a number of interesting studies and these negotiations (see: www.iprsonline.org/resources/FTAs-htm; Oxfam produced various briefing notes and briefing papers on this subject; Oxfam 2002; see also Vivas-Eugui, 2003; Abbott, 2006).

discusses the ways in which, against the odds, the access norm gained prominence and relatively widespread acceptance in the first years of the twenty-first century.

Chapter 5

˙ The HIV/AIDS Crisis:
The Rise of the Access Norm

The HIV/AIDS crisis was the single most important driving force behind the global access to medicines movement from 1999 to 2011 ('t Hoen et al., 2011). The lack of access to ARVs for the majority of HIV-infected people in developing countries constituted a moral scandal that mobilized broad-based political opposition: millions of people were facing death because neither they nor their governments could afford patent-protected medicines at prices demanded by TNPCs in the late 1990s. This chapter provides a brief introduction to HIV/AIDS medicines, describes the global political mobilization for access to these drugs, and offers an explanation for how this movement changed global norms, rules and practices, ultimately resulting in the (at least partial) solidification of a universal access norm.

(a) A brief introduction to HIV/AIDS medicines

As of 2011, there was neither a cure nor a vaccine for HIV. However, beginning with the discovery of zidovudine's (AZT) efficacy against HIV in 1985, treatment to counteract the virus itself has been available. However, HIV's ability to mutate quickly and develop resistance to existing drugs meant that individual drugs quickly became ineffective. AIDS treatment reached a turning point in 1996, when researchers announced that combining three drugs from different classes into a "cocktail" could suppress the virus to nearly undetectable levels in the body. "Triple therapy," also known as "combination therapy," "Highly Active Antiretroviral Therapy (HAART)," or "antiretroviral therapy (ART)," required patients to take multiple ARVs simultaneously to suppress replication of the virus and reduce the risk of resistance. Triple therapy transformed AIDS in the industrialized world from a death sentence to a chronic and manageable, if very difficult, condition. ART has been credited with reducing AIDS-related morbidity and mortality in the high-income countries where it has long been available; for example, in the US, AIDS-related deaths fell by 69% from 1994 to 2007, and in Europe mother-to-child HIV transmission was "virtually eliminated" (2009). Since AZT, the US Food and Drug Administration has approved 26 ARVs for HIV/AIDS in six drug classes (US Food and Drug Administration, 2011).

Though triple therapy had changed the face of the AIDS epidemic in high-income countries by the late 1990s, it remained virtually inaccessible to the 95%

of HIV-positive people who lived in the developing world (Grant and De Cock, 2001). At approximately \$10,000–15,000 per patient/year (ppy) for the drugs alone, triple therapy was prohibitively expensive (Perez-Casas, Mace, Berman and Double, 2001). Buying the drugs was simply unimaginable for most developing country governments. Cost, combined with the range of technical and medical challenges involved in delivering ART, made treatment seem a sheer impossibility in most developing countries in 1999.

However, activists and a few leaders in the academic and policy communities did not accept that treatment would remain out of reach for the majority of those in need of it. The debates over patents, drug prices, and health infrastructure became closely intertwined in the coming years. Not long after effective drugs were developed in the North, the question arose as to whether and how such treatment could be made available to people in the South.

(b) AIDS treatment and IP rules in the developing world: The special role of Brazil

In the late 1990s, IGOs active in the fight against HIV/AIDS in developing countries—basically WHO and the World Bank—concentrated their efforts on prevention, as this was seen as the most "cost-effective" strategy. This approach largely took the extremely high prices of ARVs as immutable; "treatment for all" was simply unaffordable for most developing countries and for the international community. This situation changed starting in the late 1990s: under strong pressure from Brazilian civil society, the Brazilian government had committed by law to provide free, universal access to ARV therapy for all who needed it in the country. A brief review of the evolution of AIDS treatment in Brazil provides important context for understanding later developments, particularly the influential role played by the Brazilian government and national civil society groups at the global level. In particular, during the early phase Brazilian CSOs played a significant role in pushing the government towards an active role in fighting HIV/AIDS and towards the guarantee of free access to ARVs for all PLHIV. The establishment of a new comprehensive national health system was an important element in the transition towards democracy in the second half of the 1980s leading to the proclamation of health care as a "right of all and the duty of the state" in the democratic constitution of 1988 (Calcagnotto, 2007).

Brazil was the first developing country to provide widespread access to HIV/ AIDS treatment for its population. Brazil's remarkable efforts to combat the epidemic became a powerful example for other governments: over the seven-year period from 1997–2004, the AIDS-related mortality rate in Brazil fell by an estimated 50% and inpatient hospitalization days by an estimated 70–80%; an investment in treatment of \$232 million from 1996–2001 led to estimated savings of \$1.1 billion in averted healthcare costs (Berkman, Garcia, Munoz-Laboy, Paiva and Parker, 2005). Brazil's AIDS program initially relied heavily on local production of generic ARVs, which brought it into direct conflict with the global IP regime.

In the late 1980s, the pharmaceutical company Burroughs Wellcome began marketing AZT in Brazil at $6000–8000 per patient/year (Nunn, 2009)—two to three times the per capita GNI of $2510 in 1989 (World Bank). At the time, AZT was considered a wonder-drug and reports of its efficacy in the US circulated widely in Brazil. PLHIV were well aware of the latest developments in medicine from attending international AIDS conferences and through international networks. The dense trans-border networks among PLHIV contrasted sharply with the relatively nascent networks among those advocating for access to medicines for non-communicable diseases a decade later, as we discuss further in Chapter 10. CSOs and individual leaders pushed the government to provide AZT to people living with HIV; after initial resistance, the health minister Alceni Guerra made the consequential decision in 1990 to provide HIV drugs to all patients in need.

Shortly thereafter, the government began providing AZT to patients. Initially, the government purchased AZT from the patent-holder, Burroughs Wellcome, but also encouraged efforts to produce the drug locally as a generic. Such production was legally permissible because, at the time, Brazil did not grant patents on medicines. Despite the absence of an AZT patent, local generic production of AZT sparked strong protest from TNPCs, which had been pushing for more stringent IP legislation in Brazil since the 1980s.

The government subsidized research efforts at local firm Microbiológica to manufacture AZT from raw materials and provided a purchase guarantee for the finished product, which the firm sold at about 50% of the Burroughs Wellcome price. Microbiológica's success in synthesizing AZT demonstrated that local ARV production was possible, and could make ARV treatment more affordable and sustainable in Brazil (Nunn, 2009).

In 1996, AIDS activists began filing cases through the courts for access to newer medicines, based on the right to health and the right to life, which are both contained in the national Constitution (Reis, Vieira and Chaves, 2009). Later that year, Parliament passed "Sarney's Law" (Law 9.313), which solidified government commitment to providing HIV/AIDS treatment, and strengthened the legal and political hand of activists who had been pushing for comprehensive treatment through the courts. According to one activist, "as a result of Sarney's Law, no one messes with the AIDS program, not Health Ministers, and not even our President" (Interview by Amy Nunn as cited in Nunn, 2009). Article 1 of the law guaranteed that "Individuals living with HIV/AIDs will receive, free of charge, from Unified System of Health [SUS], all medication necessary for treatment" (as cited in Nunn, 2009). Importantly, the law created a channel for *new* medicines to be included in the program as they became available, and specified that medicines would be provided to all at no cost. The inclusion of new medicines was of particular importance, since newer medicines were more likely to be eligible for patents and costlier; the uncanny ability of HIV to develop resistance to ARVs meant that many patients would need to transition to newer medicines as they became available. By the late 1990s, AIDS treatment had become well-institutionalized. The health infrastructure necessary to deliver treatment was funded by a World Bank loan, which did not pay for ARV drugs (which the Bank did not consider cost-effective at the time) but did free up national funds to do so.

The National AIDS Program, under the leadership of Pedro Chequer, had secured its position through high-level national political ties and international support, both of which were important for securing ongoing funding from the Brazilian Congress. Chequer and other high-level Brazilians in the health sector would later join UNAIDS and other UN agencies, creating a personal and institutionalized link between Brazil and influential intergovernmental organizations. A number of other key individuals similarly moved between Brazilian civil society, government, and key intergovernmental organizations—a revolving door that would help to create a "node" and strengthen international networks that facilitated the spread of knowledge on IP and public health between Brazil and the international community.

But Sarney's Law was not the only new law passed in 1996; the same year, Brazil adopted a new Industrial Property Law that began authorization of patents on medicines, several years before it was obligated to do so by TRIPS. This meant that the government of Brazil had a thorny problem on its hands: it was obligated to provide universal access to newer ARVs, which would be eligible for patents and therefore quite costly. Patents would restrict local production, which had enabled the national treatment program to begin just a few years earlier, to only a few of the drugs needed. Compounding the problem was Brazil's economic crisis in 1998–99, which dropped the value of the Brazilian real by 57% against the dollar and made imported patented medicines even costlier (Barbosa-Filho, 2008). ARVs cost about $4000 per patient/year at the time—far less than the US price of about $10,000–$15,000, but still far more than treating many other diseases in Brazil (Buckley, 2000). And the high price of patented drugs soon began to consume more and more of the ARV budget, with three patented medicines (out of a total of 17) consuming 75% of the AIDS program's drug budget at one point.

Preparations began within government to resolve this situation. Health Minister José Serra began to pursue a strategy of price negotiation and local drug production through the use of compulsory licensing. With the technical expertise of Dr Eloan dos Santos Pinheiro, a chemist and director of the national drug producer FarManguinhos, the government began R&D efforts to produce generic ARVs (Nunn, 2009). In October 1999, President Cardoso provided Serra with the legal means required with Presidential Decree 3.201. Article 71 of the 1996 Industrial Property Law had authorized compulsory licenses for national emergencies or for the "public interest," and the 1999 Presidential Decree clarified the definition of public interest to include "those facts, among others, related to the public health, nutrition, protection of the environment, as well as those of primordial importance to the technological or social and economic development of this country" (Art. 2, Para 2 in Cardoso, 1999). Less than two months later, Serra announced to the press on World AIDS Day, "There is a Presidential decree that allows for patents to be broken in the case of abusive prices, and two of our AIDS drugs are candidates for this clause. The laboratories will not be penalized if they lower their prices" (Serra as quoted in Nunn, 2009).

The stage was set for a direct confrontation between the Brazilian government and the multinational pharmaceutical industry, and between norms on the enforcement of IP and the right to health and access to medicines. These national problems quickly became international in scope.

In January 2001, the US requested that the WTO DSB adjudicate a formal complaint regarding the TRIPS-compliance of a "local working" requirement in Article 68 of Brazil's 1996 Industrial Property Law. This article allowed the Brazilian government to issue a compulsory license if the patent-holder did not manufacture a product locally (in-country) within three years of the patent grant, unless the patent-holder could show that it was economically infeasible to do so (Champ and Attaran, 2002).[1] The US complaint was perceived as an attempt to undermine Brazil's local production of generic ARVs, and by extension, its national AIDS treatment program. However, notably, Article 68 had never been used to produce generic medicines, as those used in Brazil's national program were not eligible for patents in Brazil. In response, Brazil filed the equivalent of a countersuit at the WTO DSB, challenging a provision in US patent law that required entities receiving patents on inventions developed with US federal funding to "manufacture substantially" their end-products in the US (World Trade Organization (WTO), 2010c). In doing so, it became the first developing country to file a TRIPS-related complaint at the WTO DSB.

Brazil also took its cause outside the WTO to the UN human rights system. In April 2001, the UN Commission on Human Rights passed a resolution sponsored by Brazil on "Access to Medication in the Context of Pandemics such as HIV/AIDS," by a vote of 52–0 (as mentioned in Chapter 3). The US was the sole abstention. For the first time the Commission recognized access to medicines as part of the right to health (Nunn, 2009) and called on States to promote the availability, accessibility and affordability of medicines (United Nations Commission on Human Rights, 2001).

(c) A window of opportunity: The 1999–2001 "policy crisis"

From 1999 to 2001, a series of key events took place both in key countries (Brazil and South Africa) and at the international level, which would build momentum that culminated in the 2001 Doha Declaration. Though these events were occurring at great geographic distances, social networks and communications technology effectively meant that they were taking place at a single discursive interface.

---

1   There is considerable disagreement among WTO Members and legal scholars as to whether local working requirements are permissible within TRIPS (Champ and Attaran, 2002).

South Africa

In parallel with developments in Brazil, legal challenges to IP rules were emerging in other countries as well. Most notable was the landmark court case that came to a head in 2001 in South Africa. In early 1998, 41 TNPCs had sued the new democratic post-apartheid government of South Africa over amendments made in 1997 to its Medicines Act, which aimed to lower the prices of medicines. The companies asserted that it was neither constitutional nor in compliance with the TRIPS Agreement (Cooper, Zimmerman and McGinley, 2001).

This lawsuit was brought against the backdrop of the growing AIDS crisis. While ARVs were becoming available in the industrialized countries, they remained far out of reach of most South Africans and others living in developing countries. At the time, South Africa was (and remains today) home to the largest estimated number of PLHIV in the world, with over five million people living with HIV in 2010. The court case became a rallying point for civil society groups both within South Africa and globally.

In 2001, the case was scheduled to be heard by the country's high court, and national CSOs such as the AIDS Law Project and the Treatment Action Campaign, together with international CSOs such as MSF and Oxfam, began to draw media and public attention to the lawsuit. A front-page *Wall Street Journal* article summarized the political miscalculation of the industry, when it began, "Can the pharmaceuticals industry inflict any more damage upon its ailing public image? Well, how about suing Nelson Mandela?" (Cooper et al., 2001). By April 2001, a global public outcry had tarnished the reputation of the pharmaceutical industry, and the drug companies dropped their case against the South African government. *The Guardian* described the case as "one of the great corporate PR disasters of all time" (Denny and Meek, 2001). This landmark concession marked a turning point in the political debates around IP and access to medicines, and momentum continued to gather in the ensuing months before the Doha WTO Ministerial in November 2001.

Both Brazil and South Africa represented "nodes" where critical events were taking place, actors were coming together in discursive interfaces, and informal but powerful networks were being built.

International

During this time parallel events were also taking place in Northern countries and at the international level, largely in Geneva.

In March 1999, CSOs MSF, CPTech, and Health Action International (HAI) organized a meeting for developing country government officials on compulsory licensing of AIDS medicines at the United Nations headquarters in Geneva. This meeting was intended to increase understanding among public health delegates of the health safeguards available in TRIPS and the extensive use of such safeguards in the industrialized countries. This meeting marked the informal beginning of a coordinated campaign by international and national CSOs to challenge intellectual property rules in order to improve access to medicines. At that time, topics such as compulsory licensing remained largely confined within specialized intellectual property and trade circles. During the 1990s, neither WHO nor UNAIDS nor any other UN agency had been particularly vociferous in supporting universal access to HIV medicines;[2] however, especially after civil society mobilization began to take shape, Geneva became the center of nodal governance on access to medicines due to the continuous presence of most of the stakeholders involved in this conflict. Key stakeholders included IGOs such as the WTO, WHO, WIPO and UN Human Rights Commission; CSOs observing, cooperating with, and/or protesting against these IGOs; the International Federation of Pharmaceutical Manufacturers and Associations (IFPMA) as the main voice of industry; and delegations of Member States to the various intergovernmental organizations.

Later that year, these CSO organized the Conference on Increasing Access to Essential Drugs in a Globalised Economy, which issued the Amsterdam Declaration (as mentioned in Chapter 3). The Declaration outlined the shared agenda of many civil society groups, including ensuring that TRIPS would be interpreted and applied in a manner sensitive to public health and alternate approaches to ensure sufficient R&D into the "neglected diseases" ('t Hoen, 2009). It was also in 1999 that MSF officially launched its International Campaign for Access to Essential Medicines, shortly before receiving the Nobel Peace Prize for its humanitarian aid work (Pecoul, Chirac, Trouiller and Pinel, 1999).

In the US, the AIDS activist group ACT-UP followed Vice President Al Gore on the presidential campaign trail, staging protest after protest against his support to the pharmaceutical industry in the South African Medicines Act court case. ACT-UP also staged demonstrations in Washington, at one point occupying the USTR offices and hanging a giant banner from the windows, reading "Essential Drugs for All Nations" (Cooper et al., 2001).

The access to medicines issue gained prominence at the WTO ministerial conference in 1999, during the famous "Battle of Seattle" in which CSOs concerned with a wide range of social and environmental issues effectively brought WTO proceedings to a halt through a series of street protests. Public health CSOs and developing country governments had formed a coalition to advocate for greater flexibility in IP rules for public health purposes.

The European Commission came to the Ministerial with a proposal that developing countries be allowed to issue compulsory licenses on drugs included on the WHO Model List of Essential Medicines (EML). This proposal would have severely constrained rather than promoted TRIPS flexibilities, since only 11 out of 306 EML drugs were widely-patented at the time, and no ARVs were included on the EML (One criteria for inclusion on the EML was price, and the first ARV was

---

2   In the early 1990s WHO twice sent missions to Brazil to persuade the Brazilian government to give up their strategy to freely distribute AZTs (without success) (Calcagnotto, 2007).

only included in the EML in 2002) ('t Hoen, 2009). This proposal was an early indication that industrialized countries would have to concede at least some ground on IP, but that the scope of diseases would remain a major issue of contention.

The US also came to the table with a new policy when, in a speech to the WTO Ministerial, US President Clinton declared that

> Intellectual property protections are very important to a modern economy, but when HIV and AIDS epidemics are involved and like serious health care crises, the United States will henceforward implement its health care and trade policies in a manner that ensures that people in the poorest countries won't have to go without medicine they so desperately need. I hope this will help South Africa and many other countries that we are committed to support in this regard. (Clinton, 1999)

The Clinton speech initially was not limited to a specific list of diseases or countries, but when the policy was formalized in an Executive Order five months later, it had become restricted to HIV/AIDS and sub-Saharan Africa only.[3]

By 2000, the issue of access to medicines had also drawn attention in the human rights community. In 2000, the UN Sub-Commission on Human Rights issued Resolution 2000/7, "Intellectual property rights and human rights," expressing concern regarding "restrictions on access to patented pharmaceuticals," among a range of other concerns (United Nations High Commissioner for Human Rights, 2000). The Resolution stated that

> the implementation of the TRIPS Agreement does not adequately reflect the fundamental nature and indivisibility of all human rights, including the right of everyone to enjoy the benefits of scientific progress and its applications, the right to health, the right to food and the right to self-determination, there are apparent conflicts between the intellectual property rights regime embodied in the TRIPS Agreement, on the one hand, and international human rights law, on the other. (United Nations High Commissioner for Human Rights, 2000)

At the same time that awareness of the public health implications of TRIPS was growing, so was political attention to the AIDS crisis. In 2000, under the presidency of Japan, the Group of 8 convened a meeting in Okinawa to focus on

---

3 Executive Order 13155 stated: "... the United States shall not seek, through negotiation or otherwise, the revision of any intellectual property law or policy of a beneficiary sub-Saharan African country, as determined by the President, that regulates HIV/AIDS pharmaceuticals or medical technologies if the law or policy of the country: (1) promotes access to HIV/AIDS pharmaceuticals or medical technologies for affected populations in that country; and (2) provides adequate and effective intellectual property protection consistent with the Agreement on Trade-Related Aspects of Intellectual Property Rights (TRIPS Agreement)" (Clinton, 2000).

infectious diseases and the response to HIV/AIDS, and was also the birthplace of the Global Fund.

Under increasing public pressure, the patent-holding pharmaceutical industry also began to respond. In May 2000, five pharmaceutical companies announced a joint initiative with the UN, the Accelerating Access Initiative, which involved the negotiation of discounted prices on HIV-related medicines and diagnostics to developing countries. However, even with the discounts, the prices offered through this initiative paled in comparison with the prices offered by generic producers.

This point was driven home in early 2001, when Indian generic medicines producer Cipla stunned the world by publicly offering to sell a triple-combination of ARVs for $350 per patient per year—a small fraction of the $10,000 price tag in Western countries. It was not only the low price, but also the transparency of the offer and the eligibility of all countries that marked a departure from business-as-usual. At the time, originator prices through the Accelerating Access Initiative were generally not publicly announced, and eligibility was restricted to a limited number of developing countries. (Cipla was able to produce generic ARVs legally at the time because the Indian Patents Act did not provide for patents on pharmaceutical products until required by TRIPS to do so in 2005.)

The stage was set for another major global political confrontation at the WTO Ministerial in Doha later that year.

(d) The Doha Declaration on the TRIPS Agreement and Public Health

In the conflict around IPRs and health, CSOs insisted that the problem of access to medicines could not be solved by philanthropy alone, but was more deeply rooted in the emerging legal basis of the global economy. Based on fundamental doubts on the appropriateness of patent monopolies on medicines in developing countries—and reinforced by the South African and Brazilian conflicts—there was increasing pressure from CSOs and governments from developing countries to maximize the flexibilities within the global IP system. After the failure to launch a so-called Millennium Round of trade negotiations at the Seattle Ministerial Conference in 1999, a declaration on IPRs and access to medicines which would address developing countries' concerns seemed to be an important pre-condition for the success of the following ministerial meeting in November 2001 in Doha. In early 2001, the African Group requested that the TRIPS Council deal with this problem based on documents by WHO and UNCTAD, which stressed use of the flexibilities built into TRIPS (Correa, 2002).

Debates over a potential declaration continued throughout 2001 at the TRIPS Council, with strong disagreement between two camps—the developing countries led by the Africa Group and Brazil on the one hand, and the industrialized countries, led by the US and EU on the other. Brazil in particular undertook extensive diplomatic efforts to strengthen alliances with other developing countries, including offering technical cooperation to African countries, after it had gained significant international recognition for its successful domestic HIV/ AIDS program. Brazil participated at a high level at the 2000 International AIDS Conference in Durban, at a conference organized by UNAIDS together with the health ministers of Nigeria, India, China and Russia on the issues of technology transfer and ARV price reductions, and at many other international events in the run-up to the Doha WTO Ministerial Conference. During the 2001 TRIPS dispute between the US and Brazil, the Brazilian HIV/AIDS Programme (BHAP) organized a "guerrilla like information action, with a list of international reporters and NGOs favorable to ARV treatment and the use of the telephone during several days demanding their support" (quoted from document by then-BHAP General Director Paulo Teixeira in Calcagnotto, 2007).

A major source of contention before Doha was the question of disease scope. The US had pushed for any declaration to be limited explicitly to certain infectious diseases, while the developing countries' argued for the inclusion of all public health problems. There were two main reasons for this battle over disease scope. First, any new limit on the use of flexibilities would have served the interests of industrialized countries that were keen to build a watertight, stringent global IP regime. Second, with the important exception of HIV/AIDS, there were relatively few new patented medicines for the infectious diseases responsible for the greatest burden on developing countries. Rather, the majority of investment by Western pharmaceutical firms had been into the non-communicable chronic diseases that plagued the West, such as cancers, diabetes, heart disease, and mental illness. There were many new patented medicines for these conditions, and these drug classes accounted for the majority of pharmaceutical company revenues. At the TRIPS Council meeting in September 2001, the last scheduled to take place before the Ministerial Conference in Doha, country positions remained far apart (Abbott, 2002).

However, an idiosyncratic twist of events would help bring countries closer to a consensus text. In October 2001, just weeks after the terrorist attacks on the World Trade Center in New York City, letters containing anthrax spores were sent to various members of the US Congress. In the ensuing weeks, public panic over the possibility of a bioterrorist attack mounted as anthrax was also found elsewhere in the postal system. Public concern began to grow over possible shortages of ciprofloxacin, a broad-spectrum antibiotic patented by German pharmaceutical company Bayer, as the drug was the only proven treatment for anthrax exposure. Under intense public criticism, Secretary of Health and Human Services Tommy Thompson began negotiating with Bayer for increased stocks. In nearby Canada, where anthrax spores had also been found in the postal system, the government issued a compulsory license for ciprofloxacin, authorizing local production of the drug should there be shortages of the patented version. Thompson publicly threatened Bayer with a compulsory license, though ultimately he reached agreement with the company over supply and price during negotiations. These events took place just weeks before the Doha Ministerial, and contributed to making Northern resistance to developing country use of compulsory licensing politically untenable (Abbott, 2002).

During the Doha Ministerial Conference (November 9–14, 2001), after last minute negotiations reportedly between Brazil and the United States, the so-called Doha Declaration on the TRIPS Agreement and Public Health was accepted (full text of the Declaration is in Annex 1). The Doha Declaration signaled a turning point in global debates over IP and public health, and could be seen as the culmination of several years of political contests that had taken place in Brazil, South Africa, and in intergovernmental policymaking arenas (primarily in Geneva).

The Doha Declaration made clear that the TRIPS Agreement "can and should be interpreted and implemented in a manner supportive of WTO Members' right to protect public health and, in particular, to promote access to medicines for all."

In the first paragraph, the declaration recognizes "the gravity of the public health problems afflicting many developing and least-developed countries, especially those resulting from HIV/AIDS, tuberculosis, malaria and other epidemics" (§1). The use of the general phrase "public health problems" makes clear that the Declaration applies to any health problem, not only to infectious diseases or epidemics, which are listed merely as examples in the phrase that follows. It explicitly acknowledges concerns about the effects of intellectual property protection on prices (§3).

Paragraph 4 constitutes the heart of the declaration (and implicitly refers to TRIPS Art. 8.1):

> We agree that the TRIPS Agreement does not and should not prevent members from taking measures to protect public health. Accordingly, while reiterating our commitment to the TRIPS Agreement, we affirm that the Agreement can and should be interpreted and implemented in a manner supportive of WTO members' right to protect public health and, in particular, to promote access to medicines for all. In this connection, we reaffirm the right of WTO members to use, to the full, the provisions in the TRIPS Agreement, which provide flexibility for this purpose.

Notably, the use of TRIPS flexibilities is not limited to a pre-defined set of countries. While the first paragraph recognizes the problems facing developing and least-developed countries, latter paragraphs refer to WTO members, not to a sub-set of the poorest members. Furthermore, it is worth noting that there is no formal definition of "developing country" or "developed country" within the WTO (in contrast, the WTO relies upon the UN-defined list of least-developed countries, but this is the only explicitly defined grouping of countries by level of development).

Paragraph 5 stresses the right of each country to make use of "entry points" for social concerns in TRIPS:

In applying the customary rules of interpretation of public international law, each provision of the TRIPS Agreement shall be read in the light of the object and purpose of the Agreement as expressed, in particular, in its objectives and principles. (§5a)

Paragraph 5(b–d) refers to the flexibilities in TRIPS which could be used for securing access to required medicines (as summarized above) and to members' sovereignty to determine "what constitutes a national emergency or other circumstances of extreme urgency."

Paragraph 6 of the Declaration recognizes an omission in the TRIPS Agreement: Compulsory licensing had been authorized "predominantly for the supply of the domestic market" (Art. 31 (f) TRIPS), which made it difficult for countries that had no generics industry to use this instrument. Further negotiations on compulsory licenses for supply from third countries were to be held. Finally, §7 extended the transition period for pharmaceutical patent protection in LDCs until at least January 1, 2016.

In general, developing countries and CSOs[4] recognized the Doha Declaration as a success for the access campaign and for strengthening the position of developing countries in conflicts with TNPCs and countries supporting strong IPRs.[5] Arguably, the most significant aspects of the Declaration were political rather than legal. (For detailed legal analyses of the Declaration see 't Hoen (2009); Abbott (2002); Correa (2002a).) The Declaration did launch a process that would lead to the first agreed amendment of any WTO treaty, and in that sense, a formal change in rules that carried important legal significance. However, far more dramatic was the *informal* change in rules: prior to Doha, compulsory licensing was technically legal but widely-understood as non-compliance with the global IP regime. Doha made clear that the use of compulsory licensing should be understood as TRIPS-compliant, and thereby considerably broadened the policy space to use such measures. It also provided legal grounding for arguments in support of other types of flexibilities, such as high patentability criteria, which are not explicitly authorized in TRIPS but can be said to fall under the Doha Declaration. The story of the Doha Declaration suggests that state compliance with international regimes is as much a politically-determined and socially-constructed assertion, as it is a technical or legal one.

While actual use of the flexibilities remained hotly-contested in the ensuing years, the Doha Declaration provided important legal and normative clarity to an issue that had been shrouded—in some cases intentionally—in uncertainty and fear. The following section describes the processes by which countries did or did

---

4   See Drahos and Braithwaite (2002) and the websites of CSOs such as MSF, Oxfam, HAI; also: personal interviews with people working for CSOs in Geneva (Oxfam, 3 D, CIEL, MSF).

5   See for example Abbott (2002); Abbott (2005); Correa (2002a).

not make use of the policy space afforded by Doha, and the subsequent impact on global access norms.

(e) Early debates on disease scope:
The WTO medicines (§6) decision and the TRIPS amendment

The issue of which diseases would be understood to fall within the scope of the Doha Declaration arose again during the so-called "Paragraph 6" debates. While the text of the Doha Declaration did not contain any disease restrictions and was quite clear in referring broadly to "public health problems", industrialized countries sought to recover ground lost at Doha by pushing for a narrow solution to the Paragraph 6 problem that would only apply to some diseases and some countries.

TRIPS restricts compulsory licensing "predominantly for the supply of the domestic market" except in cases of anti-competitive practice (TRIPS Article 31(f) and (k))—in other words, compulsory licenses could not be issued primarily for export. This restriction would result in potential supply shortages, since most LMICs do not have sophisticated drug production capacity and would have to rely on another country to issue a compulsory license for export (World Health Organization (WHO), 2004). The Doha Declaration recognized that this restriction needed to be loosened if poorer countries were to be able to make meaningful use of compulsory licensing.

WTO Members launched into negotiations after Doha to resolve the §6 problem, but rapidly bumped heads. Basically, three points proved to be controversial between those countries that tried to limit the use of compulsory licenses as narrowly as possible (the host countries of major TNPCs) and those that wanted to allow a broad use of it in support of public health:

The "scope of diseases"

The US used §1 of the Doha Declaration to argue that a §6-solution should be limited to the diseases specifically identified there, while developing country delegations insisted on the point that the Declaration always referred to the protection of "public health" in general.[6] At one point in the negotiations, the EU introduced a list of diseases to which the system could be restricted, which contained primarily neglected diseases that only occurred in developing countries; however, when MSF conducted an analysis showing that there were virtually no patented drugs developed for those diseases, this proposal quickly fell flat.

---

6   As Frederick Abbott stressed: "If developing countries were facing public health problems that required access to lower-priced medicines, it was not apparent why a distinction should be made between HIV/AIDS, on the one hand, and cancer, heart disease, diabetes or asthma, on the other" (Abbott, 2005: 328).

The determination of eligible countries

Paragraph 6 referred to countries "with insufficient or no manufacturing capacities in the pharmaceutical sector." As capacities vary considerably according to the medicines involved, developing countries insisted that each country should be responsible to determine whether it has the capacity to produce the needed pharmaceutical while the US and the EU wanted a more limited solution.

How simple or cumbersome the procedure would be

According to MSF, "the fundamental disagreement was over whether the solution would be simple and economically feasible," as advocated by developing countries, WHO and CSOs, "or complex and economically risky (2009)," as advocated by the Northern countries and pharmaceutical industry. CSOs and developing countries advocated for a solution based on TRIPS Article 30, which allowed for "limited exceptions" to patent rights and would have allowed a more flexible and non-bureaucratic use of the intended mechanism. In short, an Article 30 solution could have automatically authorized production for export once the importing country issued a compulsory license—in other words, only the country with the public health need would have to issue such a license. In contrast, the US, EU and pharmaceutical industry pushed for a solution based on amending Article 31, which delineated procedural requirements for a compulsory license and where the clause "predominantly for supply of the domestic market" had to be waived. Such a system would require a compulsory license to be issued in both the importing and exporting country—a significant procedural hurdle since no developing country had yet to issue a single compulsory license on a medicine as of the Paragraph 6 negotiations.

After two years of protracted and divided negotiations, on August 30, 2003, with the Cancun Ministerial rapidly approaching, WTO Members reached agreement on what would come to be known as either the "Paragraph 6" system or the "August 30th decision." The August 30th decision required both importing and exporting countries to issue compulsory licenses and notify the WTO of their intention to use the system; importing countries had to establish that they lacked local production capacity, and also inform the WTO as to the product, quantity, and duration of expected supply; producers had to export all goods authorized by the importing country under that specific compulsory license, and report on such quantities and any distinctive packaging to the WTO (World Trade Organization (WTO) General Council, 2003). While the developing countries managed to avoid restricting the system to a limited list of diseases, the industrialized countries succeeded in creating a complex, bureaucratic system that was subject to many delays.

CSOs criticized the August 30th decision, arguing that the system was economically unworkable and out of line with the realities of industrial pharmaceutical production because it required a "drug-by-drug, case-by-case, country-by-country" approval process ('t Hoen, 2009). With regard to geographical scope, the final agreement did not narrowly limit the countries eligible to use the system, but certain countries did voluntarily opt-out of using the system for imports altogether[7] while others opted out except in "circumstances of extreme urgency."[8] The Decision was accompanied by a "Chairperson's statement," which stressed the need to prevent the diversion of products from the markets for which they were intended.[9]

The August 30th Decision was implemented through a temporary waiver of TRIPS Art. 31 (f) and (h), which formed the basis for the first amendment agreed to TRIPS in December 2005 at the Hong Kong Ministerial (Article 31 bis).[10] The amendment is nearly identical to the waiver, but would be a more permanent legal arrangement, and only formally comes into force after two-thirds of WTO Members ratify it (approximately 100 Members). The US was the first to ratify, and as of November 2011, a total of 39 Members had ratified the amendment, including India, China and Brazil.[11] The original deadline for ratification, December 2007, was extended twice until December 2009 and again until December 2011, due to acceptance of the amendment "taking longer than initially foreseen" (World Trade Organization (WTO) General Council, 2009). The slow pace of ratification likely reflects dissatisfaction with the August 30th decision. By 2011, only one country (Rwanda) had used the system to import generic medicines from a producing country (Canada).

Did the August 30th Decision signal a consolidation of the access norm, or a retreat? Some have framed it as a success for the industrialized countries, since the system was bitterly criticized by CSOs and largely held to be practically unworkable (see Drezner, 2007). However, others have pointed out that the very first amendment agreed by Members to any WTO treaty was done to address access to medicines, which should be seen in and of itself as hugely symbolic of the consolidation of the access norm (Moon, 2010). Nevertheless, it should be recognized that the amendment itself was relatively minor and did not fundamentally change the obligations that TRIPS put on developing countries to provide patent monopolies on medicines.

---

7   Australia, Austria, Belgium, Canada, Denmark, Finland, France, Germany, Greece, Iceland, Ireland, Italy, Japan, Luxembourg, Netherlands, New Zealand, Norway, Portugal, Spain, Sweden, Switzerland, United Kingdom and United States of America.

8   Macao, Hong Kong, Taiwan (Chinese Taipei), Israel, Korea, Kuwait, Mexico, Qatar, Singapore, Turkey, and the United Arab Emirates. See the list at: http://www.wto.org/english/news_e/news03_e/trips_stat_28aug03_e.htm.

9   For the "General Council Chairperson's statement" see: WTO General Council, WT/GC/M/82, November 13, 2003). Note that LDCs are assumed to have insufficient manufacturing capacity; any other country must submit a notification to the TRIPS Council that it has insufficient or no manufacturing capacity for the "product(s) in question."

10   See: Implementation of Paragraph 6 of the Doha Declaration on the TRIPS Agreement and Public Health (August 30, 2003), Doc. WT/L/540 (September 1, 2003).

11   See list at: http://www.wto.org/english/tratop_e/trips_e/amendment_e.htm.

Arguably, the avoidance of a narrow list of diseases or countries eligible to use the system may have been more important than the concrete mechanism established by the Decision. The broad affirmation of the right of WTO members to make use of TRIPS flexibilities to protect *public health* and not only to fight a specific set of diseases was successfully defended in these negotiations, despite strong pressure from the industrialized countries to limit the concessions they had made at Doha. This was a critical point in the consolidation process of the universal access norm.

In March 2010 a special meeting requested by developing country Members to discuss how well the system was functioning took place, to lay the groundwork for the TRIPS Council's annual review of the mechanism in October (World Trade Organization (WTO), 2010d). This meeting was the first time WTO Members had actively discussed the August 30th decision since it was agreed upon in 2003. The August 30th decision has since been discussed at the October 2010, March 2011, and October 2011 TRIPS Council meetings, signaling that it may be re-opened for negotiation in the not-too-distant future (International Centre for Trade and Sustainable Development, 2011). The re-emergence of the August 30th decision as a contentious issue within the WTO reflects two important changes that have taken place since the decision was agreed. First, on a very practical level, India has begun granting product patents on medicines after fully implementing TRIPS in 2005; as a major source of generic medicines throughout the developing world, the implementation of medicines patents in India implies an increased need for compulsory licenses for export. Second, the growing economic and political strength of some middle-income countries (as discussed earlier) raises the possibility that a deal more favorable to developing countries could be reached should the agreement be re-opened.

(f) Improved access to medicines: Using TRIPS flexibilities

By mid-to-late 2001, international opinion had begun to shift on the question of the feasibility of ARV treatment. From 2001–2004, a flurry of new international initiatives began to make access to treatment seem for the first time like a real possibility for millions in the developing world. At the UN General Assembly Special Session on HIV/AIDS in June 2001, Member States agreed upon the goal of expanding access to treatment and creating an international fund to mobilize resources to fight the epidemic, which the G8 endorsed at its summit in Genoa shortly thereafter. By early 2002, the Global Fund to Fight AIDS, Tuberculosis and Malaria was established to channel unprecedented sums of money to hard-hit countries. In 2003, discussions that had begun under WHO Director General (DG) Gro Harlem Brundtland took on renewed life when the new DG Jong-wook Lee launched the "3 by 5" Campaign to get three million people in the developing world on ARV treatment by 2005. The same year, the US President's Emergency Plan for AIDS Relief (PEPFAR) was established, and would channel billions of dollars to AIDS treatment (Office of the United States Global AIDS Coordinator, 2008). The dramatic drop in ARV prices enabled by generic producers in India had put wide scale access to AIDS treatment as an option on the table, and helped to catalyze the dramatic increase in resources being dedicated to combat the epidemic.

At the same time, it was clear that for these new initiatives to work, countries would need access to low-cost generic ARVs. Doubts were initially raised regarding the quality of Indian-produced ARVs, and whether they would be equivalent to originator products. The WHO Prequalification Programme, first established in 2001, played a critical role in certifying that generic ARVs could meet stringent international standards and providing donors with confidence to allocate hundreds of millions of dollars for their purchase. In 2002, WHO included ARVs for the first time on the EML, which sent a clear message to governments about the public health importance of AIDS treatment and also had implications for state responsibilities to provide ARVs under their human rights obligations (Recall that General Comment 14 had specified that providing essential medicines, as defined by the WHO, was a core obligation of States in fulfilling their obligations regarding the right to health). PEPFAR initially did not allow its funds to be used to purchase generic versions of drugs still on patent in the US, citing government procurement rules. However, under strong civil society pressure, and after a US General Accounting Office report highlighted the enormous taxpayer costs of purchasing only US-made branded drugs, PEPFAR established the necessary regulatory procedures to begin purchasing generic ARVs. This regulatory change led to a dramatic increase in the purchase of generic ARVs, and significant cost-savings to PEPFAR. From 2005 to 2008, the generic proportion of PEPFAR-funded ARVS increased from 15% to 89%, with estimated savings to PEPFAR totaling $323 million over the four-year period (Holmes et al., 2010). In total PEPFAR spent hundreds of millions of dollars on generic ARVs since its inception (Holmes et al., 2010; US Global AIDS Coordinator, 2008)—a stunning turnaround for a government that had challenged developing countries' rights to access generic ARVs just a few years earlier.

The freedom to use donor funds to purchase generic ARVs gave many countries the impetus to make use of TRIPS flexibilities. While donors required that drug procurement be done in compliance with national and international IP rules, it was widely recognized that—at least for the poorest African countries—the use of compulsory licenses for AIDS drugs was indeed understood to be compliant. The use of low-cost generic drugs was a critical factor that enabled the international community to support access to ART for 6.6 million people by 2010 (2011).

After sustaining heavy damages to their public image, TNPCs realized that they needed to be responsive to social concerns in order to uphold the political support of their home countries in international trade negotiations. In the end, public pressure was so strong that TNPCs did not succeed in securing the continued support of their main political allies to prevent modifications to TRIPS.[12] When the

---

12   See for example (Thomas, 2004) on public pressures on the US government in 2000 to push for stronger IPRs in developing countries.

battle over the Doha Declaration was lost, TNPCs themselves were increasingly ready to compromise with respect to selling drugs cheaper, granting voluntary licenses to generic firms to supply some developing countries, and to refrain or withdraw from legal action to defend their patent rights in some cases. These changes happened gradually over time, in part due to compulsory licenses and other legal action at the national level in key countries.

The widespread use of TRIPS flexibilities in over 60 developing countries, together with financing provided by the international community through the Global Fund and PEPFAR, led international prices of ARVs to plummet between June 2000 and July 2001 and then decrease gradually but constantly through 2011, with the prices of some products dropping by as much as 99%. This included generic and originator products. According to MSF, which regularly produced "a pricing guide for the purchase of ARVs for developing countries," originators' prices for a WHO-recommended first-line regimen (tenofovir, emtricitabine or lamivudine, efavirenz) was offered in 2011 at about $600–$1000 per patient/year (depending on the income group of the country), while generics offered the same combination for about $140–$170 (depending on whether the drugs are combined into one pill or co-packaged as separate pills) (Médecins Sans Frontières (MSF), 2011). Countries could obtain further price reductions through various procurement strategies, such as bulk purchasing, participating in international pooled procurement initiatives, tendering, negotiating, and other measures.[13]

(g) The first developing country compulsory licenses: Zimbabwe and Malaysia

From the signing of TRIPS in 1994 through the Doha Declaration in 2001 not a single developing country made use of compulsory licensing, as discussed in previous sections. Even with the Declaration's clear language, developing

---

13   See Médecins Sans Frontières (MSF) (2005). The comparison of prices between originator and generic producers is a field of potentially unlimited manipulation. To illustrate, the Hudson Institute (a Washington-based think tank close to the industry) produced a White Paper (Myths and Realities on Prices of Drugs (Adelman and Norris, 2004)) which used MSF data to indicate that the average price of patented drugs is considerably lower than that of "copy drugs." This paper was used extensively by organizations close to pharmaceutical corporations (Glassman, 2004). The Hudson Institute analysis, a brief study of six pages, however, could be criticized in various respects, among others: (1) it is not the average price of ARV drugs that is important, but the prices of the needed triple-combinations; (2) fixed-dose combinations, which are more appropriate for use in developing countries, were not included in the Hudson study; (3) while the prices of generic products have no geographical limits, prices of originator drugs vary according to the system of differential pricing (the Hudson study used only the lower prices for the "poorest eligible countries" (Adelman and Norris, 2004). MSF stressed that the latter system excludes the poor in countries that are not eligible for differential pricing.

countries remained uncertain as to whether compulsory licensing would indeed be "permitted" by the major powers post-Doha. The first country to test the waters was Zimbabwe, which issued a compulsory license on all AIDS drugs in 2002. Zimbabwe's health minister and ambassador to Geneva had both been closely involved in previous international debates on IP issues, such as supporting the then-controversial 1998 WHA resolution mandating WHO to monitor the impact of TRIPS on access to medicines. (However, the impact of Zimbabwe's decision as an international precedent was probably discounted by its international isolation by 2002.)

Of greater import, arguably, was the Malaysian example. In 2002, the international NGO Third World Network provided technical support (including access to international experts such as KEI's James Love) to the Malaysian Ministry of Health to apply for a compulsory license (personal communication, Yoke Ling Chee, 2010). Bolstered by the Doha Declaration, the MoH received Cabinet approval to begin procedures to get a government use authorization (a type of compulsory license for public non-commercial use) for several AIDS drugs, most of which were patented in Malaysia (Chee, 2006). Upon hearing this news, GlaxoSmithKline offered to drop the price of its two-drug combination (zidovudine+lamivudine) by 57%—a significant drop, but one that left prices above the generic equivalent. Authority to grant a compulsory license (CL) rested with the Ministry of Domestic Trade and Consumer Affairs, which was, however, initially opposed to the compulsory license due to fear of its potential effect on foreign investment. Nevertheless, in November 2003, the Ministry agreed to issue the CL for a period of two years for three drugs patented by GlaxoSmithKline and Bristol Myers Squibb, which had earlier warned that this decision would reduce foreign investment and set an undesirable precedent. At this point, the Ministry of Health announced that ARV treatment would be provided free of charge once importation of the generic drugs began in February 2004. The generic drugs, imported from Cipla in India, cost about 80% less than their patented counterparts, and allowed the Ministry to increase the number of patients on treatment from 1500 to 4000. The government offered a royalty payment of 6% of the generic price, but the remuneration was not claimed by the patent-holders, possibly because it would have been interpreted as legitimating the license (Chee, 2006).

As the first country in Asia to use compulsory licensing, the Malaysian decision did indeed draw attention and set a precedent, particularly in its neighboring countries. In October 2004, Indonesia followed Malaysia's lead. In the late 1990s, very few HIV-positive Indonesians had access to ARV treatment. A local NGO, Pokdisus, negotiated with the patent-holders for discounts and managed to reduce the price from the previous level of $9600–$12,000/year to $7200 by 1999. However, the high cost of drugs kept treatment limited to just a few hundred people, and in late 2004 after a civil society campaign for government use, the Ministry of Justice announced a compulsory license for local production of two ARVs patented by Boehringer-Ingelheim and GlaxoSmithKline, with a royalty of 0.5%. According to an interview with the patent office, the patent-holders did not contest the government decision, and at least one (Boehringer-Ingelheim) accepted its royalty payment. Coverage of ARV treatment increased from about 3.5% in 2003 to 50% in 2006, supported by the lower cost of generic drugs resulting from the compulsory license and a 50% government subsidy for ARV costs (Hanim and Jhamtani, 2006).

(h) Thailand: Regularizing the use of compulsory licensing

Thailand played a central role in expanding and consolidating the universal access norm. The Thai government first yielded to external trade pressures by implementing pharmaceutical product patents in 1992 (over a decade earlier than would be required by TRIPS), but then subsequently set a precedent in 2006–7 with the number, scope, and high political profile of its compulsory licensing decisions.

IP rules have been a hotly contested issue in Thailand's foreign relations since at least the 1980s. For example, in 1988 the US-based Pharmaceutical Manufacturers' Association (PMA, later PhRMA) filed a Special 301 complaint on Thailand with the USTR over the country's 1979 Patent Law, which disallowed patents on food, medicines, and agricultural machinery (Kirchanski, 1993). In response, the US revoked preferential access to the US market on a number of goods, denying duty-free status to $165 million of Thai exports (Rust, 1992). At the time, 20–25% of Thailand's exports went to the US, making it Thailand's largest export market (McDorman, 1992). Within a year of the trade sanctions, the Thai Assembly had passed a new law that granted product patents on pharmaceuticals, despite opposition from local industry, academics, NGOs, doctors associations, and within government (MacLeod, 1992; McDorman, 1992).

However, the situation began to change at the turn of the millennium, as Thai civil society organizations—particularly HIV/AIDS groups—began developing their expertise on IP issues. With an estimated one million people living with HIV in 1999, Thailand had been struck with the worst HIV/AIDS epidemic in Asia, but had also mounted an effective and widely-admired public health response. Very few people had access to ART in the late 1990s—only 5–10% of people in need had access to any ARV drug at all, and only 1% to the three-drug combinations required to suppress HIV; triple-therapy cost about 675 USD/month (8100 USD/ year)—over five times the average office worker's salary of 120 USD (Sakboon, 1999; D. Wilson, Cawthorne, Ford and Aongsonwang, 1999). The government had provided monotherapy with zidovudine (AZT, available as a generic) since 1992, dual-therapy with the addition of ddI in 1995, and in 2000, triple-therapy— but high drug costs restricted access to such treatment to only 1500–2000 patients out of several hundred thousand estimated to be in need (Revenga et al., 2006).

Civil society groups initially focused on the ARV didanosine (ddI), which had been invented by the US National Institutes of Health and licensed to BMS. In the late 1990s, BMS sold ddI for 178 Thai Baht (THB) (3.36 USD)/day (or 1226.4

USD/year),[14] which exceeded the daily basic wage of 120 THB (2.26 USD)/day (Wisartsakul, 2004). A broad coalition of Thai actors, including the Government Pharmaceutical Organization (a state-owned drug manufacturer), the academic Drug Study Group based at Chulalongkorn University, MSF, and PLWHA groups, formed the Working Group to Challenge the ddI Patent. The Thai Network of Positive People (TNP+) also requested that the Ministry of Public Health (MoPH) grant a compulsory license on ddI, and set up camp at the MoPH offices to draw public attention to their cause. The MoPH denied their request in early 2000, after officials from both the Health and Commerce ministries "expressed great caution in pursuing the issue for fear of US retaliation" (Bhatiasevi and Maneerungsee, 2000).

However, the Working Group continued pursuing its challenge of the ddI patent, and in May 2001, the AIDS Access Foundation and two PLWHAs filed suit against the patent's validity at the Thai Intellectual Property court, becoming the first patient groups to contest a patent in Thailand (and possibly in any developing country). In October 2002, the court affirmed the right of patients to challenge patents as "interested parties"—an important decision since BMS had argued that patients did not have the legal standing to contest the patent. In addition, the court found that BMS had unlawfully omitted critical information from its ddI patent application, which comprised grounds for revoking the patent. Though BMS initially appealed the decision, in December 2003, the company reached a settlement with the CSOs: BMS would withdraw its appeal in exchange for the CSOs withdrawing their suit to revoke the patent. The practical effect was the removal of the monopoly on ddI (Ford, Wilson, Bunjumnong and von Schoen Angerer, 2004; Wisartsakul, 2004). The overturning of the Thai patent on ddI marked a major victory for public health CSOs in Thailand, and also set an important example that civil society groups would emulate in Brazil, India, and China. (CSOs in different countries often shared legal strategies, in addition to technical information, to support like-minded efforts taking place in other national contexts.) The ddI issue also built up literacy on IP issues within Thai civil society and the MoPH, which established a foundation on which Thailand's compulsory licensing decisions would build a few years later.

Thailand launched its first universal health insurance program in 2002. The newly-created National Health Security Office (NHSO) had included antiretroviral therapy (ART) among its covered services, after strong civil society reaction to the initial exclusion of ART. Significantly, the high cost of ARV drugs began directly impacting the government budget. Discussions on how to address high drug prices had been ongoing within NHSO and other parts of the government for several years. According to one official present at a January 2006 intra-governmental meeting, the question arose as to why Thailand had not made use of compulsory licensing, as its fellow Southeast Asian countries Malaysia and Indonesia had

---

14   Thai Baht converted to USD based on average January 1998 exchange rate of 53 THB/USD (www.oanda.com/currency/historical-rates).

done (Tantivess, Kessomboon and Laongbua, 2008). Precedents set in other parts of the region seemed to carry more weight than examples from Latin America or sub-Saharan Africa.

After several years of negotiations with patent-holders, in late 2006, the Thai government issued its first compulsory license on efavirenz, an ARV patented by the pharmaceutical company Merck (Ministry of Public Health (Thailand) & National Health Security Office (Thailand), 2007). The CL was one of the first decisions of Health Minister Mongkol na Songkhla, who took office after Prime Minister Thaksin Shinawatra was ousted by a military coup; Mongkol was a long-time civil servant in the health ministry and familiar with the many debates on IP and medicines prices over the years. The CL enabled the government to import generic efavirenz at half the Merck price (after Merck had offered additional discounts), which enabled the government to expand coverage with efavirenz to an additional 20,000 patients (Tantivess et al., 2008).

The international reaction was remarkable for its silence. The day after the announcement, *The New York Times*—which had closely followed AIDS drug and IP issues—carried an article about the Clinton Foundation's price reductions on pediatric AIDS medicines, with only a very brief mention of the Thai compulsory license at the tail end (Giridharadas, 2006). *The Washington Post* gave the story a few lines in its World in Brief section, squeezed between news of clashes in South Sudan and the risk of a coup in Fiji (World in Brief, 2006). The *Wall Street Journal* did not cover the story at all. The limited press coverage suggested that norms on the proper balance between patents and access to AIDS drugs had shifted so firmly that a compulsory license on an ARV in a developing country was non-news in the American mainstream and business media. The London-based *Financial Times*, the only major English-language paper to cover the announcement at any length, noted that Merck recognized "it was legal for countries to seek a compulsory licence" (Kazmin and Jack, 2006) but complained that Thai authorities had not met procedural requirements by neglecting to conduct prior negotiations with the company. What is notable about the Merck reaction is the public acknowledgment of the right to use compulsory licensing, and the limited grounds that they advanced for their complaint.

The Thai decision attracted more attention at USTR. In response to reports that USTR told the Thai government it had to negotiate with the patent-holder, James Love wrote to USTR Susan Schwab in December 2006 to clarify that TRIPS did not require prior negotiation in cases of government use. In January 2007, 22 Democratic Members[15] of the US Congress wrote to Schwab "to urge that the United States respect the decision of the Thai government to issue a compulsory

---

15   Tom Allen (D-ME), Sander Levin (D-MI), Henry Waxman (D-CA), Jim McDermott (D-WA), Pete Stark (D-CA), John Lewis (D-GA), James Moran (D-VA), Lloyd Doggett (D-TX), Earl Blumenauer (D-OR), Charles Gonzalez (D-TX), Betty McCollum (D-MN), Linda Sanchez (D-CA), Carolyn Maloney (D-NY), Hilda Solis (D-CA), Dennis Kucinich (D-OH), Barbara Lee (D-CA), Michael Michaud (D-ME), Loretta Sanchez (D-

license on the AIDS drug efavirenz" (Allen et al., 2007). The letter cited the 2002 Trade Promotion Authority Act, which specified that among the "principal negotiating objectives" of the United States with respect to intellectual property was "to respect the Declaration on the TRIPS Agreement and Public Health" (US Public Law 107–210, §2102(b)(4)(c)). Schwab replied that, "we have taken care to respect fully the Thai government's ability to issue compulsory licenses in accordance with its own law and its obligations as a Member of the World Trade Organization" and "we have not suggested that Thailand has failed to comply with particular national or international rules" (Schwab, 2007).

Meanwhile, in Thailand, the government was busy implementing its new policy. Since GPO (Government Pharmaceutical Organization) was still developing its capacity to produce efavirenz, the government use order was initially implemented by importing generic drugs from Indian supplier Ranbaxy, which sold efavirenz at about $205—or, less than half the Merck price. Ranbaxy had received WHO Pre-qualification for its drug, and supplied it to many other countries where the efavirenz patent was not in force. The NHSO estimated that the drop in price would enable it to provide efavirenz to an additional 20,000 patients with the same drug budget (Tantivess et al., 2008).

However, this relative calm dissipated when Thailand announced on January 25, 2007 that it was making government use of two more patented medicines: American firm Abbott's second-line AIDS drug lopinavir/ritonavir (Kaletra), and French firm Sanofi's clopidogrel (Plavix), a blood-thinning agent for heart disease and hypertension. In its announcement, the government noted that the ARV budget had been set at approximately $110 million to cover treatment for 108,000 patients—or, about $1000 per patient (Thailand's per capita GNI in 2007 was $3240).[16] Abbott's lowest price to the Thai government prior to the CL was $2919, or about three times the per-patient budget for one drug alone. Generic lopinavir/ritonavir was estimated to cost two-thirds less than Abbott's version, with prices expected to drop over time as competition increased; the generic version of clopidogrel would drop the price by 90%. Before the CL, high prices limited the quantities of both drugs provided by the NHSO, which did not meet the mandate of universal coverage; in total, the NHSO estimated it would save 800 million THB ($21 million) per year.

By 2007, arguably, the access norm had evolved to the point that TRIPS flexibilities could be used for AIDS drugs, but only in rare circumstances. Though the letter of the Doha Declaration was expansive, and by no means limited to AIDS drugs or to exceptional circumstances, the shared understandings regarding the use of compulsory licensing were—before Thailand—much narrower. According to an industry source,

---

CA), Janice Schakowsky (D-IL), Maxine Waters (D-CA), John Tierney (D-MA), James McGovern (D-MA).

16   Based on the exchange rate of 35.2 THB/USD on January 25, 2007. GNI data from the World Bank.

> We thought we had an agreement on how the TRIPS mechanisms should be used, but obviously we have different interpretations ... In this case [Thailand], it is one government and the entire NGO community that think this is justified ... When Italy has its next financial crisis, will it also break all the patents? (as quoted in Gerhardsen, 2007)

(One month later, the competition authority in Italy did grant a compulsory license on finasteride, a drug used to treat prostate cancer and male-pattern baldness; it was the Italian government's third compulsory license on a medicine in two years on grounds of anti-competitive practice (Love, 2007). Notably, no major English-language newspaper covered this compulsory licensing decision, and it was not mentioned in the US Special 301 reports in the years following the decision (2007–2011).)

Recognizing the new precedent that Thailand was setting, the alarmed response from industry and some Western governments to the latest announcement contrasted sharply with the relatively mild reaction to the efavirenz license. The Pharmaceutical Research and Manufacturers' Association (PreMA), which represented multinational firms in Thailand, criticized the government for not having consulted sufficiently with the patent-owners—a critique that would be reiterated by individual firms and some Western governments repeatedly. According to a Thai official,

> We have learned from our past experience that prior negotiation before announcing the use of the government use [compulsory license] is not an effective way to bring the price down and reach better access ... Our principle is that discussion is [a] must, but it is much more effective to discuss after the announcement ... Most importantly is that this is totally in compliance [with] international and national law. (as quoted in Gerhardsen, 2007)

Abbott initially responded by offering a further price cut if the government would withdraw its compulsory license (Treerutkuarkul, 2007a). When the offer was refused, Abbott announced that it was withdrawing the seven medicines it had submitted to the Thai Food and Drug Administration from the market, because "Thailand has revoked the patent on our medicine, ignoring the patent system" (Treerutkuarkul, 2007d). Notably, the patent had not been revoked, nor was the use of compulsory licensing outside the patent system; however, Abbott's discourse suggested that compulsory licensing was an extralegal measure. Among the withdrawn products was a new formulation of lopinavir/ritonavir that did not require refrigeration and was therefore particularly well-suited for use in tropical developing countries like Thailand. Other withdrawn medicines included those to treat kidney disease, rheumatoid arthritis, blood clots, pain, high blood pressure, and bacterial infection.

Abbott's move was unprecedented. Other countries had issued compulsory licenses, but no firm had ever responded by withdrawing its other medicines from the market.

The decision drew swift condemnation both within and outside the country, and may have inadvertently catalyzed new allies for the MoPH both within and outside of Thailand. Permanent Secretary for Justice Jarun Pukditanakul declared that "The drug industry is an obvious profit-oriented business. But its present business protection goes beyond the limit—to the extent that the principle of human rights has been completely forgotten" (Treerutkuarkul, 2007c). Civil society groups announced a boycott of Abbott's vitamins, milk products, and antibiotics.

Internationally, Abbott was publicly condemned by a wide range of actors, including international CSOs, national CSOs in both developing and industrialized countries, academics, investors, student groups, and political leaders (Consumer Project on Technology, 2007). An internationally-coordinated day of action on April 27 resulted in protests at Abbott offices in 16 countries, including several locations in the US.

On April 16, Abbott offered to drop its price again, from $2200 to $1000 for a list of 45 middle-income countries, including Thailand. However, it did not change its decision to withdraw products from the Thai market. Borrowing a page from the South African playbook, Thai NGOs then filed suit against Abbott for abuse of monopoly (anti-competitive practice) (S. Flynn, 2008).

Merck responded to the CL in February by offering to reduce the price of efavirenz by about half to $243—roughly matching the generic price (Treerutkuarkul, 2007b). A week later, it publicly announced a similar price reduction for other developing countries.[17] Though Merck emphasized that the announcement was its second price reduction in less than a year, and was "due to efficiencies resulting from improved manufacturing processes," others directly attributed the global price drop to Thailand's compulsory license (Merck press release of February 14, 2007, as reproduced in (Ministry of Public Health (Thailand) & National Health Security Office (Thailand), 2007). In this way, a decision in Thailand had both normative and material effects internationally.

The response from Western governments was mixed, and included concern as well as support. On July 12, 2007, the European Parliament passed a broad-ranging resolution on TRIPS and access to medicines, asking the European Council "to support the developing countries which use the so-called flexibilities built into the TRIPS Agreement and recognized by the Doha Declaration" and "Encourages the developing countries to use all means available to them under the TRIPS Agreement, such as compulsory licences" (European Parliament, 2007). However, six days later, the European Commissioner for Trade, Peter Mandelson, wrote to

---

17   Merck's tiered pricing policy for its AIDS drugs was to offer the lowest price to countries with a low Human Development Index score (HDI, a UNDP measure) and medium HDI with adult HIV prevalence of over 1%. A second-tier, higher price was offered to developing countries with medium HDI and adult HIV prevalence less than 1%.

Thai Commerce Ministry Krik-Krai Jirapaet with a different tone, "concerned by recent indications that the Thai Government may be taking a new approach on access to medicines." Mandelson wrote that "Neither the TRIPS Agreement nor the Doha Declaration appear to justify a systematic policy of applying compulsory licenses wherever medicines exceed certain prices." He urged the Thai government to "establish through constructive dialogue a partnership … in particular with Sanofi-Aventis," to address price and affordability (Mandelson, 2007 (July 10)). Despite the Doha Declaration's explicit recognition that countries had the "freedom to determine the grounds" for compulsory licensing, Mandelson's letter illustrated the ongoing struggle to define informally just how much "freedom" countries would have.

ACT-UP Paris and Aides, a French AIDS organization, responded angrily to Mandelson's letter, pointing out that the laws of EU Member States considered excessive pricing to be grounds for compulsory licensing. They accused Mandelson of acting against the position of the European Commission and European Parliament, and of attempting to re-write international law on behalf of the pharmaceutical industry (Martin and Trenado, 2007 (August 22)).

In his response to Mandelson, Mongkol repeatedly emphasized that the compulsory license did not affect the private sector market, and argued that those covered by the government's insurance program did not have access to the licensed drugs beforehand, and that therefore, the companies would not be losing a significant market. He also pointedly referred to the July 2007 European Parliament resolution, noting that "the Council was asked to mandate the Commission to refrain from taking action to interfere with these proceedings. I would like to request for Your Excellency's kind advice on how the Commission is going to react to the EP resolution and how Your Excellency's letter supports the said EP resolution" (Songkhla, 2007).

In the United States, reactions were also mixed. Former US President Clinton, whose foundation worked closely with generic AIDS drug manufacturers, declared that "No company will live or die because of high price premiums for AIDS drugs in middle-income countries, but patients may" (as quoted in (Dugger, 2007). As noted above, 22 Democratic Members of Congress had written to Schwab in January to urge that USTR respect Thailand's compulsory licensing decision on efavirenz. In March 2007, a different group of 12 Democratic Members of Congress[18] and five Senators[19] wrote to Schwab concerned that Thailand would expand its compulsory licensing policy to include medicines "to treat high cholesterol and other conditions apparently unrelated to any urgent public health issue." They urged her to do more to convince the Thai government to negotiate

---

18   Ron Kind (D-WI), Adam Smith (D-WA), Ellen Tauscher (D-CA), John Tanner (D-TN), Artur Davis (D-AL), Melissa Bean (D-IL), Joe Crowley (D-NY), Allen Boyd (D-FL), Jim Matheson (D-UT), Brad Ellsworth (D-IN), Joe Courtney (D-CT), Ron Klein (D-FL).

19   Joseph Lieberman (D-CT), Thomas Carper (D-DE), Robert Menendez (D-NJ), Dianne Feinstein (D-CA), Frank Lautenberg (D-NJ).

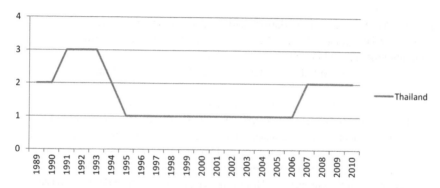

Figure 5.1   Thailand Ranking on USTR Special 301 Reports: 1989–2010
Note: 3 = Priority Foreign Country (most severe); 2 = Priority Watch List; 1 = Watch List;
0 = absent.

with patent-holders. "We do not believe that WTO members intended those rules to be used to allow compulsory licenses on any medicine whatsoever as a matter of standard government policy." Recognizing the importance of precedent, they wrote, "Without an appropriate response by the US government, we are concerned that respect for intellectual property rights worldwide will diminish" (Kind et al., 2007 (March 15)).

USTR elevated Thailand from "Watch List" to "Priority Watch List" in its 2007 Special 301 Report, citing as grounds (among other concerns) that "there were further indications of a weakening of respect for patents, as the Thai Government announced decisions to issue compulsory licenses for several patented pharmaceutical products. While the United States acknowledges a country's ability to issue such licenses in accordance with WTO rules, the lack of transparency and due process exhibited in Thailand represents a serious concern." Thailand remained on the Priority Watch List through 2010.

Responses from the UN system varied. In December 2006, UNAIDS head Peter Piot wrote to Minister Mongkol "to commend you and the Government of Thailand for your strong and steadfast efforts to provide antiretroviral treatment … Your latest decision to import generic efavirenz until Thailand is able to manufacture the drug itself, is a good example of that commitment" (Piot, 2006 (December 26), reprinted in (Ministry of Public Health (Thailand) & National Health Security Office (Thailand), 2007). He was the first UN official to support the Thai policy publicly. However, WHO's response was lukewarm. In a visit to the NHSO shortly after the January €L announcement, WHO's new Director-General Dr Margaret Chan urged the Thai government to negotiate further with patent-holders, and to moderate its use of compulsory licensing (Treerutkuarkul, 2007). In failing to provide political support for the Thai decision, Dr Chan earned swift and vocal condemnation from civil society groups around the world (Macan-Markar, 2007). Representatives of MSF, the academic Drug Study Group, TNP+, and the AIDS Access Foundation criticized Chan in an article in *The Lancet* entitled "WHO must defend patients' interests, not industry" (Cawthorne, Ford, Limpananont, Tienudom and Purahong, 2007).

Chan quickly recanted in a letter to the health minister, writing

> I deeply regret that my comments at the close of the briefing at the National Health Security Office were misrepresented in the media, and may have caused embarrassment to the government of Thailand. They should not be taken as a criticism of the decision of the Royal Thai government to issue compulsory licences, which is entirely the prerogative of the government, and fully in line with the TRIPS Agreement ... There is no requirement for countries to negotiate with patent holders before issuing a compulsory licence. (Chan, 2007 (February 7))

The MoPH requested technical support from WHO in May 2007, after the WHA passed that year Resolution 60.30 (strongly supported by Brazil and Thailand) mandating WHO to provide support to countries in making use of the TRIPS flexibilities. However, according to Suwit Wibulpolprasert (senior adviser to the MoPH), WHO delayed sending a mission to Thailand until a year after the CL announcement (personal communication, 2008).

The purpose of requesting the WHO mission was in many ways more political than technical; the mission report did not include any new information that the Thai authorities did not already have. It did, however, ultimately support the compulsory licensing policy (Velasquez et al., 2008). Securing WHO's official stamp of approval helped the Thai MoPH not only with its internal domestic political battles to defend the CL policy, but also helped to legitimate it internationally. The Thai government was able to use its institutional power as a Member State to tap into the WHO's expert and normative power, which ultimately helped to solidify international acceptance of the Thai policy. By extension, the Thai precedent broadened the policy space in the global IP regime to use TRIPS safeguards beyond HIV/AIDS.

In response to a recommendation from the Thai National Legislative Assembly that the MoPH provide a thorough public explanation for why it had decided to grant compulsory licenses, the Ministry prepared an extensive White Paper to increase understanding of the rationale behind the decision, and also to combat misinformation that the MoPH characterized as "intentional with the aim to create misunderstanding and objections to the announcements." The aim was not only "answering all the questions raised, but more importantly as a tool to inform and educate the Thai and Global Society as a whole, on the issue of pharmaceutical patent and the public health" (Ministry of Public Health (Thailand) & National Health Security Office (Thailand), 2007). In addition to discussing the legality, rationale for, process behind, and expected costs and benefits of granting the compulsory licenses, the report also contained copies of 27 related documents. These included government documents, correspondence between the MoPH and patent-holders, letters from international organizations and civil society groups, copies of legal texts, and examples of compulsory licenses issued in other developing countries for medicines.

Also included was an analysis of the legality of the government use licenses under Thai and WTO law by Sean Flynn, an American attorney and Associate Director of the American University Law School Program on Information Justice and Intellectual Property. Flynn had concluded that the MoPH had met the requirements of both domestic and international law. There was no legal analysis by any Thai or Bangkok-based legal expert included in the White Paper. When asked in an interview why an American legal opinion on Thai law was included in the White Paper, Wibulpolprasert responded that experts from the industrialized countries carried more weight both internationally and within Thailand—even if they were commenting on Thai law (personal communication, July 2008). According to Wibulpolprasert, developing country experts simply did not have as much influence.

In March 2007, Dr Wibulpolprasert presented the White Paper to the international community at a meeting organized by Love's group in Geneva. In May, he and Dr Mongkol traveled to Washington to make the case for the license directly with American policymakers. Several Thai civil society leaders came to the US as well to meet with US-based civil society groups and attend the Abbott shareholders' meeting in Chicago. In other words, the Thai government and CSOs were waging an international public-relations counter-campaign.

In December 2007, elections in Thailand restored to power a democratic government that was friendlier to business interests. Just before leaving office, in January 2008, Mongkol announced compulsory licenses for four additional medicines, all cancer drugs: docetaxel, erlotinib, letrozole and imatinib ((Limpananont, Eksaengsri, Kijtiwatchakul and Metheny, 2009). Novartis offered a donation of its blockbuster drug imatinib (Glivec), and averted the implementation of the license. The government moved ahead with the other three drugs. When his successor, Chaiya Somsab, took over in February 2008, one of Chaiya's first announcements was that he would revoke the compulsory licenses. Civil society groups reacted immediately, and within a few weeks, Chaiya had shifted his position—the government use policy would stay. Though the initial CLs had been criticized in the Western media as illegitimate, because of the military government from which they originated, the persistence of the CL policy in the new government suggested that public support for such measures was widespread.

In August 2010, the government announced it would extend the compulsory licenses on the two AIDS drugs until their respective patent expiry dates (2012 for efavirenz, 2016 for lopinavir/ritonavir). It also announced that the CL policy had enabled savings of 1.18 billion THB ($36 million), and increased the number of patients accessing efavirenz from 4539 to 29,360, and those receiving lopinavir/ritonavir from 39 to 6200; extending the license would lead to estimated additional savings of 3.2 billion THB ($99 million) and enable the NHSO to extend AIDS treatment to a population of 4.5 million ethnic minorities living in Thailand without citizenship (Treerutkuarkul, 2010).[20]

Thailand's compulsory licensing policies from 2006–2008 challenged the widespread implicit assumptions that TRIPS flexibilities should be reserved for HIV/AIDS, and set new precedents that strengthened the universal access norm. Three months after Thailand's license on efavirenz, Indonesia made government use of the same drug, and six months after, Brazil did as well. Notably, this was Brazil's first issued compulsory license, after eight years of publicly threatening to do so—a clear demonstration of the impact Thailand had on global norms. Though the Thai decisions set off a heated political battle, global networks of civil society activists and experts helped to defend and legitimate the government's decision to make broader use of compulsory licensing than developing countries previously had. International support from UNAIDS, Members of the US Congress and American legal experts also helped the Ministry of Health to win internal political battles as well. Though the fight was about a national policy decision, it took place within a global public domain and exhibited characteristics of nodal governance, with a relatively small set of globally-dispersed but tightly-networked actors on either side of the policy debate.

Overall, Thailand's decisions expanded policy space to use TRIPS flexibilities for medicines other than ARVs, increased the political acceptability of compulsory licensing, and strengthened global norms that prioritized public health over stringent IP protection.

(i) Role and character of finance for treatment

The consistent use of (or frequently, the mere threat to use) compulsory licensing and the acceptance of such practices (as explicitly justified in the Doha Declaration) was a decisive factor in the continuous reduction of ARV prices in lower-income countries. As reflected in the following figure (Figure 5.2) from the regular MSF publication on ARV prices (Untangling the Web, see: (Médecins Sans Frontières (MSF), 2011), the lowest price of a generic first line ARV regimen had reached $ 61 per person/year by 2011—less than 1% of the price in 2001.[21]

However, even when generic ARV prices were low, such prices alone could not guarantee universal access to these medicines in poor countries with a high

---

20   Based on the exchange rate of 32.3 THB/USD on August 3, 2010 (www.oanda.com).

21   However, stavudine (d4T), which forms part of the lowest-cost ARV combination, causes serious side-effects and is increasingly replaced by combinations with tenofovir (TDF): while the price of the lowest generic offer for a TDF-based combination had fallen from $422 in June 2007 to $143 in June 2011, the tiered prices of originator medicines did not change during this time ($613 in low-income; $1033 in lower middle-income countries; (Médecins Sans Frontières (MSF), 2011).

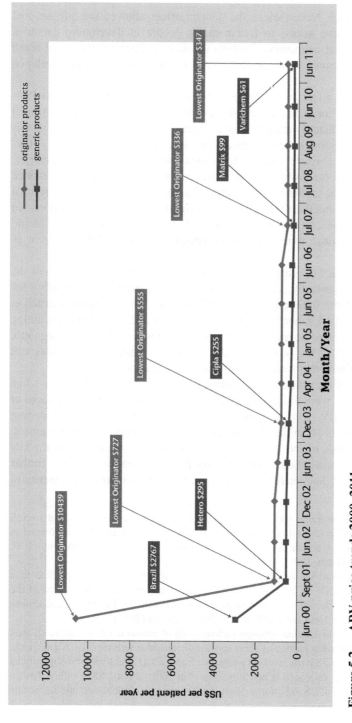

Figure 5.2 ARV price trends 2000–2011
Source: Médecins Sans Frontières (MSF), 2011.

prevalence of HIV.[22] Nevertheless, the generic prices allowed the international community to ensure access to treatment for people in developing countries through international cooperation—which would have been totally out of reach if medicines had remained priced at the level originators charged in developed countries.

The widespread attention paid by politicians and civil society to HIV/AIDS—whether as a threat[23] or as an expression of empathy—helped to mobilize financial resources that significantly exceeded the average growth of development aid; this aid was channeled through the creation of new institutions to respond both to HIV/AIDS as well as to a broader range of infectious diseases in developing countries.

As noted earlier, there was a dramatic increase in total development assistance for health from 1990 to 2010 (Murray et al., 2011).[24] Not only did total financial assistance increase, but there was also a rise of significant new types of donors—in particular foundations, NGOs and new types of hybrid actors like the GFATM and GAVI; at the same time, funding through bilateral and some multilateral agencies grew as well.

The evolution in financing for HIV/AIDS also reflected the evolution of the access norm more broadly. The first major source of international funding for HIV medicines came indirectly from the World Bank, which permitted Brazil in the 1990s to use Bank money to support the national AIDS program (excluding treatment), which freed up government funds to go towards ARVs (Calcagnotto, 2007; Nunn, 2009). This was taking place at a time when the Bank was still officially maintaining that treatment was not "cost-effective."

The next significant increase in funding had its roots in the late 1990s when the G 7/8 countries were discussing the need for a significantly higher amount of resources to fight HIV/AIDS more effectively. An important step was the founding of the GFATM in 2002, initiated essentially to support access to HIV treatment. Following the trends of the 1990s, the GFATM was not created within the UN system, but in the institutional form of a public-private partnership (see further details in Chapter 2, Section (c)), though most of the financial resources were still

---

22   One estimate found (on the basis of UNAIDS estimates for 2005) that overall resource needs for fighting HIV/AIDS in low and middle income countries amounted to US$11.592 Billion, of which only 24.8% was on expenditures for ARV therapy (Bell, Devarajan and Gersbach, 2004).

23   Various discourses in Western countries (in particular the US) pointed to a perception of HIV/AIDS at least as a double threat concerning the global spread of the disease as well as its destabilizing role in African politics (closely linked to the discourse on failing states), see: Hein and Kohlmorgen (2008); Jenkins (2007).

24   Because of the overlap between various goals of financial aid, it is quite difficult to determine exactly what portion of aid is specifically aimed at fighting HIV/AIDS. Hecht et al. concluded that within the levels of assistance from OECD countries (probably official development aid; the reference is not fully clear) "in 2006, about US$15 billion funded health overall and about US$6 billion supported AIDS programs in low- and middle income countries" (2009).

provided by states.[25] The WHO was considered too bureaucratic and insufficiently results-oriented, and was restrained by frozen budgets and little support from many of its main stakeholders;[26] thus, it became attractive to create new organizations to react quickly and effectively to pressing global health challenges. From founding of the GFATM in 2001 until October 2010 governments contributed a total of $19.26 billion and non-state actors contributed $993 million to the fund, increasing from about $1 billion/year on average between 2002 and 2004 to $3.56 billion in 2010. Though this is much less than the Commission on Macroeconomics and Health had originally proposed (about $8 billion per year by 2007), this level of funding made the GFATM one of the most significant funders of global health activities.[27]

Industrialized countries also increased their contributions bilaterally through new global health initiatives such as the US President's Emergency Plan for AIDS Relief (PEPFAR); the US government disbursed over $18 billion from 2003–8 and about $7 billion each year since then for global health efforts.[28]

Non-state actors also made significant contributions. The patent-holding pharmaceutical industry began by offering voluntary price discounts to a number of developing countries, though as the MSF graph above demonstrates, always at a level significantly above the lowest prices of generic ARVs. In addition, beyond their advocacy campaigns, many CSOs such as MSF and other CSOs (including faith-based organizations) became involved in providing access to medicines in poor countries through financial support as well as through various forms of technical cooperation and voluntary work. Foundations also made significant contributions to global health financing, accounting for close to $2 billion in 2011

---

25   This new dynamic came about because in the late 1990s UN organizations were facing major difficulties. A zero-growth strategy had been imposed on the budget of many UN organizations by the United States through the United Nations Reform Act (Helms-Biden Act, a 1999 US law), which set a number of conditions for the reform of the UN system before the US would release its total amount of arrears in payment to the UN.

26   For a more recent critique in the same vein, see for example Chow (2010).

27   See GFATM Pledges and contributions (http://www.theglobalfund.org/en/about/donors/); WHO CMH Support Unit 2003 (http://www.who.int/macrohealth/infocentre/advocacy/en/investinginhealth02052003.pdf), p. 25. In 2007, 12.3% of all global health financing was channeled through the GFATM (Ravishankar et al., 2009).

28   See e.g. the PEPFAR webpage; http://www.pepfar.gov/press/80064.htm. Since 2009, PEPFAR is part of the US Global Health Initiative, which integrates various US activities in this field, as summarized in the home page: "The Global Health Initiative, now coordinated from the State Department, is a new, integrated approach to unify our government's investments in global health. This approach draws upon the expertise and programs of the US Agency for International Development (USAID), the Department of Health and Human Services (HHS) (including the US Centers for Disease Control and Prevention [CDC] and its other agencies), PEPFAR, Peace Corps, and the Department of Defense. GHI supports better integration coordination among programs at both the headquarters and country-level with the US Government, countries, donors, nongovernmental organizations (NGOs), and all partners working in a community" (http://www.ghi.gov/).

(Murray et al., 2011). While the Bill & Melinda Gates Foundation (BMGF) is the unrivalled top donor, others focused on more specific tasks such as the Clinton Foundation, which negotiated with generic ARV manufacturers to achieve better prices for health institutions in poorer countries.

Furthermore, governments also established innovative mechanisms such as UNITAID (founded in 2006 by Brazil, Chile, France, Norway and the United Kingdom) to coordinate the financing of medicines and contribute to improving access to drugs against HIV/AIDS, malaria and tuberculosis. The majority of UNITAID's budget is financed by a "solidarity levy" on airline tickets (63% of revenue in 2010), with the remainder through regular budget allocations or (in the case of Norway) from a tax on carbon dioxide emissions from air travel. In 2010 UNITAID had 30 members: 29 (contributing) member states plus the Gates Foundation. Perhaps due to the financial crisis, UNITAID's budget has been more or less stagnant between 2007 and 2010 (between \$300 million and \$350 million), nevertheless, it has raised a significant amount of funding targeted at improving the way global markets function for better access to medicines. UNITAID finances the relevant activities of its "partner organizations" (e.g. WHO, UNAIDS, UNICEF, GFATM, Roll Back Malaria, Foundation for Innovative New Diagnostics (FIND), the WHO Prequalification Programme to help assure the quality of medicines. It also founded in 2009 the *Medicines Patent Pool* (see Chapter 8, Section (b)), originally proposed by the CSOs KEI and MSF to accelerate the availability of low-cost generic versions of newer medicines in developing countries. UNITAID also created the *Millennium Foundation* to allow individuals to make small voluntary donations when booking airline tickets.

As of this writing, many developing countries still depend on external aid for a significant proportion of their HIV/AIDS budgets—and this reliance may last for decades, in the absence of a cure or the implementation of effective prevention strategies (see Hecht et al. (2009); Sulzbach, De and Wang (2011)). Thus, the ability to sustain sufficient levels of international funding for HIV (and other) medicines remains a key component of realizing meaningful access to medicines.

(j) The rise of access to medicines:
Timeline of decisions and increased use of compulsory licensing, 2001–2010

Timelines are quite frequently used as a supportive methodology for making causal inferences—in particular in medical research, but also in a large number of other disciplines, based on the quite simple assumption that causes precede consequences (though in specific cases they might be perceived as simultaneous) (Baumgartner 2008). In complex situations, such as those we are considering here, many assumptions are implicit in the selection of relevant actors and in making guesses about the strength of their relative impact. Nevertheless, the timeline is a useful tool to direct attention to potentially important impacts of generally acknowledged important actors on the course of events in a specific field.

Figure 5.2 displays a timeline of decisions and conflicts around IPRs and access to medicines. Above the thick line are the key events in access to medicines, and below the line the main groups of actors in the field of global health governance (GHG), with supporting actors in the upper group and reluctant actors in the lower group, and NGOs/CSOs distributed all over the field. The relative impact of actors on the key events is indicated by blue (NGOs/CSOs) and red arrows, and the importance of the key events themselves is reflected in the length of the double arrows at the top of the field. These are just (certainly debatable) estimates based on research on HIV/AIDS and institutional change in global health governance (Hein, Bartsch and Kohlmorgen, 2007). For a more detailed account of important events during this conflict see Annex 2.

One of the interesting observations in this timeline is the fact that, while political conflicts in the field of access to medicines concentrated on the interpretation and modification of the TRIPS Agreement, TNPCs rather early (in 2000) began to take measures to counteract their critics with regard to AIDS drugs; some began to offer discounted prices for select developing countries through the UN-sponsored Accelerating Access Initiative. This can be seen, in part, as a reaction to the decision by the Brazilian state in November 1996 to guarantee (ARV) "treatment for all," followed until 2001 by a number of other Latin American countries,[29] the availability of ARVs as generics in 2001 and the growing strength of the relatively well-resourced civil society access campaign, which was launched in 1999. TNPCs continued to fight any modification of the TRIPS Agreement (by lobbying in the US and the EU), though they did publicly welcome the Paragraph 6 TRIPS amendment to facilitate the use of compulsory licensing by poor countries with no technical capacity to produce generics (Hein 2007).

The sequence of key events in this process and the analysis of political conflicts in the background demonstrate the basically voluntary[30] and strategic character of activities. Political bargaining concentrated on state politics and intergovernmental organizations where legally important decisions were taken. Primarily, these were the WHO and WTO (specifically, the TRIPS Council). As conflicts in Brazil and South Africa (see above, and also (Wogart, Calcagnotto, Hein and Soest, 2009) showed, the affirmation of TRIPS flexibilities in the Doha Declaration was not without political significance in the power game between the respective governments, TNPCs and the US government, but still did not fundamentally question the TRIPS regime. What is significant, however, is

---

29   In Argentina, Chile, Costa Rica, Cuba, Mexico, Uruguay and Venezuela the respective laws or regulations were in force and policies for effective supply initiated (though not everywhere fully implemented) by December 2001 (Chequer, Cuchí, Mazin and García Calleja, 2000). Legal provisions in Argentina even preceded those in Brazil, but there seemed to be considerable problems (basically lack of finance), which led to shortages in drug stocks.

30   Here, "voluntary" does not necessarily exclude reactions to public or other political pressure.

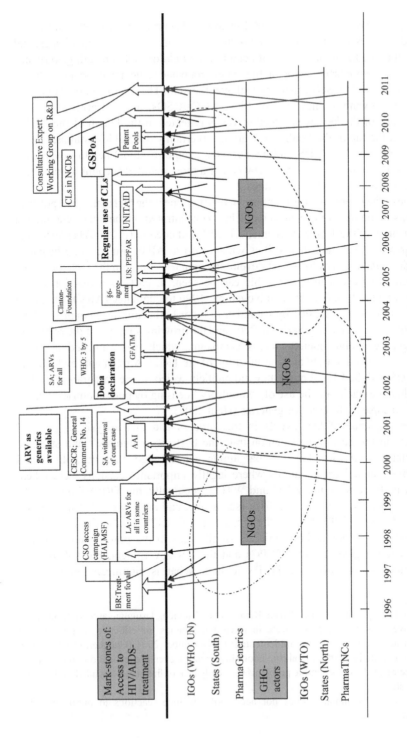

Figure 5.3   Timeline of decisions and conflicts around IPRs and access to medicines

that the positive results in greatly expanding access to ARV-treatment were not achieved by an integrated regime but by many different activities and strategies pursued by a large number of actors. Undeniably, the point of orientation was the access norm—which had not yet expanded beyond ARVs to include all essential medicines.

As indicated in Table 5.1 below, more and more developing countries began to use compulsory licensing, in particular to access generic HIV drugs. The table includes countries that made public announcements of their compulsory licenses, but is far from exhaustive. Many countries chose to issue letters to international drug suppliers such as UNICEF or the International Dispensary Association (IDA) to authorize the procurement and importation of generic versions of patented drugs, particularly for HIV/AIDS. 't Hoen analyzed these letters (which are not publicly available) and found that 65 countries had made use of TRIPS flexibilities to access generic AIDS medicines from 2004–2008 (2009). In these procurement letters, many LDCs made reference to the Doha Declaration and their extension until 2016 to enforce pharmaceutical patents. Other governments (non-LDCs) referred to emergency circumstances and/or government use, both of which were conditions under which TRIPS did not require prior negotiation with a patent-holder to issue a compulsory license ('t Hoen, 2009).

These findings were confirmed by a 2007 analysis of drugs purchased with PEPFAR or Global Fund money. The study found that many sub-Saharan African countries were procuring generic versions of drugs that were patented in their territories (Chien, 2007).

In sum, while the formal rules regarding the right to issue compulsory licenses did not change from 1994 to 2011, the informal rules—that is, the political acceptability of doing so—changed significantly after Doha, as demonstrated by the increasing and relatively widespread use of these measures. Compulsory licensing and government use not only opened up access to lower-cost generic medicines, but also pushed pharmaceutical companies to engage in other behaviors—such as price discounts and voluntary licenses—to avert further compulsory measures.

However, these normative changes did not come easily, nor were they uncontested by patent-holders. Countries such as Brazil and Thailand contributed to evolving global norms by making public high-profile announcements of their compulsory licenses, and thereby contributed to removing the "taboo" around them. In contrast, countries that merely issued non-public letters to procurement agencies benefited from these normative changes, but did not contribute substantively to making them happen.[31]

---

31 Many countries contributed to global norm-setting through their work in intergovernmental arenas, such as voting for resolutions, joining coalitions, or speaking in favor of more flexible IP norms. The key point here is that, unless challenges to norms are communicated in the global public domain, they do not make a significant impact on the global regime.

Table 5.1   Publicly-announced compulsory licenses on medicines 2001–2012

Year	Country	Drug (indication)	Patent-holder (home country)	Notes
2001	Canada	Ciprofloxacin (anthrax)	Bayer (Germany)	Government issued CL to local producer; Post-9/11 and Pre-Doha
2001	United States	Ciprofloxacin (anthrax)	Bayer (Germany)	Threatened in negotiations with patent-holder; Post-9/11 and Pre-Doha
2002	Zimbabwe	ARVs (AIDS)	Various	First country to make use of Doha Declaration to issue CL
2003	Malaysia	Didanosine, zidovudine, lamivudine/zidovudine (AIDS)	BMS (US), GSK (UK)	CL for import from India; first Asian country to use CL post-Doha
2004	Zambia	Lamivudine, stavudine, nevirapine (AIDS)	GSK (UK), BMS (US), Boehringer-Ingelheim (Germany)	
2004	Indonesia	Lamivudine, nevirapine (AIDS)	GSK (UK), Boehringer-Ingelheim (Germany)	
2004	Mozambique	Lamivudine, stavudine, nevirapine	GSK (UK), BMS (US), Boehringer-Ingelheim (Germany)	
2004	Swaziland	ARVs (AIDS)	Various	
2005	Taiwan	Oseltamivir (avian flu)	Roche (Switzerland)	Following outbreak of highly-pathogenic H5N1 avian flu in Southeast Asia
2005	Guinea	ARVs (AIDS)	Various	
2005	Ghana	ARVs (AIDS)	Various	
2005	Eritrea	ARVs (AIDS)	Various	Though Eritrea is not a WTO Member and therefore not bound by the TRIPS Agreement, it cited the Doha Declaration in its CL order

Year	Country	Drug (indication)	Patent-holder (home country)	Notes
2005–6	Italy	Imipenem/cilastatin (antibiotic), Finasteride (cancer, hair loss)	Merck (US)	To counteract anti-competitive practice
2006–8	Thailand	Efavirenz (AIDS), lopinavir/ritonavir (AIDS, clopidogrel (heart disease),	Merck (US), Abbott (US), Sanofi-Aventis (France)	
2007	Indonesia	Efavirenz (AIDS)	Merck (US)	Three months after the Thai CL on efavirenz
2007	Brazil	Efavirenz (AIDS)	Merck (US)	Brazil's first issued CL, after eight years of threatening to use CL in price negotiations. Followed six months after Thailand's.
2007	Canada	FDC of zidovudine + lamivudine + nevirapine	GSK (UK), BI (Germany)	Used WTO TRIPS Paragraph 6 system to export to Rwanda
2010	Ecuador	Lopinavir/ritonavir	Abbott (US)	The first issued CL after President Correa announced in October 2009 that nearly all patented medicines would be considered for compulsory licensing
2012	India	Sorafenib (cancer)	Bayer (Germany)	The first CL issued by India, in response to excessive pricing and a CL request from generic firm Natco

Chapter 6

Beyond HIV in Africa: Solidification and Expansion of the Access Norm

The first decade of the twenty-first century witnessed a dramatic normative shift regarding the very nature of medicines. Medicines had formerly been conceived of as private goods—or at best national public goods—with access only guaranteed for societies wealthy enough to bear the costs of R&D and patent-based monopoly prices. However, by 2010 the idea that certain medicines should be available as global public goods—that is, goods to which all populations should have access—had arguably gained relatively widespread acceptance. The norm of "universal access to essential medicines" had become a key secondary norm for implementing the primary human rights norm of the "right to health." Much of the debate and political mobilization for improved access centered on the AIDS epidemic and access to ARVs ('t Hoen et al., 2011). At the same time, many developing countries and CSOs had long insisted that access to medicines was not only about HIV/AIDS or a limited group of diseases (such as infectious or tropical diseases), but rather, about access to all important medicines. However, as of this writing in 2012, the scope and depth of the norm remained highly contested beyond the widely-accepted fields of HIV/AIDS and sub-Saharan Africa. Despite clear successes in practical implementation of the access norm in the field of HIV/ AIDS, two central questions remain: (1) How stable is the norm, given predictable fluctuations in public interest, political mobilization, and the interests of powerful actors? and (2) How inclusive is the norm, in terms of both diseases and countries covered? In other words, would the AIDS crisis in Africa prove to be a beachhead for broader gains in access to medicines, or would it remain a limited exception in a world of ever-expanding intellectual property rights? This chapter examines the evidence regarding the solidification and inclusiveness of the access norm.

(a) Solidification of the access norm

Solidification of norms is a somewhat abstract concept. It can be difficult to prove, but evidence can suggest how widespread and deeply-held a norm has become. Three types of evidence suggest that the access norm has indeed taken solid root: the discourse of major actors, the practices of major actors, and the effectiveness of monitoring systems in place to "punish" those who violate the norm.

(i) Changes in discourse: The acceptance of informal norms

One factor that suggests that the access norm has solidified is the discourse of a wide range of actors professing support for and adherence to the norm. For example, in 1999 the US government was one of the most aggressive proponents of stringent IP rights on medicines, and stated in a State Department report to Congress on South Africa's Medicines Act that "the USG would never abide abrogation of patent protection or acquiesce in parallel importation of patented medicines ... Should there be an actual violation of any US pharmaceutical patent right (e.g., patent abrogation) this Administration will respond forcefully in accordance with appropriate trade remedy legislation" (Larkin, 1999). In contrast, by 2010, the US trade office recognized the need to take into consideration health concerns, stating that "the United States respects our trading partners' rights to grant compulsory licenses, in a manner consistent with the provisions of the TRIPS Agreement, and encourages our trading partners to consider ways to address their public health challenges while maintaining intellectual property systems that promote investment, research, and innovation" (Office of the United States Trade Representative (USTR), 2010).

Similarly, the European Union trade office had noted in 1998 that "No priority should be given to health over intellectual property considerations" (European Commission, Directorate General 1, 1998). However, by 2010 the very same office was trumpeting its sensitivity to public health concerns, declaring that "The EU has also been active in the WTO debate on TRIPS and access to medicines and has been one of the main promoters of the Doha Declaration on the TRIPS Agreement and Public Health. The EU supports the flexibilities contained in the TRIPS Agreement" (D. 1. European Commission, 2010).

The pharmaceutical industry has also changed its discourse, in some cases, dramatically. The CEO of the British company GlaxoSmithKline deflected attention away from the effect of patents on drug prices in 2002 when asked about the affordability of its AIDS medicines, arguing,

> In the middle of the global AIDS epidemic, it is easy—although misguided—to assume that the cost of drugs used to treat HIV and AIDS is the primary barrier to people in poor countries having greater access to such drugs. In reality, the crux of this problem is more fundamental. The main barrier to access is the lack of adequately resourced healthcare systems. (Sykes, 2002)

Seven years later, GSK's new CEO would change track, making the case that

> We need to stop saying 'it's not our fault there is no infrastructure to deliver healthcare' and start saying 'who can we work with to ensure that the infrastructure does exist?' ... we need to make sure nothing gets in the way of access, least of all price. The children who need this vaccine are among the

poorest in the world; that is why price cannot be a barrier to access. So we need to get the price right. (GlaxoSmithKline, 2009a)

The industry association, often more conservative than individual member companies, also made a dramatic turnaround. In 1999, the head of the International Federation of Pharmaceutical Manufacturers and Associations (IFPMA) had remarked that

> Compulsory licensing benefits nobody except the fortunate commercial entity that is the beneficiary of the largesse offered by such licenses. In the medium and long-term, it is patients who will lack new treatments for serious diseases they suffer, as researchers will undoubtedly stay away from targeted disease groups subject to CL policies. Compulsory licensing seriously detracts from the purpose of the patent system. (Bale, 1999)

A decade later, in response to the president of Ecuador's announcement that he was considering compulsory licenses on over 2000 medicines patents, the Ecuadorean branch of the patent-holding pharmaceutical industry association declared, "We accept the democratic decision ... to legally implement this extraordinary measure ... No legal right is superior to the requirements of public health, especially in such serious circumstances" (Agence France Press (AFP), 2009; Industria Farmaceutica de Investigacion (IFI), 2009).

While discourse does not necessarily reflect an actor's genuine beliefs or practices, it does signal the actor's understanding of what is socially expected— that is, what is the dominant norm. The preceding examples illustrate that by 2010, some of the most powerful actors involved in access to medicines debates had outwardly stated their support for the norm—in a marked shift from a decade prior.

(ii) Practices of pharmaceutical companies

Evidence that the access norm had taken hold was demonstrated not only by the discourse, but also by the practices of pharmaceutical companies. By 2009, of the 16 medicines included in the 2006 WHO treatment guidelines for HIV/AIDS (World Health Organization, 2006), all were offered by originators at a publicly-announced tiered-price (Médecins Sans Frontières (MSF), 2011).[1] Seven of the nine companies with patents on ARVs of public health importance had issued voluntary licenses by 2009 (covering 12 different ARVs), a practice considered radical a decade earlier. Finally, some companies—notably Boehringer-Ingelheim and Roche—simply declared that they would not enforce their patents in certain territories.

---

1 In 2009 WHO narrowed the list of recommended medicines to nine, all of which were offered at publicly-announced tiered-prices (World Health Organization (WHO), 2009).

The geographical coverage of these policies varied significantly, with some companies accepting a more flexible approach to IP management in only the poorest countries, while others included middle-income country markets as well. For example, Merck included just 11 countries within its voluntary licenses, while Gilead included 95 (UNITAID Secretariat, 2009).[2] (The number of countries covered by Gilead voluntary licenses was expanded to 112 countries, the highest of any company, in the 2011 license negotiated with the Medicines Patent Pool.[3]) Some countries were excluded from all licenses, such as Brazil, China, Russia and (except for one company) Thailand. The debate over which countries should be included in special "access" programs reflected a larger contest regarding how inclusive the access norm would become (we return to this issue in greater depth below).

In general, the industry resisted mandatory measures—or even exhortatory statements such as guidelines or assertions of obligations—in favor of voluntary measures.

Notably, the relatively widespread adoption of voluntary licensing had compulsory origins. The first significant use of voluntary licenses resulted from an out-of-court settlement in 2003 after the South African Competition Commission found GlaxoSmithKline and Boehringer-Ingelheim guilty of anti-competitive practice in a case brought by the CSO Treatment Action Campaign. As one study of access policies concluded, "Companies in turn may be more motivated in part to adopt such policies knowing that a compulsory license could issue at some point. International and national efforts to bolster the legitimacy of compulsory licenses, while at times criticized, deserve some credit for encouraging the access to patented medicines that has been achieved" (Chien, 2007).

The close relationship between voluntary and compulsory measures suggests that informal norms alone did not compel changes in industry practice. Rather, the combination of normative carrots (e.g. positive public image, demonstrations of "corporate social responsibility") and hard legal sticks (e.g. the threat of compulsory licensing or other regulatory measures) shifted company behavior towards greater respect for the access norm. Nevertheless, the shift in policies—particularly with respect to HIV medicines—has been considerable.

---

2   A review of companies' voluntary licensing policies reveals significant variation. It is unclear why some companies choose to engage in more liberal licensing practices, while others are more restrictive. While there is no single variable that seems to explain such variation, it is notable that in characterizing the geographical scope of their concessions companies use different classification schemes, referring to the sub-Saharan African countries, least-developed, or low-income countries (there is considerable but not perfect overlap between these three types of country classification), while upper-middle income and Latin American countries are least often included (unpublished study carried out by S. Moon).

3   Details on the countries included in the Medicines Patent Pool license with Gilead are available here: http://www.medicinespatentpool.org/LICENSING/Current-Licences, accessed March 4, 2012.

(iii) Monitoring mechanisms for adherence to the norm

An informal but seemingly effective system has emerged to monitor the adherence of major actors to the access norm. The development of such a system suggests not only that the access norm has solidified, but that it will continue to consolidate further. Three types of monitoring activities are discernible: ad hoc watchdog activities by CSOs, more institutionalized assessments by third parties, and codification of expectations of pharmaceutical companies and governments. Notably, none of these has been formalized in changes in international law; nevertheless, they seem to function relatively effectively at enforcing the norm.

The first and perhaps most powerful systemic check on actors is the "watchdog" function played by CSOs. A well-developed global network of CSOs has emerged after ten years of mobilization, advocacy, research, education and training on complex access to medicines issues. Advocates have a solid understanding of highly-technical legal, trade, economic, medical and public health issues related to access to medicines, and keep a close eye on the policies and practices of pharmaceutical companies, key governments, and international actors such as IGOs.

An illustrative example is the international mobilization of civil society in response to the draft free trade agreement between the European Union and India, which was leaked in late 2009. The draft text contained a number of provisions that would have lengthened, broadened, or strengthened patents or other forms of monopoly protection on medicines in India. The IP provisions in the draft raised concerns not only among health advocates in India, but also in other developing countries. CSOs in other countries mobilized, it seems, both out of a sense of solidarity with Indian groups, and also because India's position as a major global supplier of low-cost generic medicines meant that the trade agreement could threaten affordable drug supply worldwide. Prior to the leaking of the text, news reports of the negotiations had pointed to labor and environmental issues as the major sticking points between the two governments—the Indian government did not appear to find the IP provisions a major problem. After news of the IP provisions leaked, national CSOs in India, Brazil, Thailand, Indonesia, Malaysia and elsewhere, along with international CSOs such as MSF, KEI, HAI, and Oxfam began pressing the EU to drop its IP demands and for India to refuse to accede. Intergovernmental organizations UNITAID and UNAIDS also issued strong public statements regarding their concerns for continued low-cost drug supply should the trade agreement proceed in its current form. The network shared information in real time through online resources such as the ip-health listserve run by KEI, a Stop the EU-India FTA Facebook page, and websites such as FTAWatch. In May 2010, the EU Trade Commissioner in response to a letter sent by MSF, denied that the EU was seeking a number of stringent IP provisions that had been contained in the earlier draft (de Gucht, Karel (DG Trade), 2010 (May 5)). In March 2011, thousands of people living with HIV from across Asia protested in Delhi; in June 2011 the Indian government officially and unequivocally declared that India would not accept certain IP provisions sought by the EU, for the sake of public health (Médecins Sans Frontières, 2011). This mobilization demonstrated the direct and powerful impact that CSOs playing a watchdog function could have on the behavior of even the most powerful governments. As of this writing, the negotiations had not yet concluded and critics have pointed to a number of other provisions that remain in the draft agreement that could be harmful for the production and export of generic medicines from India; thus, it is too early to draw any firm conclusions from this case (the EU-India FTA negotiations are also discussed in Chapter 7).

A second type of monitoring is institutionalized assessments of actors by third parties. One example of such monitoring is the *Access to Medicine Index,* first published in 2008 with a second edition issued in 2010 (Menou, Hornstein and Lipton-McCombie, 2008; RiskMetrics Group—ESG Analytics, 2010b). The Index was published by the Access to Medicine Foundation, and involved consultation with the pharmaceutical industry, WHO, bilateral development agencies and CSOs (e.g. church-based organizations, Oxfam). The report ranks TNPCs according to a number of criteria related to access to medicines and seems to have had a significant influence on the pharmaceutical industry, not least through the influence of shareholders.[4] It should be noted that the Index reflects a relatively limited interpretation of the "access norm" in terms of country and disease scope: it excludes all upper-middle income countries from its analysis, and only focuses on a fixed set of diseases (14 WHO neglected tropical diseases, and top 10 communicable and non-communicable diseases based on burden of disease) (RiskMetrics Group—ESG Analytics, 2010a). Nevertheless, the emergence of this institutionalized monitoring mechanism can be seen to reflect a solidification of the access norm.

A third type of monitoring activity is the codification of expectations of pharmaceutical companies and governments. International human rights norms clearly put binding legal obligations on governments that become States Parties to human rights treaties, as discussed in greater length in Chapter 3. With respect to the right to health and access to medicines, such obligations include the duties of governments to protect and provide such access, and to refrain from activities— such as acceding to harmful trade agreements—that will undermine access.

However, norms regarding the human rights responsibilities of private sector firms are far less clear. Efforts to delineate such norms more clearly can be seen as both a reflection of solidification of the access norm, as well as an attempt to consolidate it further. We referred in Chapter 3 to the Draft Human Rights Guidelines for Pharmaceutical Companies in Relation to Access to Medicines submitted by the UN Special Rapporteur on the Right to Health to the UN General Assembly (Khosla, Rajat and Paul Hunt, 2009). Although they were developed with the broad participation of various stakeholder groups,

---

4   See further information at: www.accesstomedicineindex.org, accessed November 29, 2011.

including TNPCs, the industry reacted negatively to these Guidelines, with both GlaxoSmithKline and Merck speaking publicly against the obligations therein (see Chapter 3, Section (c)).

Professor John Ruggie, the UN Secretary General's Special Representative for Business and Human Rights (2005–2011) developed "Guiding Principles on Business and Human Rights" to implement the "Protect, Respect, Remedy" framework that he developed during his term, also based on broad-based stakeholder consultations and endorsed by the UN Human Rights Council in June 2011. In brief, the principles outline the responsibilities of businesses to respect human rights, the state responsibility to protect human rights by clarifying expectations of businesses operating from or in their territories, and assert that remedies must be made available to people when rights are violated. They are broad principles intended to apply to all businesses, and have not specifically targeted the pharmaceutical industry or the specific question of its obligations with regard to access to medicines (Office of the United Nations High Commissioner for Human Rights, 2011). To our knowledge, the pharmaceutical industry has not yet publicly reacted to the issuance of these guidelines.

How can we explain these different reactions? One reason may be that Hunt's Draft Human Rights Guidelines were formulated in a more concrete way (closer to secondary norms) and were directly related to the pharmaceutical industry, whereas Ruggie's Guiding Principles were presented in a more general way as a new approach to human rights, that is—adapting to the role of powerful private actors in a globalizing world, they pointed to the need to extend the scope of human rights obligations beyond nation states. To some degree they can be compared to Fidler's extension of the domain of international relations from an anarchical system of nation states to a system of open-source anarchy—without, however, referring to transnational non-state actors other than "business." They can both be considered revolutionary, in the sense that they introduce norms for private actors from a position of authority—a competence that traditionally has been reserved for nation states. Further analysis is needed to understand what their implications may be for consolidation of the access norm.

(b) Inclusiveness of the access norm: Which medicines are essential?

A central and ongoing source of tension regarding the access norm is its scope—particularly along two dimensions: which medicines would be considered "essential"? In which countries?

The access norm emerged from a push by developing countries and CSOs for "access to *essential* medicines for all" and not just "access to ARVs for the poorest countries." However, the public debate has mostly focused on the latter, which was the concrete starting-point of the campaign and continues to drive forward debates and institutional innovation in this field. TNPCs and industrialized countries have consistently pushed to circumscribe the reach of the access norm as narrowly as possible. For example, pharmaceutical companies offered voluntary price discounts (also known as differential or tiered pricing) for ARVs and drugs for infectious diseases primarily affecting people in developing countries, such as malaria or certain neglected diseases. Some companies also offered donations, usually limited to a certain disease, country, or time period.[5] Finally, companies also engaged in voluntary licensing in which they authorized other manufacturers to produce generic versions of their drugs for sale in a fixed set of countries. What characterized all of these offers were their voluntary nature, the relatively small sizes of the markets at stake, and the decision-making power retained by companies in determining who received what types of discounts, where, and for how long. The countries that were usually targeted by these efforts tended to be low-income (as classified by the World Bank), Least Developed Countries (as classified by the UN), and/or in sub-Saharan Africa. In other words, the poorest countries where no sizeable markets were at stake. Middle-income countries (lower-middle or upper-middle income, according to annual World Bank categorizations) were a source of growing and potentially significant profits, particularly the "pharmerging markets" that were projected to contribute the majority of growth to the pharmaceutical industry's bottom line. The growing economic importance of the middle-income markets would mean that expanding the access norm to include such countries would entail hotly contested political battles, as discussed in the following sections.

The first major global contest over the scope of the access norm followed the 2001 Doha Declaration. The Declaration had ostensibly reflected a consensus view among all WTO Members that TRIPS "can and should be interpreted and implemented in a manner supportive of WTO Members' right to protect public health and, in particular, to promote access to medicines for all." Notably, there was no disease restriction or country restriction regarding these principles. The US and EU had pushed for such limits (i.e. to a list of diseases and only for use by the poorest countries) in the negotiations leading up to the Doha Declaration, but had not obtained them in the end (Abbott, 2002). However, the Doha negotiation left unresolved one key issue—the extent to which compulsory licenses could be issued to export medicines to countries that did not have domestic manufacturing capacity, as described in greater detail in Chapter 5. In line with the pharmaceutical industry position, the EU and US had proposed to restrict use of the system to a pre-defined list of diseases, a limited set of countries, and only in cases of emergency. The EU proposal listed the following eligible diseases: HIV/AIDS, malaria, tuberculosis, yellow fever, plague, cholera, meningococcal disease, African trypanosomiasis, dengue, influenza, leishmaniasis, hepatitis, leptospirosis, pertussis, poliomyelitis, schistosomiasis, typhoid fever, typhus measles, shigellosis, hemorrhagic fever, and arboviruses. However, either no treatments were available for these diseases, the treatments were already off-patent, or little R&D was being carried out to develop new, potentially patentable treatments for them (as cited in 't Hoen, 2009). In other

---

5　E.g. the Mectizan Donation Programme (against river blindness) and the Malarone Donation Programme (against malaria), see also Liese, Rosenberg and Schratz (2010).

words, the system would have applied to very few medicines. In the final August 30th decision, as noted in the previous chapter, there were no disease restrictions. Nevertheless, this episode reflected a persistent and continuing political contest between those advocating for more inclusive access norms (developing countries, CSOs), and those seeking to narrow them as much as possible (industrialized countries, pharmaceutical industry).

In fact, the very issue of *inclusiveness* underscores the informal character of the Doha Declaration: it did not create new international law, but rather, politically strengthened the right to use TRIPS flexibilities "to protect public health" by clarifying how TRIPS should be interpreted. Nevertheless, the exact interpretation of the respective TRIPS clauses has remained a matter of discursive power; considering the political context of 2001, there was no way to deny the legitimacy of HIV/AIDS treatment as a reason for issuing a compulsory license. On the other hand, to interpret TRIPS "in a manner supportive of WTO Members' right ... to promote access to medicines for all" still leaves some scope for interpretation (and thus conflict) regarding the relationship between TRIPS (and its supposed role in incentivizing pharmaceutical research) and access to medicines.

Efforts to push the access norm beyond HIV have met with some success but also with much resistance, and have originated largely at country-level. In our description of the Thai experience in Chapter 5, we noted that the government's use of compulsory licenses on non-HIV medicines—including drugs for cancer and heart-disease—was probably a key reason why the government met with such fierce political reaction to its decision. It was effectively pushing the boundaries of the globally-accepted access norm as it stood in 2007. Here we recount events in two other countries, India and Ecuador, where CSOs and governments pushed with some success to make the access norm more inclusive.

(i) India: Expanding and institutionalizing broad access norms—the fight begins with a cancer drug

India was one of the first countries, alongside Thailand, where access to cancer drugs became a political issue.

India made full use of the transition period allowed under TRIPS, and amended its patent law to become TRIPS compliant in 2005. In the months during which the Patent Act revision was being debated from late 2004 to early 2005, there was a massive mobilization of civil society organizations both within and outside of India. Recognizing that the majority of generic HIV medicines used in developing countries were produced and exported from India, the global HIV activist community mobilized to shape the Indian Patent Act. Indian firms had established a reputation for being able to manufacture ARVs at stringent international quality standards, but at prices just a fraction of those offered by TNPCs. Not only were Indian firms able to reverse engineer and produce many new medicines at low-cost, they also developed new formulations, such as fixed-dose combinations (FDCs) that combined three medicines into one pill, and pediatric formulations for children. By 2008, Indian firms supplied 86% (by volume) of the developing country ARV market, which included at least 111 countries (Waning et al., 2010).

Thus, the political fight over the shape of the new patent law took place at both national and global levels. Civil society groups from India, Brazil, Burkina Faso, Canada, France, Germany, Italy, Kenya, Latvia, Malaysia, Morocco, Namibia, Nigeria, Portugal, Rwanda, South Africa, Switzerland, Tanzania, Thailand, Uganda, US, UK, and Zimbabwe wrote to Prime Minister Singh asking that he take into account the widespread international reliance on Indian generic medicines when reforming the Patents Act (Health GAP et al., 2004 (December 16)). Leaders from WHO and the UN acting on behalf of a long list of Member States, implored the Indian government to take public health needs in other countries into consideration as they deliberated over the new law. IP experts within Indian academia, the legal community, CSOs and the major generic firms also lobbied Parliament for a law that would maximize the possibility of continued generic drug production (personal communication, KM Gopakumar, 2009; personal communication, Anand Grover, 2009; personal communication, Vivek Divan, 2010).

The mobilization seems to have paid off. The patent law, ultimately passed by Parliament on March 23, 2005, contained some of the most far-reaching provisions to safeguard generic drug production. While TRIPS meant that India could not avoid product patents on medicines altogether, Parliament set high standards of patentability that could reduce the number of patents granted (Section 3(d)); allowed continued production of medicines that were already on the market as generics but could become patented; implemented a relatively simple and predictable system for compulsory licensing both for domestic supply and for export under the August 30th system (Section 92(a)); strengthened the rules for pre- and post-grant opposition; and incorporated R&D exemptions for use of patents (Press Information Bureau, Ministry of Commerce and Industry, Government of India, 2005 (March 23)). Some of these safeguards were quite innovative and unprecedented in any other developing country, and critically, they applied to all medicines, not only those for HIV/AIDS.

The multinational industry welcomed the provision of product patents, but also complained that several of the above-mentioned provisions were not TRIPS-compliant (Inside US Trade, 2005). Many CSOs greeted the final law with a mix of caution and relief. For example, MSF said it was "deeply concerned" that the law would cut off affordable medicines supply, but welcomed some of the flexibilities included (Médecins Sans Frontières (MSF), 2005 (March 23)). Trade Minister Kamal Nath insisted that the new law would prevent drug price increases and protect the domestic industry. Whether the multinational industry, CSOs or Minister Nath would be proven right would depend very much on how the law was implemented.

The first major challenge to the 2005 Patents (Amendment) Act came when the Swiss firm Novartis was denied a patent for its cancer drug imatinib mesylate (brand name Glivec). Glivec is one of the most effective new cancer drugs to emerge in many years, "a miracle drug for the new century" (Strom and Fleischer-

Black, 2003), and is used for the treatment of chronic myeloid leukemia (CML) and gastrointestinal stromal tumors (GIST). CML accounts for 15–20% of all adult leukemias (Kanavos et al., 2009).

Novartis first filed for patents on imatinib, the base compound of Glivec, in 1993—when India did not grant product patents on medicines. The company filed an Indian patent application for a modified version of imatinib (the beta-crystalline form of imatinib mesylate) in 1998, which went into the "mailbox" to be examined after January 1, 2005. Novartis then began marketing Glivec in the country in 2002, which helped to boost its profits by 48% in the fourth quarter of that year, when it still had a monopoly. Several months after launching Glivec, Novartis began operating the Glivec International Patient Assistance Program (GIPAP) in India.[6] GIPAP donated Glivec to patients meeting certain criteria through a network of selected doctors.[7]

Starting in January 2003, Indian generic firms began marketing competing versions of imatinib. Novartis sold its drug at $30,000/year while the generics were sold at $2400–$3600/year. The generic drug price was still quite high for a country with a per capita GNI of $470 in 2002; however, according to Y.K. Sapru, head of the Mumbai-based Cancer Patients Aid Association (CPAA), many middle-class patients could afford the drug at the generic price but the Novartis price was simply out of reach (personal communication, October 2009). CPAA had been purchasing generic imatinib for its patients at a discounted price of about $1000/year from generic firms.

In May 2003, Novartis stopped enrolling new patients in the GIPAP program, which had operated on condition that the government would not authorize any generic competitors (Strom and Fleischer-Black, 2003).[8]

A few months later, Novartis became the first company to obtain "exclusive marketing rights (EMR)"—a government-granted monopoly required under TRIPS Article 70(9) as a transitional measure until full product patent protection would be implemented. The EMR would expire in five years or until a decision was made on the relevant patent application(s), whichever was earlier. After securing its EMR, Novartis filed suit at the Chennai and Bombay High Courts to have generic versions of Glivec removed from the market. The Chennai High

---

6   In 2003, in a highly critical *New York Times* investigation of the program, which argued that it was being used for both commercial and humanitarian purposes, Novartis admitted that GIPAP encouraged patients to campaign for inclusion of the drug in public health systems in various countries where it operated (Strom and Fleischer-Black, 2003).

7   According to Novartis, 99% of patients on Glivec in India received it through GIPAP—that is, 7100 patients received the drug through GIPAP and 45 purchased it (with reimbursement) as of end-2007 (India comprised nearly 40% of the global number of GIPAP participants, which reached 18,000 patients in 80 developing countries in 2007 (Kanavos, Vandoros and Garcia-Gonzalez, 2009).

8   In January 2005, the Chennai High Court ordered Novartis to make the drug available through GIPAP to all CML patients with an income below 7700 USD/month ($92,400/year) (Our Legal Correspondent, 2005).

Court decided in Novartis' favor, causing seven generic firms to withdraw their products from the market, while the Bombay High Court did not, allowing a few generic firms to continue selling the generic drug.

When the new patent law came into force in 2005, the "mailbox" was opened and Novartis' application for Glivec examined. The CPAA, with the Lawyers Collective HIV/AIDS Unit as legal counsel, filed their first pre-grant opposition on the application, as did generic firms Natco Pharma and Cipla (George, Sheshadri and Grover, 2009). In January 2006, the Indian patent office denied a patent on the application, arguing that the beta-crystalline form of imatinib mesylate was "only a new form of a known substance" (Rengasamy, 2006 (25 January)). The patent examiner found the application did not meet the strict patentability standards set by Section 3(d) (among other grounds), a decision that also automatically terminated the EMR (Novartis, 2007). This decision was the first major test of the new patent law—particularly Section 3(d) and the pre-grant opposition process— and demonstrated that it could indeed lead to far fewer patents being granted in India than elsewhere.

In August 2006, Novartis challenged the patent office's decision at the Chennai High Court, as well as Section 3(d) of the new Indian patent law, arguing that it was unconstitutional and did not comply with TRIPS. In the year that elapsed between the filing of the Novartis lawsuit and the final decision of the Chennai High Court, a global political mobilization that rivaled the 2001 South Africa court case got underway. Although the case concerned a cancer drug, its implications were clear for the many PLWHA who relied on Indian drug supply. Demonstrations were held at Novartis head offices in India and Basel, and international CSOs mobilized their networks in a coordinated global campaign asking Novartis to drop the case.

"The Novartis case provided a unique opportunity to build the capacity of Indian civil society in matters relating to patents" and also brought together AIDS activists with cancer patient advocates to pursue a common agenda for the first time (George et al., 2009). It also served to expand the access debate far beyond ARVs.

In August 2007, the Chennai High Court upheld the patent office rejection and the constitutionality of Section 3(d), and referred the question of TRIPS compliance to the WTO dispute settlement system. Novartis appealed the decision on its patent application, but did not appeal regarding the constitutionality of Section 3(d)—effectively letting it stand.[9] The Swiss government also declined to challenge the patent law at the WTO. (This points again to the dependence of pharmaceutical companies on governmental support to fully enjoy the advantages of strong IPR rules.) The discursive power mobilized by CSOs seems to have

---

9 It is quite possible that the heavy criticism aimed at Novartis influenced this decision. The company had posted detailed explanations of its position in India on its website. At the time, it also funded a number of meetings on the right to health (personal communication, Sofia Gruskin, September 2010), perhaps with the intention of improving its public image.

had a significant impact on the attitudes of governments as well as on the legal interpretations that prevailed.

In 2008, the case of the Glivec patent application was heard at the Intellectual Property Appellate Board (IPAB), a judicial body newly-created to manage patent disputes; in July 2009, IPAB rejected the application, upholding the ruling of the lower courts. The case has been appealed and had not yet been decided by the Supreme Court as of mid 2012.

Another key case still under consideration by India's Supreme Court as of mid 2012 also involved a cancer drug, sorafenib. The case was brought by German pharmaceutical company Bayer, and concerned the issue of "patent-registration linkage." In some countries, such as the US, the drug regulatory authority is not allowed to grant marketing approval to a generic version of a medicine if it is patented (or, in some cases, if patent litigation is ongoing). However, critics argue that it is inadvisable to "link" the drug regulatory authority (DRA)—whose responsibilities generally entail assessing the safety, efficacy and quality of a medicine—and the patent office, whose job is to assess patent applications. Generally, the DRA does not have the competency to assess patents. Economically speaking, the purpose of a linkage system is to strengthen the monopoly accorded by a patent. Linkage could delay marketing approval of a generic drug, particularly in cases where there is reason to believe a patent is invalid—an extremely relevant question in India, given its strict patentability standards. Patent linkage is not required by TRIPS, though it has been negotiated into some bilateral/regional free trade agreements (Correa, 2006).

Bayer had acquired a patent in India for its kidney and liver cancer drug sorafenib tosylate (brand name Nexavar), and marketed the drug at about $6300/month. In 2008, Indian generics firm Cipla applied for marketing approval for a generic version of sorafenib to the Drug Controller General of India (DCGI, the national drug regulatory authority). Bayer asked the Delhi High Court to order the DCGI to take patent status into consideration when assessing applications in general, and to block the application of Cipla in particular. Justice Ravindra Bhat of the Delhi High Court granted an initial interim injunction, which kept Cipla's sorafenib off the market. In August 2009, Justice Bhat rejected Bayer's petition and scolded Bayer for attempting "to tweak public policies" through the court. Bayer appealed to the Division Bench of the Delhi High Court, which upheld Justice Bhat's decision in February 2010 and noted, again, that Bayer's case "to establish a linkage cannot be countenanced," commenting that this was a question for Parliament (Mankad, 2010). As of mid 2012, the case rested with the Supreme Court.

(ii) Ecuador

Ecuador offers an intriguing example of the potential "mainstreaming" of compulsory licensing. Confronted with the high price of patented medicines, President Rafael Correa had been convinced to move forward with compulsory licensing after learning that other developing countries had already made use of the measure (personal communication, Andres Ycaza, 2010). Andres Ycaza, who would later head the patent office, was an Ecuadorean who had been collaborating with US-based CSO Essential Action, which had supplied information on the worldwide use of compulsory licensing and technical issues such as how to set royalties (personal communication, Peter Maybarduk, 2010). In late 2009, Correa announced in a radio address that two thousand patents covering nearly all medicines in the country would be considered for potential compulsory licensing. (Note that many, if not most, medicines are covered by multiple patents, and so the number of actual medicines is far lower than 2000). What was notable about the announcement was that it did not distinguish between HIV medicines and other medicines, nor did it mention infectious disease epidemics or public health emergencies. As of late 2011, Ecuador had issued one compulsory license on the ARV lopinavir/ritonavir; there are a number of cancer drugs that may also be eligible for compulsory licensing given their high prices.

(iii) Pandemic flu: Drugs and vaccines

The India and Ecuador examples provided examples of a broadening of the access norm at national level. At the global level, perhaps the most high-profile debate around access to medicines that did *not* involve HIV concerned access to drugs and vaccines for pandemic flu. Beginning in the late 1990s, a highly-pathogenic strain of an avian influenza virus (H5N1) was detected in Hong Kong, and by 2005 had spread throughout Southeast and East Asia. H5N1 was far deadlier than most influenza viruses, killing about half of the humans it had infected; while it seemed to be spreading relatively slowly, it was feared that the virus could mutate to become a highly-infectious and deadly pandemic. Around 2005 in the face of rising public concern, governments in Asia sought to increase their stockpiles of oseltamivir (Tamiflu), the antiviral drug thought to be most effective against H5N1. The patent on oseltamivir was held by the Swiss drug firm Roche, and the high cost of purchasing large quantities of the drug for national stockpiles (which might never be deployed) began to prompt familiar debates regarding patents and public health. But unlike earlier debates regarding access to ARVs, by this time the access norm had taken root and the lessons of HIV/AIDS had made a clear impact. In October 2005, then-UN Secretary General Kofi Annan in a speech at the WHO stressed the importance of "making sure that we do not allow intellectual property to get into the way of access of the poor to medication, allowing for emergency production of vaccine in the developing countries, and I wouldn't want to hear the kind of debate we got into when it came to the HIV" drugs ... "So we should be clear that in this situation, we will take the measures to make sure poor and rich have access to the medication and the vaccine required" (as quoted in Bradsher, 2005). This was a remarkably strong public statement coming from the same leader who, in 2000, had endorsed purely voluntary measures such as price discounts for ARVs through the UN-sponsored Accelerating Access Initiative.

Thailand was one of the countries hardest hit by H5N1. In October 2005, the Thai government announced that it was willing to issue a compulsory license to enable local production of oseltamivir (Nation, 2005), a decision that foreshadowed the government's use of compulsory licensing for HIV/AIDS medicines one year later. (Ultimately, the Thai government did not move forward with a compulsory license, as it was discovered that Roche held no patent in Thailand.[10]) Around the same time, H5N1 was detected in a poultry shipment from mainland China to Taiwan; the government of Taiwan promptly announced that it was willing to issue a compulsory license for local production of oseltamivir in the event of an outbreak (J. P. Love, 2007). In response to threats of compulsory licenses, Roche also negotiated voluntary licenses with Chinese and Indian firms to produce generic versions of oseltamivir primarily for the local market (Enserink, 2006; Roche Group, 2009; Wright, 2005).

Fortunately, the spread and impact of H5N1 remained limited and a global crisis in access to oseltamivir did not materialize. The threat of a global pandemic did, however, demonstrate that affected governments would be willing to prioritize public health over stringent patent protection, and thereby reinforced the access norm.

The global H1N1 pandemic that occurred in 2009 was relatively mild, and perhaps for this reason prompted fewer concerns regarding access to oseltamivir for treatment; the issue that attracted far greater political attention was the question of access to effective flu vaccines, which were concentrated in the North. However, since the primary problem was limited production capacity rather than patents per se, a full discussion is beyond the scope of this book. Similarly, complex debates over Indonesia's virus-sharing policies and its relationship to equitable access to flu vaccine have attracted considerable scholarly attention, but lie outside the scope of this book (see, for example, Fidler, 2008a).

(iv) Non-communicable diseases

The burden of disease in developing countries from non-communicable causes has been growing for many years. Of the 31 million global annual deaths from cancers, heart disease, diabetes and respiratory diseases, 80% occur in low- and middle-income countries (Mathers and Loncar, 2006). By 2030, 70% of newly-reported cancer cases are expected to come from developing countries, where two-thirds of global cancer deaths already take place (Farmer et al., 2010). Until

---

10 Patents are territorial, not international. That is, in order to receive a patent right, an applicant must apply in a particular jurisdiction for the patent. Oftentimes, companies do not file for patents in smaller countries that are not considered to be profitable markets and therefore not worth the cost of filing for and maintaining a patent. However, patent information is also extremely difficult to obtain, and it is not uncommon in developing countries for governments and or CSOs to have difficulty ascertaining the patent status of a particular drug.

recently, political attention to NCDs has been quite low, particularly relative to the burden of disease (Stuckler, Hawkes and Yach, 2009). However, NCDs reached political prominence on the global agenda in 2011 when the UN convened its first High Level Meeting on Non-communicable Diseases.[11] At the NCD summit, IP and access to NCD medicines became a thorny political issue that, at one point, threatened to derail agreement upon a consensus declaration by UN member states.[12]

Until recently, the issue of access to medicines and patents was not a prominent part of the debate on NCDs. As with HIV/AIDS, both pharmaceutical companies and health experts noted that combating NCDs would require a host of cross-sectoral measures, and that nearly all drugs for NCDs on the WHO Essential Medicines List were already off-patent. However, those familiar with these lines of argumentation from previous debates on HIV/AIDS pointed out that the EML used relative cost-effectiveness as a criteria for selection, such that the high patented price of a medicine can be a reason for exclusion from the list. A number of LMICs, such as Thailand and Mexico, have begun providing on-patent NCD drugs as part of their national health insurance programs, and will need to find ways to obtain affordable prices in order to maintain the sustainability of their national programs (Harris, 2011; Tantivess et al., 2008).

The conflict leading up to the NCD summit centered on the question of whether or not the Doha Declaration would be explicitly mentioned in the NCD declaration. Summit declarations are generally statements of political commitment and—depending on their content—may reflect and strengthen informal norms; they are consensus texts that, in principle, represent the shared views of all UN Member States and their discursive power can be considerable. Serious diplomatic maneuvering has gone into each of the declarations at the HIV/AIDS summits (2001, 2006 and 2011), and the Doha Declaration was explicitly mentioned in both the 2006 and 2011 HIV summit declarations (United Nations General Assembly, 2006; United Nations General Assembly, 2011). While the NCD summit came just three months after the 2011 HIV summit, and involved the exact same Member States—and often even the same individual negotiators—the hard-line resistance of the US to any mention of Doha in the declaration reflected a line in the sand over the interpretation of TRIPS. Developing countries, led by Brazil, India and Mexico, pushed for inclusion of language on the use of TRIPS flexibilities—which they obtained—but did not succeed in getting explicit mention of Doha, which would have strengthened the access norm in the NCD declaration. While the NCD declaration does not formally change any element of TRIPS or Doha, the absence

---

11   The June 2001 UN General Assembly Special Session on HIV/AIDS was the first UN summit dedicated to a health issue; it was followed up in 2006 and 2011 with High-Level Meetings on HIV/AIDS; the 2011 NCD summit was the first to be dedicated to a health issue that was not HIV/AIDS.

12   Confidential cable from EU negotiators, August 2011, on file with the authors.

of a mention of Doha weakens the expansion and consolidation of the universal access norm. According to Love,

> Legally, the 2001 Doha Declaration, and subsequent amendments to TRIPS, applies to any disease. But in practice, the perceptions are as important as the legal reality. By continuing to assert that the Doha Declaration is in fact limited in various ways, US and European trade negotiators have tried to discourage the granting of compulsory licenses on patents for high-priced drugs for cancer and other non-communicable diseases. (Love, 2011)

The battle over the use of TRIPS flexibilities to improve access to NCD medicines is likely to grow more heated in the future, especially as the national health systems of middle-income countries begin expanding coverage to their populations and struggling to pay for costly drugs and rising disease burdens.

(c) The inclusiveness of the access norm:
Middle-income countries as the new battlefield?

Developing countries, CSOs and experts worked together to re-shape global IP rules significantly from 1999–2011. Middle-income countries (both governments and civil society actors within them), in particular, played an extremely influential role and created benefits that extended to all developing countries. Political struggles over IP and access to medicines have usually been framed as North vs. South; however, important shifts have taken place over the past decade both in terms of the relative position of key MICs in the global political economy and within their respective domestic spheres. The extent to which the access norm will include middle-income countries is likely to be highly-contested, as there are significant markets and public health interests at stake.

The global political and economic order is shifting towards a multipolar system, as some formerly "developing" countries industrialize and exert greater weight in trade, politics, and global rulemaking. The idea is encapsulated specifically in the emergence of the so-called BRICS countries—Brazil, Russia, India, China and sometimes South Africa—as well as in the broader phrases "emerging markets," "middle-income countries" or "rising powers" (Bliss, 2010).

Concerning foreign trade, many MICs have increased their economic power in absolute terms, and decreased their economic reliance on industrialized countries in relative terms. As illustrated in Figure 6.1 below, countries that played a leading role in establishing the access norm—namely Thailand, South Africa, Brazil, India—decreased the proportion of their exports going to the EU and US from 2001 to 2009 and thus reduced the trade dimension of their economic dependence on these industrialized countries. At the same time, these countries increased their trade with other developing countries, particularly with China. These changing patterns of trade underscore a more general power shift away from the North: the

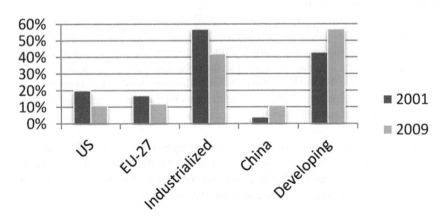

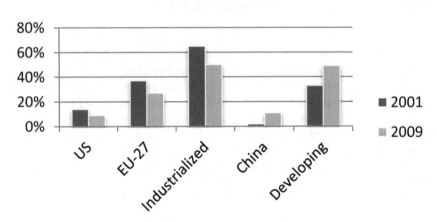

Figure 6.1   Changes in export markets 2001–2009
Source: UN Comtrade statistics (International Trade Centre (ITC), 2010.

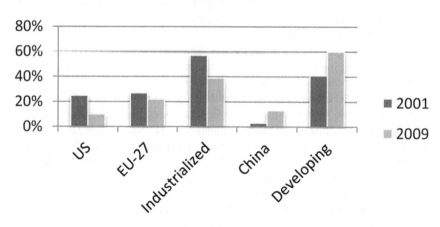

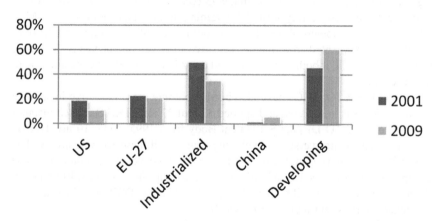

Figure 6.1   continued

older binary North-South model, in which developing countries were economically dependent on industrialized countries, is giving way to a more complex North-MICs-South arrangement in which relationships of economic dependence and power are more evenly distributed.

Simultaneously, key MICs are increasingly flexing their muscles in global IP norm-building processes. For example, frustrated by what they perceived as WIPO's promotion of ever-stricter IP rules, a group of developing country Member States who had initially established common interests in the access to medicines debates, set out at the WIPO General Assembly in September 2004 to establish for the organization a "Development Agenda". Spearheaded by Argentina and Brazil, with the Development Agenda developing countries had formally sought for the first time to institutionalize development concerns into WIPO's work program. The Argentina/Brazil proposal quickly gained support from other developing countries,[13] which formed the "Group of Friends of Development" for the negotiations. Notably, of the 13 countries that formed the group, 10 were middle-income developing countries. After three years of deliberations, in a major turnaround for the agency, WIPO Member States agreed to the Development Agenda in mid 2007. The Agenda made 45 recommendations that WIPO was to implement, and significantly shifted the framing of the organization's work (May, 2008). The Development Agenda was a codification of the notion that IP rules should be implemented in a manner sensitive to development needs, including health, and as such, it both symbolized and contributed to further consolidation of the access norm.

Within the WTO, MICs have also been becoming more proactive in shaping the way TRIPS is interpreted and applied. Out of 27 total TRIPS-related disputes brought to the WTO Dispute Settlement Body from 1995–2008, 10 involved an industrialized country versus a developing country. Of these 10, nine involved an industrialized country bringing a complaint against a developing country (the one exception was Brazil vs. US in 2001); in 2010, perhaps in a sign of shifting power dynamics, India and Brazil both challenged the EU at the DSB over the seizure of medicines in transit through the EU (see Table 6.1).

Hand in hand with the increased political and economic weight of many MICs at the global level, have come increased demands for health services at the domestic level. In many MICs, there are also high levels of inequality, and poverty often persists alongside rapidly growing prosperity (see Table 6.2 for a sample of inequality scores).

At the same time, as noted previously, the burden of disease from NCDs is expected to rise dramatically, implying a "double burden" of communicable and non-communicable diseases for many MICs (Mathers and Loncar, 2006). As disease patterns shift, increased economic development can lead to growing demands for the expansion of social insurance and improved access to a broader

---

13   Bolivia, Cuba, Dominican Republic, Ecuador, Egypt, Iran, Kenya, Sierra Leone, South Africa, Tanzania and Venezuela.

Table 6.1   TRIPS-related disputes at the WTO DSB (1995–2011)

Industrialized Member complaint against Industrialized Member (I–I)	17
Industrialized Member complaint against Developing Member (I–D) 1996: US vs. Pakistan 1996: US vs. India 1996: US vs. Indonesia 1997: EU vs. India 1999: US vs. Argentina 2000: US vs. Argentina 2000: US vs. Brazil 2007: US vs. China 2008: EU vs. China	9
Developing Member complaint against Industrialized Member (D–I) 2001: Brazil vs. US 2010: India vs. EU 2010: Brazil vs. EU	3
Total TRIPS-related Disputes at WTO DSB (1995–2010)	29

Table 6.2   Selection of intra-country inequality scores

Country	Gini coefficient	Rank	Income category
Namibia	74.3	1st, most unequal	Upper middle
South Africa	57.8		Upper middle
Brazil	55.0		Upper middle
Thailand	42.5		Lower middle
China	41.5		Lower middle
Chad	39.8	71st, median	Low income
India	36.8		Lower middle
Bangladesh	31.0		Low income/LDC
Azerbaijan	16.8	167th, most equal	Lower middle-income

Source: UNDP Human Development Report 2010.[14]

range of medicines—with serious budget implications for governments. For example, Thailand, a lower-middle income country, launched its first universal health insurance program in 2002. The newly-created National Health Security Office (NHSO) included antiretroviral therapy (ART) among its covered services, after strong civil society reaction to the initial exclusion of ART. The direct impact of high-cost ARV drugs on the government budget may have made the Thai government more willing to issue compulsory licenses in 2006, as compared

14   Statistical tables available at: http://hdr.undp.org/en/statistics/ihdi/.

to earlier in the decade (Tantivess et al., 2008). China also began implementing major health system reforms to achieve universal coverage, which has led to price controls on many medicines (D. Wilson, 2011). In 2009, in response to some of the highest drug prices in the region, the Philippines government also imposed price controls (Hookway, 2010). As more countries expand the breadth and depth of their health insurance systems, the political pressure on governments to make medicines accessible and manage high drug prices is likely to grow.

(i) Emerging markets

At the same time that key developing countries are exercising increased political influence and experiencing rising health needs, they are also becoming a critical source of market growth for the pharmaceutical industry. In 2010, the research firm IMS Health predicted that the developed markets in the US and Europe would grow by just 3–6%/year from 2010–2014, while the emerging markets—especially China, India and Russia—would grow by 14–17%/year (IMS Health, 2010). (IMS Health has defined the "pharmerging" markets as: Brazil, China, India, Russia, Turkey, Mexico, South Korea, Argentina, Poland, Venezuela, Vietnam, South Africa, Thailand, Indonesia, Romania, Egypt, Pakistan, and Ukraine.) By 2010, China had vaulted up the ranks to become the world's third largest pharmaceutical market after the US and Japan, and was predicted to become the second largest market by 2015 (Hirschler, 2010).

Simultaneously, the industry was facing a "patent cliff" as blockbuster drugs went off patent in key markets, while few promising drugs were in the pipeline. This dearth of future high-earning drugs led some pharmaceutical companies to shift their focus even more heavily towards the emerging markets to shore up revenue in the ensuing years (Wilson, 2011).

Finally, as noted, the epidemiological transition in developing countries presaged a growing burden of disease from chronic conditions such as diabetes, heart disease, cancer, and mental illness—conditions that are the most lucrative markets for the pharmaceutical industry. This shift suggested that the industry would seek stronger IP rules to protect patent rights on its most profitable products in the emerging markets.

(We return to the issue of MICs in Chapter 8, Section (c), where we also discuss the growing capacity in these countries to carry out pharmaceutical R&D and the potential shifts in the configuration of domestic interests that may result.)

(ii) Increased potential for political conflict over IP rules

The confluence of growing influence, health needs, and market size within the MICs suggested that the stakes in shaping global IP rules and access norms were high for both the pharmaceutical industry and for governments. For MICs governments, the implementation of IP rules could have a major impact on government budgets and public health, and lead to political challenges from civil society groups as well.

For industry, the way IP rules were implemented in the emerging markets could have a significant impact on revenue. The potential for continued political conflict over IP rules was high, particularly between key MICs and industrialized countries (see Chapter 4). In contrast to the North-South divisions of the past, industrialized countries and the drug industry seem to have conceded on IP issues in the poorest countries (LDCs or low-income countries); pharmaceutical company pricing and IP policies in these territories is generally more flexible, and the IFPMA in 2011 even endorsed a proposal by the UK to extend the TRIPS implementation deadline for LDCs beyond 2013 (New, 2011).[15] Thus, conflicts are increasingly characterized by North-MICs divisions, rather than North-South.

Evidence of such conflicts has arisen in negotiations over IP provisions contained in free trade agreements (FTAs). With multilateral trade talks stalled at the WTO, international IP-rulemaking has shifted to bilateral and regional arenas. Both the US and EU have negotiated free trade agreements with primarily middle-income country trade partners that require them to adopt measures more stringent than TRIPS (called "TRIPS-plus" measures),[16] further limiting the policy space available to countries (Correa, 2006). However, a number of these negotiations never came to fruition (Morin, 2009), though it is difficult to draw any firm conclusions given the ongoing evolution in trade strategies. Nevertheless, it is not a foregone conclusion that developing countries (particularly the rising powers) will agree to the TRIPS-plus provisions proposed in trade agreements, as illustrated by debates over the European Union-India FTA (see earlier in this chapter and also Chapter 7).

---

15   The Doha Declaration extended to 2016 the deadline for LDCs to grant or enforce pharmaceutical patents. Any extension of the 2013 deadline for implementing the rest of the TRIPS agreement may also lead to an extension of the 2016 deadline for LDCs.

16   This has been called the TRIPS-Plus agenda, and includes patent term extensions, data exclusivity, patent-registration linkage and other measures designed to strengthen patent monopolies.

Chapter 7
Challenges to the Stability of Informal Norms

Between the late 1990s and 2012 a relatively effective informal norm regarding universal access to essential medicines developed. Even in the absence of a detailed legal framework, political pressure was sufficient to induce voluntary acceptance of the access norm,[1] a decisive pre-condition for its successful implementation. All of the relevant actors moved towards supporting access to ARVs in a substantial manner. Because of the informality of the norm, this was done in a form that best coincided with the actors' own interests. Certainly, in terms of legal security it might be preferable to establish a well-designed regime with a clear system of sanctions. But if this is not attainable because of divergent interests concerning TRIPS and/or health-related norms, a system of informal political norms might be the *second-best solution*. However, the solution is only workable with widely-accepted and strong, stable political norms.

How strong and stable is the access norm? Beyond ARVs, the exact scope of medicines and countries subject to the access norm is still contested, in particular concerning access to medicines against non-communicable diseases and IP rules in middle income countries. In addition to the precise *scope* of a norm, the *stability* of an informal norm also merits further consideration and discussion: If stakeholders were reluctant to accept the norm in the beginning of the norm-building process, will they not work to change the norm itself and the underlying conditions that led to its emergence? And when conditions change, will those stakeholders that used their power to fight for the access norm succeed in maintaining the degree of attention and mobilization in all of the political contests that might jeopardize the norm?

While the pharmaceutical industry supported to some degree the global endeavor to improve access to medicines among the world's poor, they nevertheless continued to pursue their agenda of trying to secure stronger international IPRs. They shifted the forum of their activities towards bi- and plurilateral free trade agreements (FTAs) and other treaties, and worked to secure TRIPS-plus clauses in FTAs that restrict the use of TRIPS flexibilities. This trend was particularly pronounced in FTAs negotiated with the US, but more recently became very common in EU-negotiated FTAs. Most trade partners agreed to these demands, as their priorities were oriented towards gaining access to high-income country

---

1 Certainly, in the case of states there has been the legal obligation of the ICESCR, but this alone has often not been strong enough to provoke appropriate action by governments.

markets for their export industries. These problems have been discussed at length in relation to different US trade agreements, including those with Latin American countries, Jordan and Morocco.[2] More recently, the EU demanded TRIPS-plus provisions in negotiations with India on a bilateral FTA, as discussed in the previous chapter.[3] The following sections discuss these challenges in more detail.

(a) Challenges in access to HIV/AIDS medicines

The access norm has been strongest and most resilient for HIV/AIDS. Yet despite the significant progress in access to HIV medicines, enormous challenges remain. First, the cost of treatment began increasing again because new ARVs are likely to be more widely patented in developing countries and thus more expensive (even with the high patentability standards implemented in India). ARV prices, particularly in some middle-income developing countries, can still put them out of reach of the people who need them. Without production sources, the countries that rely on importation will find it hard to source low-cost medicines. Second, about two-thirds of people in need of treatment still did not receive first-line medicines as of this writing (World Health Organization (WHO), UNICEF, UNAIDS, 2010). In addition, increasing numbers of people will need access to new-generation ARVs as the virus mutates and develops resistance to first-line drugs ('t Hoen et al., 2011). Third, the policy space to produce or import generic versions of patented medicines has shrunk in some developing countries, as a result of the FTAs mentioned above. Fourth, as long as no effective cure for HIV/AIDS exists, every PLHIV will require the lifelong provision of medicines for survival (Bell et al., 2004)). Access to HIV medicines for people in countries dependent on international financing was still precarious as of this writing, especially amidst an economic crisis in which donors began to pull back, endangering the continuity of treatment already started. In November 2011, the Board of the Global Fund canceled its planned eleventh round of grant making, citing the lack of funds and the failure of donors to deliver on previous pledges (The Global Fund to Fight AIDS, Tuberculosis and Malaria, 2011). In July 2009, the United Kingdom All Party Parliamentary Group on AIDS called the overall situation a "treatment timebomb" and called for "political activism" to "ensure that the next generation of drugs is available to the world's poorest in future" (Oakeshott, 2009). In

---

2   There are a large number of critical texts on Free Trade Agreements with TRIPS+ provisions. The UNCTAD-ICTSD Project on IPRs and Sustainable Development presented a number of interesting studies on these negotiations (see www.iprsonline.org/resources/ FTAs-htm); Oxfam produced various briefing notes and briefing papers on this subject (Mayne, 2002; Oxfam International, 2007); see also Abbott (2006); Abbott, Correa and Biadgleng (2007); Correa (2004); Correa (2006); Vivas-Eugui (2003).

3   Other industries with a strong interest in IPRs include the information technology, entertainment and agrochemicals industries.

short, despite unprecedented progress in improving access to HIV medicines and treatment, such access still rested on shaky ground.

(b) Free trade agreements

Where multilateral attempts to achieve strict IP rules failed, Northern countries and industries turned to bilateral or regional approaches. Trade and IP law expert Frederick Abbott labeled this strategy a TRIPS II agenda pursued by "strong mercantile interests[4] seeking to increase technology and expression rents"[5] as a reaction to the change in underlying economic and technological conditions since the late 1990s (Abbott, 2006).

During the negotiation of the TRIPS Agreement, the major powers achieved formidable results through a strategy of negotiating multilaterally within the GATT while exerting bilateral trade pressure on hold-out countries outside it. The post-TRIPS era witnessed a continuation of this strategy, as the US and EU, in particular, pushed for additional concessions on IP through bilateral or regional FTAs. As Okediji has pointed out, bilateral approaches to winning IP concessions from trade partners was a "vintage strategy" for the US—with TRIPS being perhaps the multilateral exception rather than the norm (Okediji, 2004). IP norms contained in bilateral agreements may set a powerful example and serve as strategic leverage in multilateral negotiations; the bilateral-to-multilateral strategy proved its worth in the 1980–90s when IP standards contained in US agreements with South Korea, Canada and Mexico were later reproduced in TRIPS. According to Drahos, "Shifting from bilaterals to multilaterals has been at the centerpiece of US strategy for the last 20 years and has proven to be highly effective" (Drahos, 2003).

As of 2009, an estimated 205 FTAs were in force (Cooper, 2010), of which 130 were bilateral agreements. The vast majority of bilateral agreements were negotiated between industrialized and developing countries (Morin, 2008). After TRIPS came into force, the US negotiated bilateral agreements focusing on IP with Cambodia, Laos, Lithuania, Latvia, Jamaica, Nicaragua, Trinidad and Tobago, and Vietnam (Morin, 2009). In addition, as of August 2010, the US had finalized FTAs with 13 developing countries, and was in the process of negotiating an agreement with Malaysia.[6] As of 2010, the EU was negotiating agreements

---

4   This concerns the copyright-dependent audio-visual industry and the pharmaceutical and agricultural chemical industry.

5   'Expression rents': rents based on licenses.

6   US FTAs implemented with: Australia; Bahrain; Canada and Mexico (NAFTA); Chile; Costa Rica, Dominican Republic, El Salvador, Guatemala, Honduras and Nicaragua (DR-CAFTA); Israel; Jordan; Morocco; Oman; Peru; and Singapore. FTAs agreed with Colombia, South Korea, and Panama, but not yet enacted into law by the US Congress as of mid 2011.

with the Gulf Cooperation Council (Bahrain, Kuwait, Oman, Qatar, Saudi Arabia, United Arab Emirates), India, Mercosur (Argentina, Brazil, Paraguay, Uruguay), Singapore, and South Korea; agreements had been finalized with Colombia, Peru, and Central America, and signed with South Africa, Tunisia and the Palestinian Authority (European Commission, 2010). Most critical attention focused on US FTAs, since they tended to contain broader IP provisions than EU FTAs (though this situation may change) (Correa, 2006).

Trade negotiations between industrialized and developing countries were already characterized by considerable asymmetries in economic power. In bilateral, closed-door negotiations, developing countries were at an even greater disadvantage as they did not have access to the discursive power of public opinion, the institutional power of multilateral decision-making rules, or the expert resources accessible through global networks, all of which played a critical role in strengthening the access norm from 1999–2010. While developing countries still had the structural (legal) power as sovereign states to refuse an unfavorable FTA, some health advocates feared that—without health ministers at the negotiating table—trade ministries would be willing to compromise on IP in exchange for economic benefits in other sectors ('t Hoen, 2007). During the 2005 US-Thai FTA negotiations, Thai Senator Kraisak Choonhavan warned that "the only options for the government now are to pull out of the talks or sell the country down the drain on public health for dubious returns" (as quoted in Khor, 2005). Drezner has argued that, through bilateral and regional FTAs, the US had in essence regained control of the global IP regime: "In effect, the legal arrangements shift the status quo to the US-preferred outcome; one in which flexibility is only invoked in times of crisis epidemics" (Drezner, 2007).

However, as described in greater detail in Moon (2010), TRIPS-plus provisions sought in US FTAs have been softened somewhat since the 2001 Doha Declaration. Patent-related provisions in later FTAs (with Colombia, Peru, and Panama) are less stringent than those contained in earlier agreements (e.g. Jordan, Morocco, Dominican Republic-Central American FTA). Perhaps in response to criticism from some members of Congress, the World Health Assembly (Resolution WHA 57.14), the WHO Commission on Intellectual Property, Innovation and Public Health, the UN Special Rapporteur on the Right to Health, academics and CSOs ('t Hoen, 2007), the USTR initially issued "side letters" to FTAs stating that they "do not stand in the way of measures necessary to protect public health" (Office of the United States Trade Representative (USTR), 2007). In 2007, seeking the renewal of Trade Promotion Authority from a Democrat-controlled Congress, the Republican Bush Administration agreed to increase the legal weight of this commitment by including similar language in the actual text of the FTAs. Finally, in an analysis of IP provisions in US bilateral agreements, Morin found that— while the USTR expected bilateral deals to yield multilateral results, the strategy has largely failed. Instead, Morin concluded that "bilateral agreements have created instability and fragmentation among WTO members and within the US

Congress, which could ultimately damage the bargaining position of the USTR" (Morin, 2009).

The FTA strategy—while still a sizeable threat to the access norm—is not invulnerable. Perhaps reflecting dissatisfaction with FTA demands, talks that were initiated with Thailand, the Southern African Customs Union (Botswana, Lesotho, Namibia, South Africa, Swaziland), and the United Arab Emirates were later considered "dormant" (Cooper, 2010). The Thai-US FTA talks had spurred massive street demonstrations in Chiang Mai in 2005, and may have contributed to the ousting of Prime Minister Thaksin Shinawatra in 2006. South Africa's chief negotiator halted talks with the US in 2004, citing differences in IP standards (among others) that "may not be appropriate for a developing country" (as quoted in Morin, 2009). And at the 2006 World Health Assembly, a group of South American health ministers[7] issued a declaration committing themselves to "the successful implementation of the safeguards and flexibilities included both in the TRIPS agreement and in the Doha Declaration" (Public Citizen, 2006). This declaration reflected the conflicting interests within developing countries, since some of these countries had already accepted TRIPS+ rules in FTAs with the US (e.g. Chile, Ecuador, Peru), and they did not commit themselves to renegotiate the FTAs that were in contradiction to their own declaration.

Despite the pushback, the Obama Administration, however, continued and even strengthened the US drive for tighter IP rules in industrialized and developing countries through negotiations over a Trans-Pacific Partnership trade agreement; analyses of negotiating texts leaked in November 2011 suggest that the Obama-led USTR is seeking even more stringent IP measures than its predecessor (American University Program on Information Justice and Intellectual Property, 2011; Public Citizen, 2006). Close monitoring of FTAs by CSOs and experts may blunt initiatives seeking major concessions beyond TRIPS standards, but economic stagnation in the US also strengthened domestic pressure on USTR to protect US economic interests.

There has been parliamentary and civil society push back on the pursuit of TRIPS-plus measures by the European Commission's Director-General for Trade (DG Trade) as well. For example, the 2007 European Parliament resolution on access to medicines called for the EU "to restrict the Commission's mandate so as to prevent it from negotiating pharmaceutical-related TRIPS-plus provisions affecting public health and access to medicines" in trade agreements (European Parliament, 2007). The resolution had been supported by European public health CSOs and a group of MEPs (Members of the European Parliament) interested in IP, health and development issues. More recently, DG Trade came under fire from MEPs, and international and Indian CSOs—including being subject to an activist protest at the 2010 Vienna AIDS conference—for pursuing TRIPS-plus measures in FTA negotiations with India. Indian generic firms have also strongly opposed

---

7   Argentina, Bolivia, Brazil, Chile, Colombia, Ecuador, Paraguay, Peru, Uruguay, and Venezuela.

the potential agreement. Though the negotiating text remained confidential as of this writing, Trade Commissioner Karel de Gucht had confirmed that the EU was seeking certain measures that went beyond those required by TRIPS (de Gucht, Karel (DG Trade), 2010 (May 5)). Because India played such a central role in supplying low-cost generic medicines to other developing countries, the global health stakes of this FTA were particularly high (Waning et al., 2010). As mentioned in Chapter 6, the public outcry over the EU-India FTA seems to have had a strong effect on the Indian government, which announced in June 2011 that in order to protect public health it would not accept certain IP provisions sought by the EU (Médecins Sans Frontières, 2011). Political mobilization from legislators, Indian industry, and global and national civil society had raised the political costs to both the EU and Indian governments of agreeing to TRIPS-plus provisions. As of mid 2012, the provisions of the EU-India agreement remain unclear as the text is still under negotiation and talks are carried out behind closed doors.

(c) WTO accession agreements

WTO accession agreements may offer another channel for undermining the access norm. Despite being couched in a multilateral context, these agreements mirror the asymmetrical power dynamics of FTAs—many negotiations are carried out bilaterally and behind closed doors, privileging economic power over discursive and institutional power. Each country wishing to join the WTO must gain the assent of all existing WTO members. Industrialized countries have capitalized on their *de facto* veto power by extracting concessions beyond those required by WTO agreements. The most vivid example of this dynamic was illustrated in China's 2001 accession, which included TRIPS-plus provisions such as six years of data exclusivity and patent-registration linkage, among others (Moon, 2010, chapter 5.2.5). Nor were smaller countries exempt from similar demands—when LDCs Cambodia and Nepal joined the WTO in 2003, their accession agreements did not take advantage of the WTO extended deadline until 2013 for LDCs to implement TRIPS, and the Doha Declaration's 2016 extended deadline specifically for pharmaceutical patents, among other TRIPS-plus measures (Abbott et al., 2007). Acceding WTO Members have also committed to joining a wide range of other IP treaties, such as the International Convention for the Protection of New Varieties of Plants (UPOV), that contain provisions more stringent than TRIPS.

The extent and strength of TRIPS-plus provisions varies by country. In some cases, countries implemented TRIPS-plus provisions in their national laws prior to being accepted into the WTO; in others, countries made specific binding "commitments" enforceable by the DSB, while in yet others, countries did not make binding "commitments" but rather indicated their intention to implement certain policies. Therefore, in some cases, it may be legally permissible for countries to change their legislation after acceding to the WTO to remove TRIPS-plus provisions, while remaining compliant with TRIPS. (Such changes will be easier to implement if the long-standing moratorium on non-violation complaints with respect to TRIPS continues.[8]) However, in practice such legal distinctions may mean very little. As Abbott and Correa point out, "more important from a practical standpoint, the acceding country faces the prospect of diplomatic representations from economically important WTO Members regarding its failure to maintain the legislation adopted or announced during the accession process... that diplomacy may be combined with threats relating to suspension of trade preferences or economic aid packages" (Abbott et al., 2007).

The impact of accession processes on the global IP regime can be considerable. As of this writing, the WTO included 153 Members and 30 Observer governments. Observers are generally countries that have indicated their interest in joining the WTO, and must begin accession negotiations within five years of becoming Observers. Of the 30 current Observers, 27 are developing countries (non-high-income). It is unclear whether the access norm has had an impact specifically on the WTO accession process. This is an area where ongoing monitoring and further research are required.

(d) Alternate channels for IP rulemaking

There were several other channels through which the access norm could be challenged in IP rulemaking. Industrialized countries pushed for tighter IP rules through bilateral pressure, interpretation of existing treaty law, and negotiating new treaties, as detailed below.

First, the US continued to threaten trade sanctions for IP practices it deemed unsatisfactory through the annual Special 301 report. Since 2001, up-front criticism of countries for using compulsory licensing for public health purposes has nearly disappeared from the 301 reports (though some unclear language referring to Thailand's compulsory licensing remained) (Moon, 2010, Chapter 5.1.6). In addition, the report made explicit mention of the USTR's support for the Doha Declaration. However, the 301 report continued to highlight medicines-related concerns, particularly in the emerging markets such as China and Brazil. Health GAP (Health Global Access Project), together with 18 other organizations and individuals (including those based in the US, Costa Rica, Egypt, India, Kenya,

---

8 Non-violation complaints are complaints that a WTO member may bring against another at the DSB when it has been "deprived of an expected benefit because of another government's action, or because of any other situation that exists" (World Trade Organization (WTO), 2011), without having to allege that the defendant has actually violated an agreement. Non-violation complaints are perceived to privilege more economically powerful, well-resourced countries that may use the threat of launching such legal complaints as a pressure mechanism to shape the implementation of TRIPS domestically. For more information, see: http://www.wto.org/english/tratop_e/trips_e/nonviolation_background_e.htm, accessed March 4, 2012.

Malaysia, and Thailand), filed a complaint with the UN Special Rapporteur on the right to health in mid 2010, arguing that use of Special 301 to restrict access to medicines constituted an international human rights violation (Health Global Access Project (Health GAP), 2010). Despite a campaign-trail statement from President Obama in 2008 that he would support "the rights of sovereign nations to access quality-assured, low-cost generic medication to meet their pressing public health needs under the WTO's Declaration on the Agreement on Trade Related Aspects of Intellectual Property Rights" (The Office of the President-Elect, 2009), an analysis of 301 Reports found that Special 301 pressure on the middle-income countries under the Obama Administration had not significantly abated (Flynn, 2010). Such pressure may not necessarily lead to changes in developing country IP policies, however. In Ecuador, for example, the government weighed the potential trade losses against health gains and decided to move forward with its compulsory licensing policy (personal communication, Andres Ycaza, March 2010).

Second, significant North-South differences remain in the interpretation of existing IP rules. An enduring disagreement relates to TRIPS Article 39.3, which concerns protection against "unfair commercial use" of data submitted for regulatory approval of pharmaceuticals or agricultural chemicals.[9] While the US argued that TRIPS required Members to provide data exclusivity, several developing countries and the WHO contended that *exclusive* rights were not required (other forms of protection were permissible), and that such exclusivity was explicitly excluded from TRIPS during the negotiations (Correa, 2002b; Watal, 2001)). Data exclusivity could create monopolies and thereby function as the economic equivalent of patents for their duration (usually five to six years). While some countries had adopted data exclusivity through FTAs and WTO Accession Agreements, many others refused to do so on the grounds that it was not required by TRIPS.

Another conflict arose over what IP rights apply over goods in transit. From 2008–2009, customs authorities in the Netherlands, France and Germany seized 20 shipments of generic medicines in transit from India to other developing countries, on suspicion that they infringed patents in the transit countries (i.e. Dutch, French and German patents). For example, in December 2008 Dutch authorities seized a shipment from India to Brazil of generic losartan (a blood pressure drug), which was transiting through Amsterdam's Schiphol airport. Losartan was patented in neither India nor Brazil, but Merck held a patent in the Netherlands (Abbott, 2009). In May 2010, the governments of India and Brazil each filed a formal complaint

---

9   TRIPS Article 39.3, in its entirety, reads: "Members, when requiring, as a condition of approving the marketing of pharmaceutical or of agricultural chemical products which utilize new chemical entities, the submission of undisclosed test or other data, the origination of which involves a considerable effort, shall protect such data against unfair commercial use. In addition, Members shall protect such data against disclosure, except where necessary to protect the public, or unless steps are taken to ensure that the data are protected against unfair commercial use."

at the WTO DSB challenging the EU and Dutch policies regarding the repeated seizures; notably these challenges were only the second time that developing countries had complained against an industrialized country on a TRIPS-related matter at the WTO DSB. In a reflection of its far-reaching implications, the case garnered widespread attention from the media, CSOs, and trade and IP policy experts, and the governments of Canada, China, Ecuador, Japan and Turkey subsequently joined the consultations (World Trade Organization (WTO), 2010a; World Trade Organization (WTO), 2010b). A win for the EU could seriously undercut the supply of generic medicines from producing to importing countries, and more broadly, could dramatically impede the free flow of goods in global trade. Alternatively, a win for India and Brazil would improve the security of supply of generic drugs and signal a more muscular role for these two countries in using the WTO mechanisms to defend their own interests. Though the case is still pending, the robust political response to the seizures from India and Brazil suggested that this avenue would not result in significantly tightened IP rules.

Third, agreements negotiated outside of TRIPS or the WTO may provide another channel for proponents to achieve tighter IP rules.

Bilateral investment treaties (BIT), which numbered nearly 2400 in 2005 (United Nations Conference on Trade and Development (UNCTAD), 2005), protect the rights of foreign investors but may simultaneously constrain the ability of national governments to regulate health, safety, environment and labor conditions when doing so is interpreted as decreasing the value of an investment (Correa, 2004; P. Drahos, 2001; International Institute for Sustainable Development (IISD), 2010). BITs often contain clauses defining IP as investments, and provide some protections to foreign investors against expropriation or other economic losses. There is considerable lack of clarity on whether an investor could claim that certain TRIPS-compliant measures, particularly compulsory licensing or patent revocation, constituted *de facto* or indirect expropriation under a specific BIT. Even if BITs did not block compulsory licensing, Correa warned that use of this measure could be weakened: "given the grey area that overlapping protections of investment and IPRs create, investor's rights may be used to dissuade governments from using compulsory licenses or to challenge their decisions" (Correa, 2004). However, as of mid 2012, no medicines patent-holder had publicly raised a dispute under investment rules over compulsory licensing or similar measures. However, since many BITs provide for confidential dispute settlement, such disputes may have been raised outside the public eye.

Critics also raised concerns that the Anti-Counterfeiting Trade Agreement (ACTA) could erode flexibilities in global IP rules. Closed-door negotiations began in 2007 "to provide an international framework that improves the enforcement of intellectual property right laws" (European Commission, 2009). The negotiating parties were primarily high-income countries.[10] Developing country governments

---

10   Australia, Canada, European Union, Japan, Republic of Korea, Mexico, Morocco, New Zealand, Singapore, Switzerland, the United States.

and CSOs raised fears that rich countries might establish stringent IP norms through ACTA that they later press developing countries to accept through multilateral treaties, in a process Braithwaite and Drahos have labeled an "upward ratchet" (Braithwaite and Drahos, 2000). Indeed, the European Commission's DG Trade asserted that "the ultimate objective is that large emerging economies, where IPR enforcement could be improved, such as China or Russia, will sign up to the global pact" (European Commission, 2009). However, it was unclear whether the treaty would offer sufficient inducements for BRICs or other developing countries to join. Negotiations concluded in May 2011 with eight countries signing onto ACTA in October 2011 (United States, Australia, Canada, Republic of Korea, Japan, New Zealand, Morocco, and Singapore); three negotiating parties did not join at the signing ceremony (Mexico, European Union, Switzerland) (United States Office of the Trade Representative (USTR), 2011).

In addition, strong support for anti-counterfeit laws and treaties from the patent-holding pharmaceutical industry, conservative think tanks, and industrialized countries, raised concerns among CSOs that a broad-based attempt to re-frame generic drugs as a public safety issue was underway.[11] In particular, an overly-broad definition of "counterfeit" risked including legitimate, quality-assured generic medicines, a fear raised by legislation passed in 2008 in Kenya[12] and under debate in other East African countries. Tightening IP rules through the anti-counterfeit laws raised a new kind of challenge for health advocates—a re-framing of such measures in terms of public safety, which made it difficult for opponents to criticize publicly. As Outterson and Smith concluded in their analysis of the anti-counterfeiting push, "Nobody in the A2K [access to knowledge] movement wants tainted heparin or deliberately toxic counterfeit drugs. All the misleading data and rhetoric is geared to winning broad political support for much more stringent IP enforcement measures" (Outterson and Smith, 2006). The counterfeit effort was the first major attempt by proponents of stringent IP rules to reframe IP since TRIPS came into force, and the strategy had some success. According to Sell, "the discourse animating this push for higher standards of protection and enforcement echoes the 1980s focus on 'competitiveness' but also has added a 'security'

11   For a thorough collection of resources on ACTA, see: http://keionline.org/acta.

12   The Kenyan bill defines counterfeiting as: "taking the following actions without the authority of the owner of any intellectual property right subsisting in Kenya or elsewhere in respect of protected goods—(a) the manufacture, production, packaging, re-packaging, labelling or making, whether in Kenya or elsewhere, of any goods whereby those protected goods are imitated in such manner and to such a degree that those other goods are identical or substantially similar copies of the protected goods; (b) the manufacture, production or making, whether in Kenya or elsewhere, the subject matter of that intellectual property, or a colourable imitation thereof so that the other goods are calculated to be confused with or to be taken as being the protected goods of the said owner or any goods manufactured, produced or made under his licence; (c) the manufacturing, producing or making of copies, in Kenya or elsewhere, in violation of an author's rights or related rights; ..."

narrative. Introducing a security frame for IP has allowed these IP maximalists to enlist new actors, law enforcement agencies, in their cause" (Sell, 2008).

Nevertheless, the Kenyan case demonstrated the push-and-pull dynamics at work in IP rulemaking. The Kenyan law, backed by the Kenyan association of multinational pharmaceutical companies, defined counterfeiting as (among other acts) manufacturing or packaging "without the authority of the owner of any intellectual property right ... whereby those protected goods are imitated in such manner and to such a degree that those other goods are identical or substantially similar copies of the protected goods" (Article 2). Parallel imports of medicines or those produced under compulsory license, for example, could be prohibited by this definition. In contrast, the WHO defined a counterfeit as "a medicine which is deliberately and fraudulently mislabeled with respect to identity and/or source." The Kenya Treatment Access Movement and HAI-Africa proposed amending the law to clearly define generics as distinct from counterfeits, a proposal opposed by the multinationals. In April 2010, a Kenyan High Court blocked implementation of the Anti-Counterfeit Act, in response to a challenge filed by three PLWHA who argued that the law threatened their access to generic medicines and their right to life. In a victory for health advocates, the court struck down key parts of the law in April 2014, arguing that it could undermine access to affordable generic medicines. (Kenya Treatment Access Movement (KETAM) & Health Action International Africa (HAI-Africa), 2009; Parliament (Kenya), 2008; Sukkar, 2010; Intellectual Property Watch, 2012).

In summary, there was no shortage of initiatives by industrialized countries and IP-holding industries to tighten IP rules across a range of policy areas. As would be expected in an evolving complex system, actors adapted their strategies in response to setbacks and sought new channels to achieve their goals. As Sell pointed out, "now that developing country governments and Non-Governmental Organizations (NGOs) are active in intellectual property governance in multilateral forums such as WTO, WIPO, and WHO, the intellectual property maximalists are looking elsewhere to ratchet up intellectual property protection" (Sell, 2008).

However, in most cases, CSOs, developing country governments, and experts also adapted their strategies, and pushed back and/or proposed new alternatives to these initiatives. As in the past, countering the push for more stringent IP rules was more feasible where these actors had access to discursive, institutional and expert power. Such power was undermined, however, when negotiations were carried out behind closed doors and/or bilaterally. While outcomes in particular arenas were difficult to predict and likely to vary, there was an overall counter-balancing effect exerted by CSOs, developing country governments and experts. Direct, easily understood threats—such as seizing drugs in transit or threatening trade sanctions under Special 301—were likely to generate commensurably large political reactions from opponents. However, new avenues and unfamiliar terrain, such as ACTA (which involved new actors, rules, and terminology), seem to have generated a slower or more subdued response. In addition, the re-framing of IP as a public safety or security issue suggested that the counterfeit approach could pose a significant threat to the access norm.

In summary, the stability of the access norm was under steady attack from TNPCs and the industrialized countries, which both found it in their interests to continue pushing for stringent IP norms in the developing world. The emergence of the access norm tempered these efforts somewhat, due largely to the political mobilization of CSOs, parliamentarians and experts who monitored the negotiation of new trade agreements. While the access norm remained somewhat stable in the area of HIV/AIDS, it remained highly contested in other areas. Greater stabilization is only likely to occur through the formalization of the access norm (either through national or international law), and/or the re-framing of the norm to incorporate innovation, as the following chapter discusses.

Chapter 8

Re-framing the Access Norm: Incorporating Innovation

HIV/AIDS was the beginning and catalyst of a push by some health advocates to conceptualize medicines as global public goods (see Chapter 4, Section (a) for further discussion of this concept)—that is, goods that should be available to all as a core component of realizing the right to health. Public debates have focused primarily on how the IP regime could be reformed to make medicines more affordable (or, less excludable). However, the same actors that challenged high medicines prices also launched efforts to amend the IP system to generate R&D that better met the needs of people in developing countries. These efforts originated in the late 1990s in the critique regarding neglected diseases, in which it was argued that the patent system failed to incentivize R&D targeted at diseases that exclusively affected the poor (Pecoul, Chirac, Trouiller and Pinel, 1999). However, the issue of innovation did not attract the same political attention as the issue of access until later in the decade when civil society groups began a concerted effort to reframe the "access norm" as an "innovation and access norm." Such a reframing had significant implications both for the meaning of the norm itself, and for pathways to its formalization in international law. That is, by focusing on both innovation and access as important social goals, it could become possible to move beyond the political deadlocks over IP that prevented formalization of the access norm, and open up new spaces for negotiating formal rules for the global governance of innovation, as this chapter describes.

For many years, the dominant discourse around IP policy centered on how to "balance" or manage the "tradeoff" between providing incentives for innovation via IP-based temporary monopolies, against the high prices and restricted access that could result. More recently, however, experts and CSOs asserted an alternate discourse, asking how IP rules and other public policy instruments could be managed to generate innovation and widespread access simultaneously in order to meet public interest objectives such as the improvement of health, food security, and education. This idea was captured concisely by the concept of "innovation *plus* access,"[1] as distinct from the concept of balancing innovation *against* access. This critical, if subtle, shift in how the social purpose of IP was understood could have much broader implications. According to Ellen 't Hoen, "If the debate moves from IP to R&D this is likely to affect countries' abilities to change the dynamics

---

1   The phrase "innovation plus access" or "I plus A" seems to have been first coined by James Love of KEI.

in trade agreements. When the talks are no longer about how high IP standards should be but rather how can each contribute to essential health innovation the power dynamic is likely to change" ('t Hoen, 2007). The shift in framing from "access" to "innovation plus access" undercut the most powerful critique leveled against the use of TRIPS flexibilities—that it would undermine innovation. In doing so, this shift redefined and reinforced the universal access norm, and also had the potential to transform the IP system in more fundamental ways.

While political conflict continued, debates over approaches to R&D were characterized by a relatively sober assessment of the pros and cons of various policy options—in contrast to the high-octane politics of access debates a decade prior. Despite the understated political tone, it should be recognized that this project to reform the R&D system may have much greater impact—and imply a more fundamental challenge to the status quo—than the use of TRIPS flexibilities alone, as the following sections discuss.

(a) From expert commissions to global strategies

In modern societies, if there are normative conflicts between various regulations in different but interdependent sectors, it is the role of the state to deal with these conflicts and to strive for policy coherence. For example, in relatively wealthy societies, health systems are able to moderate the effects of the high medicines prices enabled by patents by using a number of policy tools to ensure that patients have access to the medicines they need.[2] In contrast, at the global level, mechanisms for achieving similar levels of policy coherence are missing. Indeed, in systems of global governance, such coherence is much more difficult to achieve due to the conflicting interests of sovereign states, and a far lesser degree of the mutual trust and social solidarity that is required to generate major resource transfers. The gap in per capita health spending between the richest and the poorest countries is extreme ($9 vs. $7300, see Chapter 1); the transfer payments from rich to poor countries that would be needed to guarantee universal access to all essential medicines at unified international prices would be exorbitant. Effective international regimes were required to resolve this tension between high medicines prices (enabled by the global IP regime) and the limited ability of the majority of the world population to pay such prices. However, taking into account the huge differences of interests, identities, principles, and resources between various societies and the existing "structural disarray" between subsystems of secondary norms to different fields of primary norms,[3] it was quite difficult to reach agreement on such a regime, even if

---

2 Examples of such policies include public or private insurance systems, price negotiation by governments or other large purchasers, reference pricing, bulk procurement, the use of pharmaco-economic principles to reimburse medicines, and compulsory licensing.

3 As in the case of of "human rights" vs. "international trade rules"; see Marschik 1998, footnote 26.

there were widespread agreement on the overarching principle of universal access to medicines.

One important vehicle for bridging major differences of opinion are expert groups, such as commissions, networks, working groups, or advisory groups, which have sometimes helped make progress towards the agreement of international regimes by clarifying facts, providing authoritative interpretations of knowledge, and advancing policy options. Such groups frequently play a role at national level in linking civil society and other stakeholders to the formal political system. But also in other fields of global governance, expert commissions have played an important role in linking various groups of actors and in bridging political rifts either as catalysts in regime building (such as the Brundtland Commission for international environmental regimes) or as a permanent institution (such as the Intergovernmental Panel on Climate Change (IPCC)). Such expert groups may be even more important when they are not immediately linked to coordination processes within and between governments and intergovernmental organizations, but are free to take up various old and new concepts, to refer to existing conflicts and to propose innovative solutions.

High-level global commissions are one type of expert grouping that has been increasingly used over the past two decades to develop global consensus on a number of important issues. They often consist of members representing stakeholders of quite diverse political and cultural backgrounds, and are established for a limited period of time to produce a substantial report on a topic of far-reaching importance; generally they are supported by a budget that allows for "commissioning" the production of a large number of papers produced by experts to shed light on many different aspects related to the central task of the respective commission. International high level commissions have a rather long history; some of them undoubtedly had an important impact on (at least) discourses in the field of global governance. (Important examples include the Brandt Commission, the Brundtland Commission, and the Commission on Global Governance). There are a number of studies on specific cases,[4] but little scientific research on the phenomenon of "international high level commissions" as a type of global governance mechanism.

In the context of this book, we refer to the two commissions most directly relevant to IP norms and access to medicines: the UK Commission on Intellectual Property Rights (CIPR) and the WHO Commission on Intellectual Property Rights, Innovation and Public Health (CIPIH). These commissions became important tools of policymaking that helped coordinate the multiplicity of actors in GHG, leading to influential policy recommendations and, at times, set the groundwork for inter-state negotiations.

---

4 See (Thakur, Cooper and English, 2005) with one general contribution by Cooper and English on "International Commissions and the Mind of Global Governance (1–27) and 13 others on specific commissions"; see also among others, Falk (1995).

The United Kingdom Commission on Intellectual Property Rights (CIPR) was tasked by the UK Department for International Development (DFID) in May 2001 "to consider whether the rules and institutions of IP protection as they have evolved to date can contribute to development and the reduction of poverty in developing countries" (United Kingdom Commission on Intellectual Property Rights (CIPR), 2002). The six commissioners came from diverse intellectual backgrounds, including biomedical science, economics, ethics, and law, and from the public, private and academic sectors. It included two commissioners from developing countries[5] and four from industrialized countries.[6] The commissioners visited a number of developing countries, organized workshops and consultations in London, and commissioned working papers from a range of experts. Though established by one government, the choice of individuals and the method of work reflected the global nature of the Commission's purpose to generate a global-consensus view on a thorny global problem. As the Foreword notes, "the Commission was set up to offer as impartial advice as possible" on a highly-polarized issue. "Its provenance and makeup should encourage all those to whom it is directed to take its recommendations seriously" (United Kingdom Commission on Intellectual Property Rights (CIPR), 2002).

Published in September 2002, the CIPR report "Integrating Intellectual Property Rights and Development Policy," recognized the beneficial role that IP rules could play in generating innovation, but also called for caution in the push to expand IP rights, and greater attention to developing country needs in formulating IP policy. The Commission also called for greater policy space for developing countries on IP, arguing that "Just as the now-developed countries moulded their IP regimes to suit their particular economic, social and technological circumstances, so developing countries should in principle now be able to do the same" (United Kingdom Commission on Intellectual Property Rights (CIPR), 2002). The CIPR report was a landmark event for several reasons. First, it added the gravitas and legitimacy of "impartial" expertise to a position that developing countries and CSOs had long espoused—the need for greater policy space and development concerns in the making of global IP policy. The expert power wielded by the CIPR contributed to embedding the global regime in a distinct way from the normative power exercised by civil society. Second, it had been commissioned by an arm of a powerful country, and held the *potential* to sway UK government policy—in other words, it was expert power possibly tapping into the state's structural and institutional power. Third, because it had been issued by an industrialized country whose government officials had previously pushed for tighter IP rules, it signaled an important normative shift.[7] If the report had been written by the same individual

5   Dr Ramesh Mashelkar, India, and Professor Carlos Correa, Argentina.

6   Professor John Barton, USA; Mr Daniel Alexander, UK; Dr Gill Samuels, UK; Dr Sandy Thomas, UK.

7   As in many governments, there is likely to be some internal disagreement between various ministries on controversial issues; as the development arm, one could argue that

experts but commissioned by Brazil, for example, it is unlikely to have carried the same weight.

Following on the heels of the CIPR report, in 2003 the World Health Assembly tasked WHO to establish an international expert commission "to produce an analysis of intellectual property rights, innovation, and public health, including the question of appropriate funding and incentive mechanisms for the creation of new medicines and other products against diseases that disproportionately affect developing countries" (WHA 56.27 as quoted in (Commission on Intellectual Property Rights, Innovation and Public Health (CIPIH), 2006)). Ten commissioners (including Ramesh Mashelkar of India and Carlos Correa of Argentina, who had both served on the CIPR) were chosen from varying backgrounds and geographic regions, and from government, industry and academia. Compared to the CIPR, the CIPIH represented a broader global spectrum of individuals and enjoyed the expanded legitimacy of a UN-mandate, while focusing on a much narrower set of issues: intellectual property rules and their impact on innovation and access to medicines. It also expanded the debate beyond the issue of the impact of patents on the affordability of existing medicines, to examine whether and how the global IP regime would stimulate R&D to meet the needs of those too poor to constitute an attractive market for commercial investment.

Over a two-year period, the CIPIH commissioned background papers, held consultations, accepted submissions from the public, and opened an online forum for comments—in other words, it engaged the global public domain in an extended debate on IP, innovation and access to medicines. As such, it was in and of itself a critical discursive interface for various actors engaged in policy debates around access to medicines. The CIPIH report was published in April 2006, after several months of delays, attributed to the inability to find consensus among the commissioners. Ultimately, five of the ten CIPIH commissioners submitted letters explaining their reservations with the report's contents. (In contrast, the CIPR had contained no such reservations.) These reservations fell along North-South lines, with two commissioners from the South (Carlos Correa [Argentina] and Pakdee Pothisiri [Thailand]) calling for stronger endorsement of measures that would enable generic competition through, *inter alia*, compulsory licensing, and three commissioners from the North (Trevor Jones [UK], Fabio Pammolli [Italy], Hiroko Yamane [Japan]), arguing that patents were not the main barrier to access.

DFID would be more likely to take the perspective of developing countries, but that other government departments would maintain their own distinct positions. Even if the CIPR did not wield influence within the UK government beyond DFID, however, it seems to have shaped DFID's own work in the area. DFID has played an important role in global access to medicines debates, in particular by supporting the development of a body of analytical work through the Health Resource Centre (see for example Gehl Sampath (2008); Grace (2004); Grace (2005); Mackay (2009)). Other bilateral development agencies, such as USAID, have not played this type of role.

Nevertheless, the CIPIH provided 60 policy recommendations and an authoritative set of conclusions regarding the empirical question of how the global IP regime impacted the public health needs of developing countries. The CIPIH distinguished between the status of the availability of treatment for three types of interventions (Type I: diseases with large number of vulnerable population in rich and poor countries; Type II: substantial proportion of cases in poor countries; Type III: overwhelmingly or exclusively incident in poor countries). It referred to the lack of affordability in poor countries of existing interventions against Type I and II diseases, and the general non-existence of effective interventions for Type III diseases occurring only in developing countries.

It further solidified the conclusions offered by CIPR that the existing global IP regime was not working to stimulate R&D targeted to the needs of developing countries, and called for new approaches to ensuring that such innovation took place. Taken together, the CIPR and CIPIH put to rest the pharmaceutical industry's justification for TRIPS on the grounds that stronger IP protection in developing countries would lead to increased R&D into the diseases of the developing world: "There is no evidence that the implementation of the TRIPS Agreement in developing countries will significantly boost R&D in pharmaceuticals on Type II and particularly Type III diseases. Insufficient market incentives are the decisive factor (Commission on Intellectual Property Rights, Innovation and Public Health" (CIPIH), 2006). Of particular importance, the Commission offered "a reconceptualized definition of innovation as encompassing discovery, development and delivery, thereby including access as an integral part of innovation" ('t Hoen, 2009). Though the report was criticized by CSOs as not going far enough in calling for systemic change, and by industry for calling for too much change to a system that worked well, overall, the report served the function of consolidating the post-Doha norm that the global IP regime should be implemented and interpreted to take into consideration health and development needs.

These commissions demonstrated their capacity to take into account the views of stakeholders with conflicting interests, and to produce a meaningful focus for strategic debates and follow-on decision-making by key actors such as WHO Member States. Intergovernmental organizations—such as the CIPIH Secretariat within the WHO—not only provided the infrastructure for such a commission, but also developed nodal functions regarding specific issues relevant to GHG.

(b) Innovation and access: I+A

The CIPIH report set the intellectual groundwork for action. Under the leadership of Brazil and Kenya,[8] the 2006 World Health Assembly decided to establish an Intergovernmental Working Group on Public Health, Innovation and Intellectual

---

8   Though not covered in depth in this book, important political battles over patent rules and access to medicines had taken place in Kenya, particularly in 2001 over the

Property (IGWG)[9] to decide on how to implement the recommendations of the CIPIH. The two-year IGWG process of regional and global consultations was essentially a political negotiation among Member States on which policies would generate the necessary R&D, how the burden of financing such R&D should be shared, and how access to the fruits of scientific progress could be ensured. In other words, it was a debate on the global governance of medicines development and production. Seen in another light, it was also an attempt to build alongside the global "IP regime," a global "access to medicines regime"—a set of shared rules, norms and understandings regarding what role various actors, from governments to companies to scientists, would play in addressing global health needs in the field of medicines. Critically, the debates incorporated considerations of both access and innovation, and was premised on the understanding that the existing global IP system was not delivering on these objectives.

The IGWG process signaled an important *forum-shift* and *regime-shift* for pharmaceutical policy debates, away from the WTO and back into the WHO. By May 2008, after eleventh-hour negotiations, the WHA adopted as the final outcome to the IGWG talks a *Global Strategy and Plan of Action on Public Health, Innovation and Intellectual Property (GSPoA)* (World Health Assembly (WHA), 2008). Some issues that remained unresolved in bracketed text were left for finalization in a 2009 WHA resolution.

Though IGWG did not succeed in establishing a definitive new global framework for financing and managing health R&D, it considerably advanced debate on policy proposals to reform the current system. Notable proposals included the establishment of a prize fund (submitted by Bolivia and Barbados), a Medical R&D treaty, support for public-private product development partnerships, and patent pools to facilitate upstream research and downstream access to end-products. The IGWG process reflected an important normative shift in the framing and discourse of the IP/access issue. First, it re-framed the issue to make public health rather than intellectual property the central concern; this shift is subtly reflected in the deliberate change in wording and word order of the various commissions from "Commission on Intellectual Property Rights" in 2002, to "Commission on Intellectual Property Rights, Innovation and Public Health" in 2006, to the IGWG's "Public Health, Innovation and Intellectual Property"—note the omission of "rights" and the placement of "public health" first in the title. Second, the key forum for multilateral negotiations had shifted, to some degree, from WTO to WHO. Third, WHO's mandate to involve itself in IP issues was widely-accepted, though political struggles over the exact role and boundaries of WHO's work in this area would continue, as well as its relationship to work

---

revision of the country's Industrial Property Bill, which authorized the importation of generic versions of patented medicines. See 't Hoen 2009, p. 54 for details.

9   The discussion of IGWG draws from the author's (Moon) experience as a participant-observer at a national consultation on IGWG in Beijing, China in September 2007, and at the final IGWG negotiations in April 2008 in Geneva.

at WIPO and the WTO, which were both perceived as friendlier to the interests of IP-owners. These intellectual developments and discursive changes were both a reflection of increasing acceptance of the access norm, as well as influential factors in further solidifying that norm.

A key follow-on process from the conclusion of the IGWG in 2008 was the question of how R&D focusing on the needs of developing countries ought to be financed. In January 2009, the Executive Board discussed the completed plan of action, including the costing of implementation, estimated at about $149 billion between 2009 and 2015 (national and international spending); this was to increase the percentage of R&D for "diseases which disproportionately affect developing countries" from 3% to 12%. The 2009 WHA "noted" the funding needs, and in response to WHA Resolution 61.21, the WHO Director-General appointed an Expert Working Group on Research and Development: Coordination and Financing (EWG) to "examine current financing and coordination of research and development, as well as proposals for new and innovative sources of funding to stimulate research and development related to Type II and Type III diseases and the specific research and development needs of developing countries in relation to Type I diseases, and open to consideration of proposals from Member States" (World Health Assembly (WHA), 2008).

However, when the EWG reported back to the 2010 WHA, it had been discredited by suspicions of undue industry influence after it was discovered that the IFPMA had had the opportunity to submit comments on the draft report before it was shared with Member States (*The Lancet*, 2010). It was also criticized for taking an overly-cautious incremental approach. *The Lancet* described the draft report as "pathetically short of the strong, decisive plan necessary" (*The Lancet*, 2010) and the governments of Bolivia and Suriname commented on the final report that, "By choosing to ignore transformative solutions to the R&D needs of developing countries, the EWG was largely an exercise in protecting the status quo" (Governments of Bolivia and Suriname, 2010). Sharing Thailand's view that the EWG "no longer has legitimacy," many developing countries refused to accept the report at the 2010 World Health Assembly (Mara and New, 2010). Instead, with Resolution 63.28 the WHA mandated the creation of a new "Consultative Expert Working Group on Research and Development: Financing and Coordination" to take up the work tasked to the original EWG (Mara, 2010), with the significant addition of the term "consultative" to the title of the expert group. The CEWG conspicuously engaged in more open public processes than its predecessor, including periodic status reports updating the public on its progress. The CEWG published its report in April 2012, and concluded with the recommendation that Member States consider launching negotiations over a binding R&D convention to improve financing and coordination of R&D (WHO Consultative Expert Working Group on Research and Development (CEWG): Financing and Coordination, 2012). As of this writing, the extent to which Member States would act upon this recommendation remained to be seen.

Would negotiations on large-scale funding take place under the auspices of the WHO, in contrast to previous shifts away from the WHO as a primary arena for global rulemaking on health (signified most clearly by the decision of the US and other industrialized countries to establish the GFATM outside of the UN system)? The prospects of negotiating a "Medical R&D Treaty" remain unclear, as so far this move to establish formal norms on medical R&D have been opposed by the pharmaceutical industry. Nevertheless, the Global Strategy has kept the access norm on the agenda and is expected to contribute to mobilizing more resources for research on neglected diseases and for supporting health research capacities in developing countries. So far, the consultative process has demonstrated fairly strong support from some Member States for the treaty idea. If governments do decide to begin interstate negotiations over a legally binding R&D treaty, it may be the single most important step towards the formalization of the access norm since the TRIPS Agreement.

As discussed above, the hard-fought GSPoA called for new approaches to medical R&D and measures to ensure globally-equitable access to the fruits of scientific progress. As such, it reflected the codification of an informal norm that access was a fundamental component of the innovation process, and that the two ought to go hand-in-hand. Indeed, over the past decade, an increasingly rich debate has arisen regarding how to ensure and maximize innovation that meets public needs, including those of the world's poorest and most vulnerable. In the "traditional" pharmaceutical R&D model, investments were driven by potential market size, and end-products designed to be used in high-technology settings (such as hospitals in industrialized countries), with relatively little consideration given to affordability.[10] In contrast, a new global normative consensus has emerged that the products of pharmaceutical R&D should address the health needs of the poor, even when they do not comprise a profitable market (Commission on Intellectual Property Rights, Innovation and Public Health (CIPIH), 2006; United Kingdom Commission on Intellectual Property Rights (CIPR), 2002; United Nations Development Programme (UNDP), 2001; World Health Assembly (WHA), 2008).

Parallel to intergovernmental negotiations, various policies and practical experiments to improve innovation for global health have been proposed and/or are being tested by governments of both North and South, CSOs, experts, and pharmaceutical companies.

A full analysis of the various reform proposals is beyond the scope of this book, but a brief review of the main types may be useful to paint a picture of the potential scope of change. Proposals generally fall into four categories: public-private product development partnerships (PDPs), regulatory incentives, patent pools, and inducement prizes.

---

10   This discussion of R&D norms and proposals has benefited and draws from collaborative work conducted with Nicole Szlezak for the S.T. Lee Project on Global Governance at the National University of Singapore.

First, PDPs are a type of "push" mechanism, in which donors fund non-profit entities to harness public and private sector capacity in R&D to achieve public ends: affordable new products that are well-adapted to developing country health needs (Moon, 2008; Moran et al., 2009; Moran, 2005). Twenty-six PDPs had been established as of 2005, with examples including the International AIDS Vaccine Initiative, Drugs for Neglected Diseases Initiative, and the Global Alliance for TB Drug Development (Ziemba, 2005).

Another type of policy tool is accelerated regulatory review. The US Congress passed legislation creating "priority review vouchers (PRV)" in 2008. A PRV may be awarded by the US FDA to an entity that develops a new product for a neglected tropical disease. The voucher from the tropical disease product can then be applied to another product—such as a potential blockbuster cardiovascular drug—to receive priority consideration for approval by the FDA. The voucher can also be sold to another firm, with a value that has been estimated at up to $300 million (Ridley, Grabowski and Moe, 2006). In a reflection of the strength of global health norms, the initial list of diseases eligible for the PRV is limited to tropical diseases that occur primarily in developing countries—that is, outside US borders.[11] In February 2012, the US Patent and Trademark Office announced the launch of a one-year pilot program that would award vouchers to firms that managed their patents in a manner conducive to meeting the needs of "impoverished populations" in the areas of medical technology, food and nutrition, clean technology and information technology.[12]

A third approach involved managing patents to improve public welfare, such as through the use of patent pools. In 2010, a medicines patent pool with an initial focus on HIV drugs was established by UNITAID, a new intergovernmental global health initiative supported by 29 high, middle-, and low-income countries and the Gates Foundation. The Medicines Patent Pool has asked companies that have developed HIV drugs to issue voluntary licenses for patents to authorize competitive production of generic medicines for use in developing countries. The Pool is designed both to decrease prices through enhanced competition, and to lower the barriers that patents may pose to follow-on innovation (such as pediatric, heat-stable, or fixed-dose formulations of medicines) (Bermudez and 't Hoen, 2010; UNITAID Secretariat, 2009).

Finally, inducement prizes, which function as "pull mechanisms" to increase the level and diversity of actors conducting R&D in a particular problem, have gained attention in a broad field of technologies (Travis, 2008a; Travis, 2008b). Examples include the Advanced Market Commitment for vaccines (Berndt et al.,

---

11   Having caught the attention of advocates for rare and orphan diseases in the US, draft legislation proposed by Senators Sherrod Brown, Al Franken and Sam Brownback was introduced in August 2010 that would add rare pediatric diseases that affect Americans onto the PRV eligibility list (Taylor, 2010).

12   Further information is available at: http://patentsforhumanity.challenge.gov/, accessed March 5, 2012.

2007), Prize4Life, a prize fund targeted at Lou Gehrig's disease, and Innocentive, a multi-prize platform that awarded $40,000 to two "solvers" who developed an improved method of synthesizing a promising new TB drug (Global Alliance for TB Drug Development (GATB), 2008). Proposals to establish more systemic prize funds to reward a broad range of new health technologies include Love and Hubbard's proposal for a global prize fund (Hubbard and Love, 2004b; Love and Hubbard, 2009); US Senator Bernie Sanders' proposed legislation to create a prize-fund for US patients (Wei, 2007); Pogge, Hollis and Banerjee's design for a Health Impact Fund (Banerjee, Hollis and Pogge, 2010; Pogge, 2009); and Finkelstein and Temin's US prize fund (Finkelstein and Temin, 2008). Depending on how they are structured, a prize could replace the need for a patent-based monopoly by providing a risk-adjusted reward that would allow investors to recoup their R&D costs and earn a fair profit; at the same time, the end product could immediately be produced by multiple, competing manufacturers so that price would approach the cost of production in a competitive market. Prize fund proposals have been critiqued as being untested and risky, for being vulnerable to political manipulation and underfunding, and for expected difficulties in setting accurate prize amounts to generate a certain degree of innovation, among other concerns (Baker, 2004; DiMasi and Grabowski, 2004; Wei, 2007). Pilot projects are ongoing, and implementation of prize-like mechanisms such as the Advanced Market Commitment for pneumococcal vaccines (Cernuschi, 2009; GAVI Alliance Secretariat, 2010), promise to generate additional evidence to drive forward policy debates.

The breadth of new proposals for how to generate innovation to meet global health needs—whether by managing, amending or bypassing IP rules—reflects an important reframing of the access to medicines debate and, in some ways, a fundamental challenge to the status quo. In earlier years, the human costs imposed by stringent IP rules could be justified as necessary to generate innovation; with these assumptions coming under increasing scrutiny, and various alternative incentive mechanisms being proposed and tested, the door may be opening to far more systemic change. These proposals are pushing to solidify the access norm further—but in new directions and in new ways. However, establishing new institutions may prove more challenging than reacting against and changing informal norms. The dynamic evolution of this issue domain suggests, nevertheless, that the contours of the access norm may appear quite different and more expansive than simply the policy space to use TRIPS flexibilities.

(c) Changing expectations for the MICs: Contributions to R&D

Any new global arrangements for how to ensure both innovation and access are likely to involve expanded and evolving roles for the MICs, due to two factors. First, growing wealth and technological capacity in the MICs suggests that they will be expected to contribute somehow to sharing the global burden of financing medical innovation. Second, growing R&D capacity in key developing countries suggests that domestic calculations of the national interest may also shift, as these countries generate higher numbers of patents. This section discusses these two trends and their implications for the access norm.

(i) Medicines as global public goods

There is evidence of emerging political demands for access to medicines far beyond HIV/AIDS, though the majority of political attention, mobilization, and change have occurred in this area ('t Hoen et al., 2011). For example, the Cancer Patients Aid Association in India joined forces with HIV/AIDS organizations and other health groups to defend the flexibilities in the country's new patent law when drug company Novartis challenged key provisions in a lawsuit related to the cancer drug imatinib (Glivec) (Cancer Patients Aid Association (CPAA), Lawyers Collective HIV/AIDS Unit, Delhi Network for Positive People (DNP+) and Médecins Sans Frontières, 2007 (August 7)). When new vaccines came on the market in high-income countries, such as those against the human papilloma virus and pneumococcal disease, it was not long before actors pushed to make those products available to the world's poorest. Finally, in the case of some infectious diseases, such as pandemic flu, global access to a vaccine may be considered necessary for reasons of both efficacy (i.e. to stop the spread of the virus) as well as for equity (i.e. to ensure that all people have access to lifesaving vaccines). In summary, global norms regarding *who* should have access to new medicines have expanded considerably in the past decade.

   However, if certain types of medicines are understood as global public goods, the question arises as to how the financing of such goods should be globally distributed. TRIPS can be understood as one model for sharing the global burden of R&D finance—countries implement certain IP standards that lead to rents being paid to patent-holders to compensate them for their R&D investments. Hubbard and Love have proposed a medical R&D treaty as another approach to solving the problem of globally-equitable burden-sharing (Hubbard and Love, 2004a). As innovative capacity grows, an increasing number of patent-holders are originating from developing countries: for example, in only six years between 2005 and 2011, the proportion of patent applications filed by China, India, South Korea and Brazil under the international Patent Cooperation Treaty process grew from 5.96% to 15.77%, with China ranking fourth among sources of international patent applications (World Intellectual Property Organization (WIPO), 2012). What does rising innovative capacity in the MICs imply for global IP rulemaking?

(ii) India & China: The R&D centers of the future?

Of all the developing countries, India and China have received by far the greatest amount of attention in the pharmaceutical sector for their production and innovative capacities.

India's generic pharmaceutical industry is one of the country's major success stories. As the "pharmacy of the developing world," it plays a central role in the global supply of low-cost generic medicines, and is steadily increasing its share of high-income markets as well. Indian "generics" firms that formerly focused on production are beginning to invest more in R&D. In the 1990s, Indian firms spent on average 1.5% of revenue on R&D, largely to develop new formulations or improved process chemistry for generic drugs. Since then, spending among the larger firms has steadily increased: for a sample of 37 of the largest firms, R&D spending increased from 1.39% of sales in 1992–93 to 3.89% in 2001–2, to between 7 and 8% for the period from 2004 to 2008. While much of this spending still focused on generics-related R&D, an increasing amount was also going into new chemical entity research (Chaudhuri, 2010). The Indian government also invested in domestic R&D through, for example, the Indian Council for Medical Research (ICMR) and Council of Scientific and Industrial Research (CSIR).

In China, the government has made investment in R&D a high priority: it was seeking to attract 2% of global pharmaceutical R&D spending, was successfully courting multinational firms to establish partnerships and research centers in country, invested heavily in the eight life sciences research centers that are subsidiaries of the Chinese Academy of Sciences, and adopted a range of tax, subsidy, procurement and other incentives to promote R&D (Kingsbury, 2007; Linton, 2008; Reynolds, 2007). China's pharmaceutical investments should be seen within the broader context of its Medium to Long Term Plan to Develop Science and Technology (S&T Plan) issued in 2006, which sets a number of goals to transform China into an innovation center, including: dedicating 2.5% of GDP to R&D by 2020 (the OECD average); reducing reliance on imported technology; increasing technology's contribution to economic growth; ranking among the world's top five countries in patents granted and citations in international scientific papers; and generally promoting indigenous innovation (Linton, 2008).

Multinational firms were also investing in partnerships, mergers & acquisitions, and joint research centers in India and China. For example, AstraZeneca established a tuberculosis drug research center in Bangalore, India in 2003 (AstraZeneca, 2010); Novartis established the Novartis Institute for Biomedical Research in Shanghai in 2009 (Novartis, 2009), along with research centers in Hyderabad, India and Shanghai and Changshu, China (Novartis, 2010); GlaxoSmithKline set up a research center in Shanghai in 2007 focusing on neurodegenerative diseases (GlaxoSmithKline, 2007); Sanofi-Aventis also established research centers in Shanghai and Beijing (Martino, 2010; Sanofi-Aventis, 2008).

For countries with little to no innovative capacity in pharmaceuticals, the choice seemed clear—more flexible IP rules would likely maximize social welfare by keeping medicines prices low. However, for countries with increasing R&D capacity, the calculation was more complex—how would individual countries both increase R&D capacity and ensure end-user access to medicines? Some might argue, as the multinational pharmaceutical industry has, that countries like India should adopt Western-style IP systems, based on the rationale that stricter, longer monopolies lead to greater profits that fund more R&D and therefore result in more innovation (International Federation of Pharmaceutical Manufacturers and Associations (IFPMA), 2005 (22 March)). Others, such as the head of the Indian generics industry association, have argued that developing country innovators should seek patents in high-income markets, while allowing for flexible IP policies in their home countries where health needs remain immense (personal communication, Shah, October 2009).

While developing countries were expected to be home to an increasing number of patent-holding individuals and firms, the high prices enabled by patent monopolies would continue to pose problems for countries with sizeable populations living in poverty, and/or where health safety nets were nascent or relatively weak. In addition, many developing countries were unlikely to match the technological capacities of the industrialized countries in the coming decades, and therefore were likely to continue losing from the existing IP system. How would developing countries with growing innovative capacity position themselves regarding global IP rules?

(iii) Reconciling innovation and access?

Rather than adopting Western-style IP systems, countries may instead experiment with new alternative models for drug R&D that do not rely on stringent patent monopolies as the driving incentive. An example of this approach is the Indian government's $35 million investment to support the Open Source Drug Discovery project, which aimed to accelerate the development of new drugs for TB. In 2010, the project announced the completion of a collaborative exercise to annotate the *Mycobacterium tuberculosis* genome, drawing on the efforts of a team of about 400 researchers contributing from all over India (*Open Source Drug Discovery* 2012). In the event that a drug results from the project, it will not be patented nor will royalties be charged for its use; however, credit is to be given to all who contributed to the development process (Datta, 2010). India was also the site of the first successful product developed by the public-private product development partnership Institute for OneWorld Health (IoWH), which was primarily funded by the Gates Foundation. In partnership with Indian researchers, IoWH successfully tested the efficacy of paramomycin against visceral leishmaniasis (kala azar), a neglected disease prevalent in India, Africa and the Middle East. Paramomycin is an older, off-patent drug that could be produced generically.

Another alternative R&D incentive mechanism was proposed by the governments of Bangladesh, Barbados, Bolivia, and Suriname, who proposed the creation of a prize fund to reward developers of innovative drugs, diagnostics or vaccines for Chagas disease (Governments of Bangladesh, Barbados, Bolivia and Suriname, 2009). The prize would be given in lieu of monopoly rights. A key argument underlying their proposal was that market-driven incentives, such as those provided by patents, were unlikely to stimulate innovation targeted to the needs of the poor due to insufficient market pull.

Regardless of the R&D models they adopt, however, it is likely that rising MICs will be expected to contribute a greater amount to pharmaceutical R&D—whether through prices, contributions to public research efforts, or innovative capacity. This expectation was clear in the pricing policies of pharmaceutical companies with respect to HIV medicines and vaccines: often, the lowest global price was offered to the low-income countries and/or Least-Developed Countries, while a (sometimes hefty) premium was charged to middle-income countries (Médecins Sans Frontières (MSF), 2011; Wilson, 2010). MICs were also being asked to make greater contributions to international collective efforts such as the Global Fund to Fight AIDS, Tuberculosis and Malaria, and were making new contributions through initiatives such as UNITAID.

Individual MICs may choose to meet these expectations in different ways. Arguably, contributing to medicines R&D as a global public good may provide MICs with greater political capital to simultaneously advocate for more flexible global IP rules.

From 1999–2010, key middle-income countries played an influential role in reshaping global IP rules to take into greater account the health needs of developing countries as a whole. As some MICs evolve into rising powers, their capacity to reshape global IP rules in their favor is likely to increase. Given increasing health needs and expected growth in demand for medicines, MICs governments will have a strong incentive to adopt more flexible IP rules that minimize the impact of patent monopolies on medicines prices. However, these same countries are also emerging markets and expected to be the major source of growth for the global pharmaceutical industry. These competing interests set the stage for increased political contestation over the shape of the global IP regime.

However, whether all MICs will advocate for greater flexibility in IP rules remains unclear. Overall, most developing countries are not yet at the stage where they will become net exporters of IP-intensive goods and services. However, some MICs, most notably India and China, were developing considerable innovative capacity and understandings of the national interest in particular countries may change as some transition from being net-importers to net-exporters of IP-intensive products. Given the multiple competing forces at play, the role of particular countries in shaping global IP rules is likely to be determined in national arenas, with strong influence exerted by global actors such as firms, CSOs, experts, and intergovernmental organizations. Political contestation over how the national interest gets defined is likely to sharpen, with deep divisions within governments—for example, between ministries of health and ministries of trade or science and technology. At the same time, the international community is increasingly expecting these countries to contribute to global collaborative efforts, such as for the production of global public goods. The more that key MICs are seen to be doing so, the greater the political space they are likely to have to push for more flexible IP rules.

This analysis suggests that the rise of MICs will not automatically lead to a more stringent or flexible global IP regime. Rather, the outcome of national debates regarding the national interest—whether defined in economic or health terms, or some negotiated compromise between the two—is likely to shape how a particular state engages with the global IP regime. Simple North-South categorizations, which have long characterized IP debates and shaped loosely-networked global coalitions, no longer offer the useful conceptual clarity they once provided. Protecting the hard-won policy space that allows countries to adopt domestic IP systems that meet public health needs will require ensuring that health concerns have a voice in national policymaking debates.

Chapter 9

The Impact of Non-state Actors on Informal Norms: Nodal Governance and Global Democracy

This analysis of the inclusiveness and the stability of the access norm has drawn a complex picture: On the one hand, the access norm has been accepted as an important dimension of the human right to health, on the other hand (a) the inclusiveness of the norm is still contested, particularly in the field of non-communicable diseases and (b) attempts at formalizing the norm e.g. through developing alternative forms to finance R&D, have thus far met with limited success. The root causes behind the evolution of the access norm have not always been obvious; in particular, the scope and impact of actors in these conflicts merits further exploration and explanation. How could a group of CSOs in coalition with a number of low and middle income countries successfully assert a new access norm in the global arena, against apparently much more powerful opponents such as TNPCs and the governments of the US and EU? At the same time, why has it been so difficult for the WHA to agree on a scheme to finance the formally-accepted GSPoA? Why has it been so difficult to make formal changes to international agreements such as TRIPS to reflect a norm that has been informally accepted by all actors concerned? What has prevented the actors involved from starting negotiations to resolve the more fundamental problems around IPRs and health (such as through a Medical R&D Treaty, as proposed in the IGWG process) after having agreed in Doha on the legitimacy of putting public health before the protection of intellectual property?

In chapters 4 to 8 we discussed the interests and positions of the most important actors in global debates on access to medicines. In this chapter we examine more closely the impacts of non-state actors and hybrid actor constellations on global norms, focusing on the phenomenon of nodal governance, how non-state actors wield influence, and the implications for global democracy.

(a) Nodal governance and informal norm-building

In this book we discussed the idea that informal norms emerging from processes of nodal governance might not only be easier to agree upon in situations when changes in formal norms and rules are impossible due to diametrically opposed and entrenched interests, but that they also might be comparatively stable. How informal norms interact with formal norms (interpretation of TRIPS flexibilities by stakeholders, constellations of power at concrete interfaces;[1] negotiations on Doha Declaration and Para 6) is apparently dependent upon the specific case and specific political constellations. Formal norms are not all-powerful nor permanent. For example, formal norms may be amended when constellations of power change, such as when they lose popular support, which can sometimes occur to the point at which laws are no longer applied. Still there is a basic difference that might give formal norms an important advantage over informal ones: They are, in principle, justiciable (at least at the national level and in some cases also through international courts or through a dispute settlement body). International law, when ratified, in most countries becomes national law,[2] though, as we have argued in Chapter 3, some broad norms such as international human rights law need to be further specified in the form of secondary norms in order to allow the application of legal sanctions.

Norms have the function of reducing *transaction costs*. Informal norms exist in large varieties of social relations. Related to the "governance" of customary behavior, norms are expressions of moral codices, and can also be linked to social status and the acceptance of hierarchies; they may also include rules about how to deal with specific situations, such as conflicting interests between different actors. The formalization of norms into laws, however, entails costs and creates reliable, but inflexible rules, which is an advantage, e.g. an asset in negotiations on more specific issues, for those who benefit from these rules. If conflicts between important stakeholders and institutional arrangements, however, make it difficult to agree on formal rules, though a basic consensus exists on some fundamental principles, nodal governance processes might help to develop informal norms and to implement them based on these principles.

The flexibility of nodal governance as well as its insertion in wider social processes plays an essential role in norm-building processes. A governance node can be created in many different ways; for example, it can develop by transformation of a specific organization that attracts a great variety of actors, because it had started a successful initiative in a specific policy field. Frequently nodes also develop around existing IGOs, as stakeholders link with each other and/or with representatives/officials of that organization. Compared to the importance of nodal governance in today's global politics, research on the impact of this mode of global governance has been minimal (see Hein et al. 2009). There are no in-depth studies of the "nodal governance of the access to medicines issue" although most scholars examining this case accept the paramount importance of networks like the MSF Access Campaign, Health Action International, the People's Health Movement, of

---

1   Cf. TRIPS disputes Brazil-USA; South African court cases (Chapter 5).

2   Depending on the specific legal tradition, ratified international law may automatically become national law ("monism") or may be transformed into national legislation ("dualism"), which usually does in fact take place. See Henkin (1995).

KEI as a communication network, of WHO scientific working groups,[3] of informal communication networks among them, or the annual World Health Assemblies (Kickbusch, Hein and Silberschmidt, 2010). Furthermore, numerous workshops, conferences and congresses dealt with this issue and frequently brought together participants from CSOs and the pharmaceutical industry.

Below, a brief sketch of the "Geneva Connection" indicates the close links between these networks, including issue-oriented links between CSOs and the respective departments of IGOs. Nodal governance is primarily based on discursive interfaces, but—depending upon the participating actors—it might also be linked to organizational (WTO, WHO) and financial interfaces (governments, health initiatives).

Beyond the Doha Declaration there were almost no formal agreements on how the access norm should be implemented. Rather, the access norm was solidified and implemented through the linking of various nodes, and processes of formal and informal norm-setting; nodal governance reflected the complexity of social relations, and allowed for the creation of new, specific expressions of power in the structure of the network.

The "super nodes" of specific normative fields are places of extensive communication; stakeholders who are not present in these nodal systems have few chances to have their positions become part of the solution to the problem. For a comprehensive analysis of the system of nodal governance in global health, more research needs to be done and another book written. For the link between health, human rights and intellectual property rights, Geneva definitely is *the* "nodal city" in norm-building processes, while other places certainly do play a role—New York, Washington, Brussels, London, and increasingly also cities in influential developing countries, such as Brazil, India, South Africa, and Thailand (though still not rivaling Geneva and the other traditional centers). The list of places points to the importance of not forgetting states as actors in nodal governance. Even if they are not able themselves to produce effective solutions to specific problems, they do not cease to matter: they played an important role in the conflicts analyzed in this book.[4]

What has developed over the decades in Geneva we might call the "Geneva Connection." When considering the results of over 10 years of conflicts in IPRs and access to medicines, it is important to realize that CSOs not only succeeded in mobilizing support for a stronger role for social rights in global governance, but

---

3   WHO scientific working groups are formal technical meetings of WHO, governed by certain rules and regulations in an attempt to produce high quality output. To consider all available evidence in their debates they use inputs from external experts.

4   For example, they played a key material role in implementing the access norm by financing (through bilateral aid and/or hybrid arrangements such as the GFATM) treatment programmes for low-income countries with a high incidence of HIV/AIDS, which would not have been in a position to finance treatment even with ARVs at the lowest generic prices.

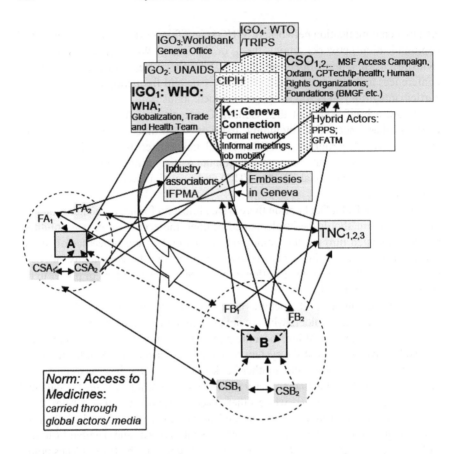

Figure 9.1   Nodal governance—Geneva as a super-node in GHG

Note: FA_1 = Firm in industry 1 in country 1; CSA_1 = Civil society organization in policy field 1 in country 1; Hybrid actors = Organizations which integrate state and non-state actors; IFPMA = International Federation of Pharmaceutical Manufacturers and Associations; CIPIH = Commission on Intellectual Property Rights, Innovation and Public Health.

that the whole framework of perceptions on this issue—and on the importance of global health in general—changed. What we call the "Geneva Connection" can be seen as a microcosm of the whole complex of interfaces that moved the process of global health governance: it is a centre of communication producing at least elements of a common understanding of affairs, which are then reintroduced into command centers of political action (WTO, WHO, the capitals of powerful nation states, and also important CSOs like MSF).

IGOs in the fields of social and economic development and human rights are concentrated in Geneva:these include WHO, ILO, UNCTAD, UNHCHR, UNAIDS, WIPO, WTO, to list only the most important; in addition, UNICEF has its regional office for Central and Eastern Europe in Geneva, there is a World Bank liaison office, and many countries have diplomatic missions in Geneva. (Though, surprisingly enough, this physical proximity did not guarantee close communication and coordination between these various IGOs.[5])

Things seem to have changed with the strengthening of global civil society and the development of global governance structures, which have created networks of communication and at times also cooperation between various types of actors in specific policy fields, and may also function as catalysts for cooperation between IGOs. Certainly, a network consisting of CSOs encompassing the health, development and human rights sectors (e.g. MSF, Oxfam, Knowledge Ecology International, Third World Network, Health Action International, CIEL, 3D), can be seen as a complex organizational interface between CSOs in the access to medicines movement.[6]

The development of a CSO network has not just led to a strengthening of CSO campaigns in this field. We find communication on strategies and on interpreting "facts" between groups and organizations with opposing political positions, discussion on compromises, selective cooperation and so on, in a field of many different options for strategies, actions, and institution-building. We find flexible relations between individuals working in different organizations (sometimes changing employers), constituting not a formal network, but linked into networks that facilitate access to media and to groups organizing campaigns, as well as to national and international institutions in Geneva and elsewhere (with access to important information, but also people closely linked to CSOs working in IGOs as experts for specific topics).

A decisive basis for the concrete functioning of this "Geneva connection" is a certain common ground of norms—basically referring to a rather broad understanding of support for global health[7] and certain forms of political and personal respect—beyond sizeable differences in concrete goals and strategies. We find all kinds of communication between CSOs in different fields, CSOs and delegates from industrialized and developing countries, CSOs and IGOs, market-creating IGOs and welfare-oriented IGOs, CSOs and the pharmaceutical industry, and so on.

---

5   The joint study on "WTO Agreements & Public Health" (WHO and WTO 2002) indicates that there are a few fields where there has been some long term institutionalized cooperation, as in the field of the SPS Agreement and the role of the Codex Alimentarius. In many other areas, however, the authors identify "potential for complementing each other's work" (WHO and WTO 2002, 143) and "increasing opportunities for taking of synergies" (WHO and WTO, 144), which implicitly recognizes that there has been little concrete cooperation in the past (as seen in 2002).

6   For the development of the movement since 1996 see Helfer (2004); Mayne (2002); Sell and Prakash (2004).

7   See also Fidler's "open-source anarchy" and his "source-code" referred to in Chapter 2, Section (e) (Fidler 2007).

At first glance, the resulting system of interactions looks like a "network of networks." But this term is not really accurate: some of them are formal IGOs, others are in fact networks (CSO networks), but in many cases the interactions are informal and interpersonal, and the participants are frequently not specifically legitimized representatives of their respective organization. On the other hand, not all of these interactions are even interfaces in the sense of recurrent interactions; some informal meetings might become ritualized but many are just onetime occurrences. There is no network in a narrower sense of implying a certain organizational effort for the exchange of information or joint activities.

A number of interviews with Geneva-based organizations focused on this communication system.[8] Most of the organizations interviewed were members of formal networks extending beyond Geneva (like the ESCR-net, the Access Campaign, Biomedical Advisor Group or WHO scientific working groups, WHO stakeholder meetings), but all ascribed a great importance to regular and occasional informal meetings in Geneva. These included regular coordination meetings with other CSOs, briefings, workshops, and conferences organized by many Geneva-based organizations mostly with broad-based participation from all sorts of agencies, including national delegations in Geneva. In addition, there were many personal contacts at the margin of organized events (including receptions and parties, or "national days" organized by the country missions) or just in the form of private meetings. Certainly, in general, people met more frequently with colleagues from similar organizations, but all of them stressed the importance of meetings "across the board" of all Geneva-based organizations. CSOs also referred to meetings with delegates from Southern countries and the role of the South Centre in this context.

Job mobility among the Geneva-based organizations can be seen as one important element intensifying communication between different organizations, also by facilitating contacts between old and new colleagues. There seems to be job mobility between all kinds of organizations present in Geneva, but, according to some of the interviewees, the most frequently observed paths are from CSOs to IGOs and from national delegations (in particular of the South) to CSOs; quite frequently people move from IGOs to CSOs after retirement. There are also no absolute ideological barriers to job mobility; thus, in one case, a person moved from IFPMA to MSF. Thus, the "Geneva connection" might be seen as a nodal center for approaching a common understanding of global health problems. A common understanding of problems certainly does not imply a change of actors' interests and ultimate goals, but it does confirm the importance of discursive interfaces in conflicts between global "market creation" and the proponents of global social rights.

---

8   These interviews covered different types of CSOs (ICTSD, MSF, and 3D, the Quaker UN Office), IFPMA, and WHO (12 interviews between June 2004 and January 2006).

The importance of these governance structures merits further consideration. They do not just reflect institutional developments to be seen as constitutive elements of the governance of a specific sector of global politics, but they also reflect processes of global socialization that are "in search" of adequate political institutions to combine effective regulation with democratic representation. Nodal governance has the potential to link the various forms of power, but tends to give more weight to discursive power. On the other hand, we should not forget that financial power can have a strong impact (via the media, via financing think tanks etc.) on discursive processes. Nevertheless, due to the historicity ("orders") of discourses, one should assume that even financially strong media—being embedded into a deep-rooted web of perception and convictions—are not in a position to "engineer" a fundamental revision of norms and values in a very short time (Fairclough, 1993).[9]

(b) Nodal governance: Interfaces between IGOs, governments and non-state actors in global politics

Coming back to our specific issue of access to medicines, we observe contestation between group interests (TNPCs vs. CSOs, developing countries vs. industrialized countries) based primarily on a moral codex. From the lay perspective, the concept of "human rights" can be seen as a widely accepted codex on what governments should do and should not do. This is strongly influenced by a specific aspect of discursive power, the power of experts (if they remain uncontested) to control the "meaning" of social and political concepts and the interpretations of strategies to solve conflicts. The supposed knowledge about what "makes sense" in order to reach "health for all," to improve the lot of the poor, is produced in a huge complex of communicative systems, which is expanding and deepening in the process of the construction of a global society (see Chapter 2). This trend constitutes the complex backdrop from which solutions to global problems may emerge if inter-governmental agreements cannot be reached. In the case of access to medicines, there seems to be a broad-based, deep-rooted moral conviction among social actors that creates space for informal norm building. Nodal governance creates paths of communication to approach a common understanding of problems and to solve problems through informal governance arrangements to implement informal norms. This can also include informal paths to building formal norms, as we discuss further in Chapter 10.

---

9   The concept of the "Geneva connection" as a supra-node in GHG came out as a kind of side-result from research on "Global Health Governance and the Fight against HIV/ AIDS" (see Hein et al., 2007). It would be interesting to concentrate a research project of its own on this topic.

Nodal governance as a platform for contestation:
CSOs in global health governance

The open character of nodal governance leaves more space for contestation than formal structures of representation and decision making in states (see Fidler's open access metaphor)—and its very existence is an expression of the possibility of discourses and negotiations on rules and norms between established stakeholders (such as the pharmaceutical industry) and contesting actors, who may be advocates for the implementation of human rights, social equity, or other interests.

In the second half of the 1990s global civil society took the lead in organizing protests against the lack of access to HIV treatment for people in developing countries and finally galvanized the political processes that led states to issue the Doha Declaration as an interpretation of the TRIPS Agreement from a public health perspective. From 1996 onwards, Health Action International (HAI) successfully developed a campaign against the TRIPS Agreement's impact on access to patented medicines. This campaign was picked-up and supported by MSF, whose normative power and influence over global public opinion was significantly boosted after receiving the Nobel Peace Prize in 1999. In early 1999, the *MSF Campaign for Access to Essential Medicines* was launched, which has since assumed a central role among civil society actors in this field. These organizations worked closely with groups of PLHIV, including national organizations such as South Africa's Treatment Action Campaign or Thailand's Thai Network of Positive People (TNP+), and international networks such as ACT-UP and the Global Network of Positive People (GNP+). Different CSOs brought varying and often complementary resources to the campaign, and adopted different strategies to effect change.

CSOs organized to put pressure on Northern states by influencing public opinion. The rising media coverage of the access issue was an important development that increased pressure on governments and the pharmaceutical industry, as mentioned by many political actors.[10] The access issue had a strong presence in specialized information networks (for instance in ip-health mailings, or in the kaisernetwork), while general media attention to the global HIV/AIDS epidemic also grew during this period.[11] US opinion polls demonstrated that (a) there was considerable awareness of HIV/AIDS as a general threat to global health and (b) there was skepticism about the effectiveness of governmental responses but at the same time (c) there was support for government policies to improve access to affordable drugs.[12]

---

10   This was pointed out in several interviews carried out in Geneva in 2004 and 2005.

11   The growth of the number of articles in major newspapers related to AIDS and Africa from 500 in 1997 to 1000 in 2000 (Busby 2006: 28) can be seen as an indication of a growing media attention to HIV/AIDS issues in poor countries.

12   See three polls taken since 2002: Kaiser Family Foundation Survey of Americans on HIV/AIDS (www.kff.org/kaiserpolls/7513.cfm), accessed June 15, 2006; Health News

Protests of CSOs against high drug prices and the impact of TRIPS can be seen as part of the tradition of contention of global social movements against GATT and the WTO and their schedules for international economic liberalization (see, for example, O'Brien, Goetz, Scholte and Williams, 2000). During the 1990s, however, CSOs became increasingly engaged as cooperating experts in policy-making processes and as actors in international negotiations. They also gained importance as advisors to developing country members of the WTO.[13] In this way, CSOs assumed an important role more or less as midwives for the development of formal and informal global norms.

Similar to the development of national civil society structures that filled the public space that opened with the decay of feudal institutions, global civil society filled the space that arose with the increase of transnational social relations beyond the nation state and formal inter-state relations (Hein 2005). As within a nation state, global civil society was involved in the construction of opinions, the formation of social norms, and the expression of political critique and demands as part of the process of agenda-setting in political institutions. We witness the development of a complex field of civil society activities and structures, which, to some degree substitute for non-existent state-based structures. Their hybrid character is also expressed in the fact that they are more or less recognized as legitimate representatives of underprivileged groups in a particular political field (for example OXFAM and MSF in health politics) and have a significant impact on negotiations between representatives of states in another political field that has attained a higher degree of formal organization on the international level (e.g. trade/WTO).

New types of political relations between CSOs, private corporations, and IGOs are themselves embedded in a changing public understanding of specific issues. Linking global social movements to constructivist analysis, Sidney Tarrow (2005) discussed the origins of establishing a specific political issue and of constructing the perceptive field in which it is interpreted. This social definition of a problem feeds back into politics through the changing perception of an issue by political actors themselves. Tarrow referred to "framing" as follows: "Proposing frames that are new and challenging but still resonate with existing cultural understandings is a delicate balancing act, especially since society's 'common sense' buttresses the position of elites and defends inherited inequalities" (Tarrow, 2005). He stressed the need for "convergence," defined as "existing political streams that combine with long-standing bundles of ideologies, practices, values, and targets" (Tarrow,

---

Index Poll; survey by Henry J. Kaiser Family Foundation, Harvard School of Public Health; conducted by Princeton Survey Research Associates, July 18–21, 2002, and a Harris Poll conducted in July 2004 for the Wall Street Journal's Health Industry Edition (www. harrisinteractive.com/news/printerfriend/index.asp?NewsID=831), accessed May 18, 2006.

13   The South Centre has played an important role in organizing communication between health CSOs and Southern national delegates to the WTO (interviews of the author (Hein) with representatives in Geneva on §-6-negotioations).

2005). Joshua Busby has shown the importance of AIDS advocates framing their arguments "to tap into moral and religious attitudes" (Busby, 2006) and analyzed the conditions for "framing" created by culture (i.e. the need for a "cultural match") and politics (i.e. shaping the interest of "policy entrepreneurs" to take up a specific issue, framed within a specific rhetoric).

The political conditions of "framing" also relate to a situation in which the generally more powerful actors in a conflict feel threatened by the potential social and political instability arising from situations of great inequality. Busby (2006) discussed the role of threats as part of the framing process of the HIV/AIDS issue. Feeling threatened by particular developments (e.g. the reemergence of infectious diseases; political instability and so on, see Chapter 1) increased the readiness of the US government to reconsider its own short term interests in relation to an "enlightened self-interest" in fighting the causes of these threats.[14]

Nodal governance as a platform of defense and negotiations:
The pharmaceutical industry as actor(s) in informal norm-building

In modern societies, business is highly dependent on norms regulating many aspects of market relations (ranging from weights and measures to product standards to competition law); depending on specific conditions in different industries, some firms might strongly lobby for government support and protection while others might participate in nodal governance processes to prevent extensive state regulation. Beyond trying to introduce their specific interests (such as protectionism) into policies to "govern the market" (Wade, 1990), however, firms also have an interest in benefitting from positive social relations (avoiding labor conflicts; providing good education and training; ensuring a healthy environment; and also contributing to the company image), as long as it does not significantly harm profits. To pursue these goals, firms frequently participate in discourses and conflicts on social norms, as well as contribute to philanthropic endeavors.

Many publications on private actors in global norm-building focus on forms of self-regulation among private enterprises, such as standards in international business from ISO norms to environmental standards of tourism enterprises to the self-regulation of drug promotion (Appelbaum, Felstiner and Gessner, 2001;

---

14   On the link between aid, philanthropy and political compromises from high income countries on the one hand, and the question of global security on the other hand see (Hein and Kohlmorgen, 2008; Jenkins, 2007). Motivations for aid in health issues were manifold: One could argue that the tradition of aid from North to South was established post-WWII in the era of decolonization, both out of a desire by former colonial powers to retain influence in their former colonies, and out of a feeling of guilt or obligation after an era of exploitation. Certainly, streams of aid from wealthy countries to poorer ones far predated the access to medicines movement. Concerning the issue of access to medicines, for the US right wing the motivation was primarily religious (including George Bush), for others it was ethical (secular), for others it was about the public image of wealthy countries in poor ones.

see, for example, Braithwaite and Drahos, 2000; Ronit, Karsten and Volker Schneider, 1999; Ronit, Karsten and Volker Schneider, 2000; Schneider, Volker and Karsten Ronit, 1999). In the case of access to medicines, there are few norm-building or standard-setting private activities,[15] but one can observe the successive development of a consensus that pharmaceutical corporations must respond to the evolving global access norm, and adopt policies that will allow medicines to be sold at much lower prices, at least in the poorest countries.

The access to medicines problem wove together the concept of CSR (see Chapter 2) with the basic norms of the international trade regime, human rights norms, civil society influence on norms, and state power. The industry adopted a number of practices and access policies targeted at developing countries, including: donation programs, voluntary price discounts (differential or tiered pricing), voluntary licensing, covenants not to sue to enforce patent rights, and R&D activities for neglected diseases (either as standalone company activities or in partnership with public-private product development partnerships (PDPs)). Notably, many of these strategies were voluntary in character, with companies retaining considerable control over the depth, breadth and impact of their access policies. The IFPMA, which at first heavily fought against any compromise on TRIPS, finally expressed its full support to the results of the Paragraph 6 negotiations (following the Doha Declaration of 2001) on a revision of the TRIPS agreement and boasted itself of having played the decisive role in reducing prices of ARVs. More recently, the IFPMA quickly endorsed a proposal put forward by the United Kingdom to extend the 2013 deadline for Least-Developed Countries to implement TRIPS (New, 2011).

What explains this shift in policies? The high price of HIV medicines in 1999–2001 had threatened to undermine the legitimacy of the TRIPS Agreement, and by extension, the legitimacy of the WTO as well. The pharmaceutical industry and the industrialized countries had a shared interest in addressing the access issue in order to preserve the broader TRIPS system. Thus, when TNPCs cooperated in the field of access to drugs in poor countries, an underlying basic objective may have been to prevent any amendment of internationally accepted IPR rules over the longer-term.

Informal norm-building and human rights

In Chapter 3 we discussed the need for the implementation of secondary norms as a basic precondition for realizing human rights. While many of these secondary norms have entered the social legislation of many countries, there are still important aspects of the human rights agenda where accepted subsidiary norms

---

15   The Access to Medicine Index (discussed in Chapter 6) is a notable exception. It ranks TNPCs according to a number of criteria related to access policies. This kind of activity can be seen as intended to prevent free-riders within the industry concerning an accepted norm.

concretizing broadly defined primary norms are missing. Examples in addition to "health for all" are freedom from hunger or the right to work. In both cases, an analysis of the impact of informal norms and nodal processes could be instructive, focusing in particular on the impacts of nodal processes on formal institutions and their norm-setting processes, and the contribution of nodal governance itself to norm-building and norm-implementation processes.

To what extent can we generalize the access to medicines example to other fields of social policy? Certainly, the case of access to medicines, particularly with respect to HIV/AIDS, has several unique characteristics—in particular, the contrast between the availability of lifesaving drugs and the suffering of millions of people living with HIV/AIDS was quite dramatic. However this could be also said for the fight against hunger, as globally there are enough resources to end all starvation. Why didn't scandalizing other dimensions of poverty, such as the lack of access to clean water and sanitation, chronic hunger and starvation, and so on, lead to such a great shift in global awareness as the case of access to medicines? One reason may be that the fight against one single disease such as HIV/AIDS and/or the focus on the medicines issue is much more concrete and tangible than fighting against poverty in general or against hunger in all poor countries. In addition, global AIDS activist networks have proven to be especially powerful. These groups were distinct from MSF, Oxfam, HAI, etc, which were more generally focused on health and pharmaceutical policy in developing countries. Many observers have remarked that AIDS activists are one of the most powerful CSO networks operating worldwide on any issue (Epstein, 1996; Smith and Siplon, 2006).

However, these are just preliminary explanations. A comparative study of civil society activities and the constellations of interests in different fields of global social policy could contribute to answering the question of how different conditions affect various attempts to build norms around economic, social and cultural human rights. For the case of health, we can assume that the densification of global social relations and the strengthening of global civil society have played an important role in increasing the impact of human rights norms.

(c) Role and power of non-state actors in global norm-building

In Chapter 2 we introduced the concept of a transformation from a Westphalian system of international relations to a post-Westphalian system of global governance. This transformation was part of the considerable growth of transnational social interactions, which might be seen as part of the process of forming a global society. Globalization has reduced the governance capacities of nation states within their territories and at the same time increased the need for trans-national governance. There is, however, no transnational state authority, let alone a legal system. Beyond the UN Security Council (with its well-known problems of decision-making, legitimacy and implementation), in a few areas, international courts do exist (International Criminal Court; The International Tribunal for the Law of the Sea) as well as assertive instruments for dispute settlement (WTO). Most other fields of international law, however, are still frequently characterized as "soft law"— institutional mechanisms to interpret, adjudicate or enforce them are weak or non-existent. Thus, societal (non-state) actors can be expected to play a growing role in the building and implementation of global norms, in fact expressing the primordial character of society in relation to the state. In abstract terms, there would be no need for a state, if there were a full consensus among social actors about norms and procedures to develop, implement, interpret, adjudicate and enforce new norms. So, is global governance by a creative and consensus-oriented process of social self-organization, i.e. based on informal norm-building, an effective alternative to a formal legal framework negotiated among governments? Reconsidering the conflicts around access to medicines against the background of the literature on the importance of the state's role in enforcing laws (as the sole institution with a monopoly on the legitimate use of force), the role of informality in implementing the universal access norm seems to be primarily the expression of an exceptional situation due to the lack of a global authority. Furthermore, the informal norm is embedded in the legal framework of nation states and the existence of TRIPS flexibilities in international law, reaffirmed by the Doha Declaration.

In most of the literature, the impact of civil society on global norm-building refers primarily to framing specific issues in the public debate and exerting pressure for the acceptance and the implementation of specific norms by states (e.g. abolition of slavery; ban on landmines etc.). Keck and Sikkink's (1998) famous "boomerang effect" has played an important role in explaining the impact of transnational/global discourses and norm-building on the behavior of governments and firms in specific conflicts (e.g. Nestlé Baby Milk; Brent Spar Oil Platform) as well as more generally in the implementation of human rights. We also have encountered that effect in this book concerning the impact of transnational CSOs on the position of governments on the Doha Declaration and on other dimensions of access to medicines.

Public pressure can exert formidable power as it transforms *discursive* (*normative and expert*) power into *political/institutional* (e.g. votes, or: expectations on voting behavior) and *economic power* (e.g. impact on consumer behavior; impact on decisions concerning public procurement and subsidies). This clearly has far reaching implications for the scope and potential impact of non-state actors in inter-/transnational affairs. In the formal context of IGOs, the role of non-state actors has not basically changed: they can officially participate as "observers" and they are *elements in the processes of interest aggregation at the nation-state level*. This entails a complicated two-stage process with uncertain results, while processes of informal norm-building allow open discourses among concerned actors, and flexible forms of acceptance and, thus, informal norm-building allows flexible, often partial forms of implementation in contrast to the "either-or" situation that arises in attempts to formalize a norm legally. The latter situation will frequently lead to a long delay in decision making, which in many cases will be worse for the issue at hand than a more or less "soft" approach to implementation.

In an open world that resembles Fidler's metaphor of open-source anarchy (2007), a logical result of blocked decision-making processes at the IGO level is an organization of interests and political resources and possibly also of compromises concerning issues to be urgently handled, outside the sphere of interstate relations and IGOs. This poses the question of how issues are settled and norms are developed and implemented in social processes outside institutionally fixed procedures.

A high degree of flexibility and the reduced role of formal decision-making procedures, however, do not erase significant powerful differentials between actors: the following paragraphs summarize our analysis on the ways in which power was exercised in the nodal structures that governed the process of informal norm-building and implementation in the access conflict. This will lead the way to some reflections on the democratic character (and the limitations of democracy) in informal norm-building or, in Rosenau's terminology, how authority was exercised in this particular sphere of global governance.

In Chapter 2 we introduced the concepts of *interfaces, types of power* and *nodal governance* at a more abstract level as tools for analysis. Instead of focusing their attention on lobbying national governments to represent their positions in a relatively fixed set of international institutions, actors sought direct interfaces with other relevant actors at various institutionally and geographically diverse "nodes."

Closely linked to the concept of interfaces is Barnett and Duvall's (2005) argument that actors wield different types of power in processes of global governance. Adapting their typology, we argue that five types of power played an important role in shaping the informal universal access norm: *normative, expert, institutional, structural,* and *economic*. These multiple forms of power were used in varying degrees by all the actors: governments, groups of countries, IGOs, CSOs, TNPCs, and experts.

Looking specifically at conflicts around the access norm, we see a complex set of impacts resulting from different types of power:

Normative power (as a specific form of discursive power) can shape understandings regarding what is appropriate and/or morally acceptable behavior, and in doing so, influence behavior itself (Barnett and Duvall, 2005; March and Olsen, 1998). CSOs and public figures of moral standing (such as the Archbishop Desmond Tutu) exerted normative power to problematize the TRIPS regime, and to convince the public that prioritizing access to medicines over stringent IP rules was the appropriate course of action.

Expert power has an impact on understandings of what is empirically true, or technically correct, and thereby shapes the choices available to and courses of action taken by various actors. It was particularly important for CSOs and developing country governments to have access to expertise on complex matters of trade law, intellectual property law, the economics of the pharmaceutical industry, and medicine, in order to mount credible critiques of the TRIPS regime and to argue for the use of TRIPS flexibilities.

Institutional power (the influence exerted through the rules, norms, and processes of existing institutions) enabled developing countries to use the one country-one vote rule within the UN system—particularly at the WHA and WIPO—to air debates and advance resolutions that supported the establishment of the access norm. Within the WTO, the norm of consensus-based decision-making, rather than one country-one vote, resulted in different distributions of institutional power that usually privileged the industrialized economies. A key exception to this rule was the negotiation of the Doha Declaration, in which developing countries used their ability to block progress in launching a new round of trade talks in order to gain concessions on IP and public health. Not having rights of active participation or decision-making in IGOs, non-state actors such as CSOs are not able to agree to TRIPS amendments or Doha Declarations; they can lobby, go to the media, and demonstrate publicly, but ultimately decision-making power over these instruments rests in the hands of states. Indeed, states continue to enjoy a unique type of *structural power* vis-à-vis non-state actors. Perhaps most importantly for this case study is the power of states to regulate private companies that operate within their borders, to make national laws and use TRIPS flexibilities, and finally, to negotiate and implement changes to formal international law. Every state, no matter how poor or how small, has the power to engage in these activities merely by virtue of their structural position as states.

Nevertheless, the exercise of this structural power is clearly constrained by other forms of power wielded by non-state actors. *Economic* power has been an important factor in shaping the access norm—particularly the economic power of large states and TNPCs, and the internal power of trade and finance ministries vs. health ministries. Governments of industrialized countries and TNPCs wielded economic power through trade negotiations, the threat of trade sanctions, or the shaping of "investment climate" to discourage the use of TRIPS flexibilities and thereby discourage the solidification or expansion of the access norm.

In summary, various types of power came into play in the formation and evolution of the access norm. CSOs largely relied upon normative and expert power, while states used institutional, structural and economic power, and TNPCs used economic and expert power to pursue their various interests. Notably, the creation of formal international law requires considerable institutional and structural power—that is, it can only be created by states, and states must have a conducive framework of institutional rules in order to do so. CSOs and developing countries could exercise the power at their disposal to assert a progressive informal norm on access to medicines, but the distribution of structural and institutional power did not allow for the creation of formal norms. More concretely, major changes to formal law such as substantive amendments to TRIPS would have required a condition that has proven impossible to fulfill: a consensus among states on what such substantive amendments should be. The institutional requirement of full consensus to amend WTO treaties resulted in a situation in which they became extraordinarily "sticky." That is, even when the conditions and rationale underlying their creation had changed—as has been the case regarding understandings of the relationship between IP and public health—the formal laws themselves were extremely difficult to amend. At the same time, the extraordinarily strong worldwide reaction to the implications of TRIPS for public health in developing countries demanded a response.

Structures of nodal governance are produced by the ability to organize transnational networks of cooperation among non-state actors pursuing specific interests in the context of a global society on the one hand, and the growing need of IGOs for expertise and support by transnational actors on the other hand. Non-state actors and representatives of IGOs create issue-specific working groups or commissions to promote specific goals or to create solutions to a specific problem by mobilizing not only normative and expert power, but also the financial power of private actors (foundations or TNCs) and state actors (outside the regular schemes of member fees for IGOs).[16] As long as the solutions coming out of nodal processes are not adopted by IGOs or through an international agreement, however, they remain informal, though they may still be effectively implemented. Sanctions produced through public processes can indeed be severe, depending on the size and force of public action. The emergence of the access norm through processes of nodal governance can be seen, at least in part, as an adaptive reaction to the constraints posed by the difficulties of changing formal international rules governing IP and public health.

(d) Transnational democracy: Problems of legitimacy, accountability, power and authority in the open-source anarchy of global politics

As we have seen, processes of nodal governance involve a large number of different actors. They are open to all stakeholders to participate in complex norm-building processes, but the outcome depends on power relations. They are also open to quite different forms of power, creating the possibility to contest economically powerful actors as well as the institutionalized decision-making and legal power of conventionally dominant coalitions such as that between governments of high-income countries and TNPCs. But is the outcome of such processes of nodal governance more democratically legitimate than the politics of conventional intergovernmental organizations?

---

16   The extreme dependence of WHO on extra-budgetary resources serves as a good example (see Kickbusch et al. 2010: 558).

What is a global demos?

Theories of democracy and the modern state have always been concerned with the idea of the "general will", that is, how the collective will of a society can be determined—this reaches from populist ideas ascribed to "the people" (from simple ideas of justice to "national destinies") to elaborate concepts about the best system of representation.[17] In effect, however, the concrete outcome of political strategies—even within a national society—can never be fully controlled by representative political bodies. Incentives can be given that hopefully move social and economic processes in a collectively chosen direction. This is "governance", defined as the "management of the course of events in a social system." Societies are complex: already at the *government* level, the analysis of the question of which concrete strategy will foster a democratically chosen aim in an optimal way, is complex and always influenced by lobbyists trying to direct the "course of events" according to their specific interests. Nevertheless, the authority of governments is based on *formal rules that define their accountability and their legitimacy.*

In the case of global issues, the distance between democratic processes that allow the expression of the "popular will" on the one hand and the actual "course of events" on the other, is considerably larger. Due to the fragmentation of global governance processes, the "popular will" is mostly expressed by distinct constituencies and related to specific issues. In Westphalian international relations, *national governments* are supposed to express the national interest. Concerning international issues of great overall importance, government positions will be discussed in the media and by national CSOs, and if the respective countries are heavily engaged in global political processes, they will also be in a powerful position to influence the opinions (and possibly, conflicts) within global civil society. *Experts* also frequently play an important role in informing government positions as well as the positions of CSOs; in the case of more technical issues, experts will be of particular importance.

The denser the social relations in a global society, the closer *global civil society* will approach something like a "global popular will"—at least related to issues where collective preferences are the result of "the interconnectedness of its members in a sufficiently closely knit network of communicative interactions or 'discourses'" (List and Koenig-Archibugi, 2010).[18] *Transnational private*

---

17 According to Swenson, Rousseau's idea of the "general will" is most appropriately expressed in the Declaration of the Rights of Man and the Citizen of 1789: "The law is the expression of the general will. All citizens have the right to contribute personally, or through their representatives, to its formation. It must be the same for all, whether it protects or punishes" (Swenson, 2000).

18 List and Koenig-Archibugi discuss various conceptions of a "global demos" and propose an "agency-based approach" linking compositional questions ("Which collection(s) of individuals should be considered as candidate(s) for a demos for a given policy area or set of issues?") with a performance question ("… what functional characteristics must it

businesses are generally more attuned to lobbying governments, but might also invest considerable resources (e.g. through the financing of CSOs, influence on media, etc.) to impact civil society opinions. There is no formal institution for popular representation at the global level and there are hardly any cases where majority decisions of intergovernmental organizations are interpreted as equivalent to the "global popular will." In spite of the growing density of global civil society relations, they are still too "thin" (and generally biased towards positions of Western CSOs) to be interpreted as being representative of a global public. Still, as in the case of the access norm, the aggregation of various positions of transnational actors can be observed, mediated by processes of nodal governance. List and Koenig-Archibugi do not use the concept of nodal governance, but their analysis of the establishment of the International Criminal Court (ICC) described a process which can be subsumed under that term:

> The United Nations provided a broad institutional framework that facilitated repeated communication and interaction, and this forum was supplemented by the activities of a large number of government officials, international civil servants, experts, and NGO representatives who created and used many opportunities for formal and informal, open and closed deliberation. (List and Koenig-Archibugi, 2010: 109)

There are a number of parallel characteristics between the global demos supporting the ICC and the global demos supporting the access norm. A "demos" as understood by List and Koenig-Archibugi (List and Koenig-Archibugi, 2010: 78) is democratically organized and is capable "to function as a state-like group"—that is, is able to set specific norms, devise strategies to solve a problem, and is in a position to implement them through sanctions (such as blaming and shaming).[19] However, there is an important difference between the ICC and access examples: While the ICC has been established as a formal international institution, the access norm remains informal and only partially implemented.

What about legitimacy, accountability and power?

We showed in Chapter 6 that informal norms can well be strongly implemented and relatively stable—thus, concerning the access norm, the access to medicines movement can well be seen as a "state-like group agent". But what about their quality as far as democratic governance is concerned? Do they represent a "global popular will?"

---

exhibit in order to guide collective decision making and to enable coordinated actions on the given set of issues?") (2010).

19   See also Rosenau's definition of global governance referring to "systems of rule" and "exercise of control" (see Chapter 1, fn. 6) and his concept of "spheres of authority" (Rosenau, 1997).

Generally, in democracies, civil society is seen as an essential institution for the organization of participation, but informal norms in public policy imply problems regarding the legitimacy and accountability of the protagonists. A full discussion of these concepts is beyond the scope of this book (with reference to global health, see (Bartsch, Huckel Schneider and Kohlmorgen, 2009), but a brief treatment of the question is warranted here. While the *legitimacy* of democratic governments at national level is based on elections and parliamentary control according to the rules set by a duly adopted constitution, the situation is much more complex in global governance processes. Whereas IGOs are at least formally legitimized by clearly-determined lines of representation by member countries (with due regard for reservations concerning the rules of representation and the lack of democracy in many member countries, see, for example, (Huckel Schneider, 2009b)), in the case of self-organized nodes, the legitimacy of any decision is open to contention. To a certain degree, the wide-spread acceptance that fully democratic governance is difficult to reach in a global society might imply a shift towards output- or "result"-oriented legitimacy combined with the explicit or implicit recognition that a high level of participation might compensate for the lack of formal legitimacy.

Regarding accountability, it is important to distinguish between internal and external accountability. Internally, organizations generally have some kind of accountability mechanism of their leadership towards their members. More difficult, however, is to determine the external accountability of non-state organizations concerning people affected by their operations. In the case of CSO advocacy there are no clear mechanisms of accountability between populations affected by the advocacy and the advocates themselves; the impacts are not always positive.

While it is difficult enough to assess the legitimacy and at least the external accountability of specific global governance actors, the issue of *transnational democracy* is much more complex, as its analysis has to take into account questions of power and the control of power, as well as the "state-likeness" of processes in which political goals, strategies and potentials of various actors interact and aggregate to create the position(s) of a global demos and (informal) norms as outcomes of global politics. These outcomes depend on processes at interfaces between various actors wielding different types of power; in chapters 3 to 8 we analyzed the rise and implementation of the access norm as a complex process of nodal governance where the economic power of transnational enterprises and mighty states, having shaped international law basically according to their interest, could not prevail over an alliance between CSOs and developing countries. Importantly, this was not due to majorities of developing countries in UN institutions but to a large degree to the discursive mobilization of normative and expert power.

Global popular will

Establishing informal norms without a formally legitimized political process raises the question of what other forms of legitimization and accountability might be developed that allows us to talk of a "global popular will" (extending Rousseau's "general will"), expressed by a "state-like" global demos. Certainly, legitimacy is derived from the reference to existing international law, such as the TRIPS Agreement on the one hand, and human rights and especially the right to health on the other hand. Legitimacy is also won by the general social reputation of organizations involved (such as MSF, recipient of the Nobel Peace Prize), and sought by TNPCs through their successes in developing new medicines and their access policies.

As is the case within national societies, there are on-going discourses between the networks directly included in political processes and their engaged and well-informed constituencies. Individuals consciously supporting positions in transnational conflicts after having been informed by the media also contribute to the formation of a global popular will.

The media, often called the "fourth power," play an important role. It is an increasingly global institution that transcends national boundaries as well as state-based governance-processes. The media have the potential to influence all groups of actors (states, firms, CSOs) and to be influenced in turn by all three. As such, internationally active media constitute a new form of linking human rights norms to broad public discourses, economic interests and political institutions.

Nevertheless, it merits mentioning that the media is not necessarily an ally of economically weaker groups, nor proponents of global solidarity. Many influential media are frequently financially dependent on the economic power of large enterprises and other affluent groups in their respective societies. The media can take implicit or explicit positions in political conflicts, and also transport the dominant world view to all levels of society from the local to the global. Also, within a democratic national polity, public opinion does not always reflect the presumed interests of the people but may instead tend towards maintaining the stability of an institutionalized and accountable system of rule.[20]

Popular will, democratic governance and the control
of power by "open source anarchy"

The formation of the popular will is irrevocably linked to the human rights of freedom of expression and of association as central elements of civil and political rights. This is recognized as an essential aspect of democratic political systems and it is also essential for the activities and further strengthening of

---

20   See the link between democratic governance and economic liberalization in the concept of "neo-liberal governmentality" based on Foucault's concept of "governmentality" in (Dean, 1999).

global civil society. However, the "popular will" not only needs instruments of aggregation and articulation, but also of a corresponding system of management; in democracies, this is basically through democratically elected governments and an institutionalized control of power. Furthermore, civilized control of power in a global society is fundamentally dependent upon norm-building processes allowing social control of conflicts where formal, legally binding agreements and rules cannot be achieved.[21] While most of the legitimizing mechanisms of the democratic state do not exist in global politics, "open source anarchy"[22] may be much more flexible and productive in terms of social self-regulation than a "coordinated anarchy" of nation states closed to independent initiatives from non-state actors. If the legitimized representatives of the "popular will" of nations are not able to produce a solution to an urgent and serious high-profile political issue, non-state actors may pursue this issue, legitimized by the reference to popular will and accountable to a global public which is able to organize itself against violations of broadly accepted norms. It is the democratic process and thus procedural legitimacy, then, that imbues "popular will" with the authority to produce the "rule of the demos."

In this context, authority is not based on formal decisions of institutions in charge of a specific issue area through a specific constitutional act—such as the authority of WHO for world health mandated in its Constitution of 1948. Authority is seated in the norm itself, based on some kind of procedural acceptance by global society, which refers to overarching norms (such as human rights) and the continuous scrutiny of this norm by stakeholders in nodal governance processes. As we have seen, such informal norms are contested with respect to their inclusiveness as well as their stability, and—depending on the depth and strength of their normative foundation in global society—might in the long or medium run also lose acceptance. Thus, there will always be a drive to formalize the informal norm, which we discussed in Chapter 8 and will take up again in the conclusion.

---

21   This perspective also puts the unending demands for better coordination in all fields of global governance (as reflected, for example, in the Paris Declaration on Aid Effectiveeness) into a more critical light, as they tend to forget the classical arguments for the productivity of pluralism and open competition between new ideas, as well as the important balancing role of opposition to the over-centralization of power.

22   David Fidler (2008b; 2007) develops his concept of "open-source anarchy" to distinguish new developments in international relations (IR) from the realist conception of IR as an anarchical system of sovereign nation states. Here we stress primarily the difference between "open-source pluralism" in a democratic nation state and in global governance.

Chapter 10
Conclusions

(a) Formal and informal norms

Over the past decade, we observed an on-going conflict in global politics around the issue of international intellectual property rights. The stakeholders involved and their basic interests remained largely unchanged, but their concrete political positions on IPRs and access to medicines underwent a surprising evolution during the first decade of the twenty-first century. Whereas during negotiations on the Doha Declaration and even thereafter on the Paragraph 6 decision,[1] the pharmaceutical industry and a number of high-income country governments fought hard to keep the use of TRIPS flexibilities as limited as possible, a few years later, the industry publicly recognized the legitimacy of the Ecuadorean government's compulsory license announcement. Instead of publicly threatening retaliation after the announcement of a compulsory license, at the end of the decade the USTR took a far more muted approach—at least as far as medicines against HIV/AIDS were concerned. We documented these changing attitudes in Chapter 6. We also observed cooperation between CSOs and TNPCs on concrete projects to improve access to medicines, for example, through patent pools and non-profit product development partnerships with CSOs or governments to stimulate R&D into neglected diseases.

What changed during these years? A few years after the TRIPS Agreement came into force in 1995, the Doha Declaration reinforced some articles of the agreement—the so-called TRIPS flexibilities—and led to a relatively small change to the treaty itself (the Paragraph 6 agreement). However, the truly significant changes in IP norms cannot be explained by predominant theories of international law: a powerful but informal norm emerged and solidified regarding universal access to essential medicines. Many of the most important changes took place at discursive interfaces, where normative power and expert knowledge were particularly influential. Developing countries and CSOs successfully framed the discourse on access to medicines as an essential component of fulfilling the human right to health, and mobilized public opinion against the policies of TNPCs and industrialized countries regarding strict IPR protection. These discursive interfaces occurred in the mass media, over specialized listserves, at the annual World Health Assembly, biannual WTO Ministerials, at academic conferences, and in many other

---

1   Notably, as discussed in Chapter 5, this amendment has not come into force as of 2011, since two-thirds of WTO Members must first ratify it and developing country Members in particular seem to have been hesitant to do so.

arenas. This debate successively integrated legal and technical experts from the health, development and trade communities, including individuals within IGOs, universities, bilateral aid agencies, and those serving on international commissions especially created to address this debate. Collectively, these discursive interfaces opened up new spaces for health concerns within the traditionally state-bound trade negotiations on intellectual property rights. More generally, support was mobilized for stronger public responsibility with regard to medical innovation and access to essential medicines, which has arguably strengthened norms of social solidarity at the global level. All these elements allow us to speak of a global demos expressing a global popular will.

These changes were not restricted to the level of norms, but had concrete, measurable impacts on individuals and communities. As of 2011, access to ART in developing countries had improved dramatically to reach 6.6 million people, enabled by major increases in both external and domestic financing to support access to these drugs (WHO, UNAIDS, UNICEF, 2011). Over 60 countries had made use of TRIPS flexibilities to access generic ARVs, and nearly all major ARV-producing TNPCs had offered either discounted pricing and/or voluntary licenses for the generic production of ARVs for use in developing countries (Médecins Sans Frontières (MSF), 2011).

As discussed in previous chapters, major changes in informal norms were possible due to increasingly flexible forms of global governance. By transcending various governance systems in the process of a successive intensification of global social relations, influential non-state actors—at least in the field of access to medicines—successfully mobilized discursive power. This resulted in the reinforcement of actors fighting for global social rights in spite of the strong position the supporters of global market creation had won with the foundation of the WTO and the hard legal norms underpinning it.

Through manifold processes of self-organization, the need to link different systems of governance (global health, human rights, the world trade order, the intellectual property system) led to more intense communication and to the rise of new institutional forms to solve specific problems. These trends have shifted the core of global health politics away from IGOs ("international health governance") to a complex system of global health governance. The system borders are fluid and constantly shifting, with many areas of overlap with other systems in global governance; the system is also open for new actors at all times.

Yet, while substantial and significant changes took place in the realm of informal norms, the prevailing constellation of state interests and power prevented any major *formal* changes to the TRIPS regime—in spite of a pervasive crisis in global health. A fundamental change concerning access to medicines was the result of an informal norm superimposed upon the formal norms of the TRIPS Agreement regarding patents as the central mechanism for financing the R&D costs of the pharmaceutical industry. Only after the dramatic impact of the informal norm had manifested itself did a slow process of negotiations on changing formal norms on health R&D begin within the global health community.

Changes in formal laws did take place at the national level in some key countries. As discussed in greater detail in previous chapters, the patent laws of India, Cambodia and the Philippines were revised to afford greater public health protections, and key court cases in Brazil, Thailand and South Africa set important legal precedents for a pro-public health interpretation of national laws. At the international level, in addition to the Paragraph 6 TRIPS amendment, the WTO TRIPS Council also formalized the extension period to allow LDCs up until 2013 to come into compliance with TRIPS and up to 2016 to grant or enforce pharmaceutical patents, with the possibility of further extending these deadlines.

These changes in formal norms (i.e. laws or binding rules) have been significant, but—it must be said—quite limited if one takes a macro-level view of the system. It is only in a handful of developing countries that changes in formal laws had taken place to protect access to medicines. The Paragraph 6 system has consistently been criticized by CSOs and developing country governments for being unworkable in practice. And many LDCs failed to take advantage of the extended deadlines for TRIPS compliance. In summary, as MSF stated, "in 2011, globally equitable access to medicines is non-existent or at best precarious."[2]

Reliable access to patented medicines still depended on the use of special provisions ("flexibilities") and exceptions to TRIPS. Public health was not, in and of itself, a core objective of TRIPS, and access to medicines remained on the margins of the Agreement. The Doha Declaration was an attempt to rectify this situation, but it remains an informal norm in the sense that its principles and language were not incorporated into TRIPS itself. At the same time, bilateral trade and other treaties with IP provisions (investment, ACTA) eroded the policy space for public health protection within the IP regime. Indeed, since 2001 there has been a proliferation of formal norms that require more stringent IP protection in the form of bilateral or regional trade agreements and bilateral investment treaties, and the national laws that must often be changed subsequent to these treaties.

Communicative consensus-seeking among actors with very different material interests could only be expected to achieve so much. TNPCs and industrialized countries accepted and even pro-actively supported the goal of achieving affordable medicines for the poor and greater research into the neglected diseases, but they did not surrender the use of their political and economic resources to fight for stronger IPRs in international law.

The contrast between significant health-oriented changes in informal norms, and the near absence of such changes in formal norms has been a central focus of this book. Having now reviewed in detail the experience in the field of access to medicines, what conclusions can be drawn regarding the relative importance

---

2   This statement was made in the context of the launch of an "Ideas Contest" on revising TRIPS on the occasion of the 10-year anniversary of the Doha Declaration. Full announcement available at: http://www.msfaccess.org/content/msf-launches-revising-trips -public-health-ideas-contest.

and the specific political role of informal and formal norms for protecting and promoting the right to health?

There was, to our knowledge, no conscious political decision to privilege informal norm-building over the formal codification of the right to universal access to essential medicines and of the necessary regulatory statutes e.g. as an addendum to TRIPS. As primary norms, human rights norms (such as the human right to health, education etc.), constitute international law, but can only be effectively implemented if there exist clearly defined secondary norms that can be implemented as formal, judiciable law at the national level. There are, however, inherently transnational issues that arise e.g. when the pursuit of primary norms depends on globalized social contexts. In this case, secondary norms either must be formulated and implemented in formal international law (which is, by definition, negotiated and agreed upon by states) or be based on a sufficiently coherent and strong set of informal norms supported by a wide range of non-state actors. The General Comments to the UN human rights treaties try to give an "authoritative but not binding" interpretation of human rights norms, which essentially aim to break down primary into secondary norms, but there is no institutional power to enforce such norms.

In the case of access to medicines we have the case of a well-defined secondary norm, which was not formalized in international law due to the vested interests of strong actors, and because of the sector-related character of most international law, which makes it difficult to integrate trade and health norms. Nevertheless, in reflecting upon the chances of guaranteeing universal access to medicines through formalized international law, we should not forget that formal norms need a basis in informal social norms and values, and thus, that a deepening of an informal norm improves the chances for a process of formalization in the future.

As we have seen, informal norms offer tremendous potential for practical, concrete change to be achieved in a situation in which there is no agreement on changing formal norms, and the negotiation of new international laws within the sector (e.g. R&D treaty) can be expected to take many years. The process described in Chapter 8 illustrates the cumbersome path that needs to be paved to prepare the international community for creating new law.[3] Therefore, a strategy to strengthen informal norms as a foundation for the implementation of secondary norms on a global or transnational scale has a number of advantages compared to lengthy negotiations of formal rules:

a. Faster change is possible. There was no need to wait for changes in formal norms to mobilize record amounts of money and political attention for access to HIV drugs. Doubtless, shifting informal political interpretations

---

3   The 2006 CIPIH report launched the 2006–2008 IGWG process, which resulted in the 2008 GSPoA, which launched the EWG and then the CEWG, which recommended the start of negotiations over a formal convention on health R&D in 2012 (see Chapter 8).

of what flexibilities were permissible under TRIPS was faster than a re-negotiation of the agreement itself would have been.

b. Flexibility. The access norm, which was articulated most clearly in the 2001 Doha Declaration, evolved and strengthened gradually over time through national practice and on-going normative work at the international level, such as through expert commissions. Informal norms can change subtly to adjust and adapt to changing underlying conditions, power distributions, and technological possibilities.

c. Open to stronger influence by traditionally weak actors. Actors traditionally considered weak in the international system, including developing countries, CSOs, and experts, have relatively greater influence over informal norms. At discursive interfaces, the normative and expert power wielded by CSOs, experts and the media, are particularly influential, and can counteract the greater economic resources of industry. At institutional interfaces, the power of developing countries vis-à-vis industrialized countries can be greater, depending on the institutional setting, rules, and norms (e.g. institutional rules are favorable to developing countries in the UN system, but favorable to industrialized countries in the WTO).

d. Informal norms can lay the ground (based on growing attention and support for a specific issue; increased expertise on related questions) for later negotiations on a formal agreement (albeit without any guarantee for success).

Our research has shown the potential of informal norms in today's global society. It has, however, also pointed to the limits and risks of relying largely on informal norms for fulfilling the right to health. Stakeholders interested in strengthening IPRs without much intrinsic[4] motivation to support global health, have pursued a number of goals that do not coincide with the access norm, such as the insistence on data exclusivity, the support of FTAs with TRIPS-plus-clauses, strong IPR clauses in WTO accession agreements, and the possible erosion of TRIPS flexibilities in ACTA. With the exception of data exclusivity these issues are not specifically related to health R&D, but to general problems of the protection of intellectual property. In the long-run, another risk is that CSOs pay less attention to the issue of access to medicines. This creates pressure to move towards formal norm-setting, linking the issues of IPRs, medical innovation and universal access.

The negotiation and effective implementation of formal norms would have the following advantages, which of course depend on the concrete institutional context in which the norms would be formalized:

---

4 We do not deny that—for whatever reason—TNPCs accept a certain degree of responsibility (in the sense of CSR, see Chapter 2, Section (c)) for the health impact of their activities, but we assume that this is not one of the primary drivers of their international strategies.

a. More predictable, reliable, stable. Formal norms offer greater predictability, reliability and stability precisely because the threshold to change them is so high. In the WTO, for example, unanimous agreement among Members is required to amend a treaty.
b. Stronger. The same norm will exert greater force when it is codified into international law than when it is not, ceteris paribus. (e.g. if Doha language were written into TRIPS itself, its importance as a legal document would not be open to challenge as it was at the 2011 UN NCD summit). Explicitly formulated trade or IP norms can, for example, be enforced through the Dispute Settlement Body of the WTO, which authorizes trade retaliation when Members are found to be out of compliance with WTO agreements.
c. More enforceable at national level. Formal international norms are likely to carry greater legal weight within national systems, and therefore stand a greater chance of being enforced through the structural power of the state, either through national laws or the courts.[5]

Access to medicines norms would be stronger, more predictable, more reliable, and more stable, if they could be formalized in international law, for example, through a revision of the TRIPS Agreement. However, as long as states remain the sole authority able to negotiate and agree upon formal international laws, and as long as powerful states oppose major revisions to the global IP regime, any major formal changes to TRIPS will be extremely difficult to achieve. These difficulties illustrate the limits to current global governance processes. They also underscore the importance of ongoing efforts to strengthen, expand, and consolidate informal norms, without losing sight of the benefits of formalization.

In the absence of major changes to international IP rules, what other types of normative changes might be on the horizon? Three non-mutually-exclusive possibilities present themselves:

First, we could see new civil society mobilization to expand and solidify the access norm beyond HIV and the neglected diseases—to, for example, NCDs. Thus far, moves in this direction remain nascent, and the success of such mobilization will depend on the strength of CSO networks advocating for this expansion and the degree to which developing country governments dedicate political capital to the effort. For a number of reasons, NCD groups are unlikely to resemble HIV activist organizations, many of which developed in reaction to strong social stigma, purposefully incorporated socially-marginalized groups, and included many members with years of healthy life available to dedicate to activism. Cancer patients' organizations, for example, do not share these traits. Yet, to the extent that

---

5 The relationship between national and international law depends on national legal systems, with some countries automatically adopting international laws as equivalent to domestic laws when they ratify treaties, while others require the elaboration of specific national laws to implement international agreements.

NCD groups can join with and build on the successes of the HIV movement, they are likely to improve their chances of expanding the access norm.

Second, we could see a greater push for formalization of public health protections at national level in the patent laws of "leading" states; these prospects are complicated by the rise of MICs as attractive markets for TNPCs and the trends towards increasing patenting in some developing countries. Nevertheless, increased formalization at country level would further solidify the access norm, both within the countries involved and through broader discursive effects at the global level.

Finally, we could see a move to change the global system for generating and disseminating health-related innovation (a legal change at a higher level), either through amendments to TRIPS (which is improbable, as we have seen) or the creation of a stand-alone biomedical R&D treaty. As discussed in Chapter 8, political support for an R&D treaty has begun to gather force, first among civil society groups and more recently among some influential governments as well. The CEWG recommended in its April 2012 report a binding convention under article 19 of the WHO constitution for R&D related to Type II and III diseases and the specific R&D needs of developing countries in relation to Type I diseases (WHO Consultative Expert Working Group on Research and Development (CEWG): Financing and Coordination, 2012). It will be important to formulate the treaty in such a way that it will generate effective support for strengthening medical R&D and for equitable access to medicines in developing countries. It remains to be seen whether such a convention with far-reaching commitments can really be achieved in intergovernmental negotiations. Possible conflicts with TRIPS will certainly constitute an important issue in these negotiations. Nevertheless, there are examples of partially conflicting international agreements in different sectors of global governance that have been applied with some success (for example, the Convention on Biological Diversity, which interacts with a number of international agreements, including TRIPS (Rosendal, 2006)).

None of these developments is likely to occur without strong political contestation from those whose interests are threatened by such moves. Though international agreements create international obligations that are formally independent from each other (with the important exception of the WTO treaties), the growing network of agreements means that many of them in practice do affect each other in one way or another. Since international law may attempt to regulate inter/transnational interactions in an increasingly comprehensive way, the occurrence of such conflicting situations is likely to increase in both frequency and significance. As long as there is no such thing as a global state, informal norms linked to more general primary norms will remain important.

The access norm seems stable enough that a major push to tighten global IP standards through changes to TRIPS seems unlikely in the near to mid-term. Given the growing economic power of some developing countries, the normative shifts of the past decade, and the close monitoring by CSOs and experts of international IP policymaking, any efforts to tighten IP rules within the WTO or other multilateral arenas would be met with stiff resistance. The high threshold for changes to formal WTO rules prevents major shifts towards more stringent IPRs, just as it prevents any moves towards substantially greater flexibility. The formal IP system is stable, and therefore fundamentally biased towards the status quo. Thus, we have seen TNPCs and industrialized countries focus their efforts on developing new formal rules through bilateral and regional law-making efforts, rather than through the WTO.

Patent-holding companies still stand to gain from stringent IP protection, and are likely to continue advocating for rules that promote their economic interests. In this context, the flipside of the rise of the MICs as emergent powers in global politics is their increasing importance as export markets and locations for direct investments or joint ventures for the industrialized countries and their IP-intensive industries. This trend raises the commercial stakes for IP rulemaking, and increases the incentive for patent-holders to push for stronger, broader and longer patent monopolies in these countries. In the medium run we can also expect that pharmaceutical research conducted by local firms in MICs will increase, and shape evolving positions towards global IP rules.

On the other hand, MIC governments also cannot ignore the ongoing need to guarantee access to affordable medicines for their populations by making use of TRIPS flexibilities when necessary; the situation is particularly acute in MICs characterized by high income inequality with large populations still living in extreme poverty, particularly at a time when the incidence of non-communicable diseases is rising, along with the cost of drugs needed to treat them. This complex situation may bolster the motivation and engagement of MIC governments to achieve reliable formal rules to support access to affordable medicines for their populations, while at the same time strengthening local R&D capacities. In particular, the governments of many MICs find themselves in a complicated situation: on the one hand, they continue to further strengthen their power as states in multilateral institutions, capitalizing on a certain neglect of these institutions by the more powerful industrialized countries, and still view the power of international CSOs with a certain suspicion. On the other hand, in recent times they have frequently benefited from alliances with these CSOs, as we have seen in conflicts over IP, and it is not difficult to imagine that—concerning the inclusiveness of the access norm with regard to NCDs, for example—they might need to continue cooperating with CSOs to assert their interests in multilateral fora.

(b) Implications for health and implications for global governance

As we have documented in this book, the development of the access norm has played a significant role in establishing global health as an important issue in global politics. The fight against HIV/AIDS has arguably strengthened, in particular, worldwide solidarity (demonstrated by growing social pressure for transfer payments to help solve problems of global inequality), transnational responsibility (including extraterritorial obligations in the negotiation of international agreements, in particular those affecting human rights), and the overall awareness of global interdependence. Universal access to essential medicines is a central issue in this context, in particular, as it has opened the doors to changes beyond HIV/AIDS. Access to ARVs has become a paradigmatic case for more inclusive, complete efforts to ensure access to all essential medicines.[6] More broadly, the response to HIV/AIDS has also reflected fundamental systemic changes in global governance linked to the broader processes of globalization and the development of a global society.

This point touches on the central topic of this book: the relationship between formal international rules (i.e. international law) and informal norms in dealing with global challenges. The global legal system is becoming increasingly dense and complex (consisting of concerted and compatible national law; international law; international private standards, etc.). This trend is to a large extent due to the "legalization" of more and more issue areas in inter- and transnational relations and to the deepening of regulation (i.e. creating rules or rule harmonization that increasingly affect daily activities), but also due to processes of regime shifting in attempts by specific actors to improve their institutional position.[7]

The global legal system, however, remains incoherent and without an overriding system of global coordination (unlike at national level, where sovereign nation states can provide at least some measure of intersectoral and inter-issue policy coherence). We are confronted with a "reality that ... international governance occurs via a multitude of nested, partially overlapping, and parallel trans-border agreements" (Alter and Meunier, 2009). Alter and Meunier offer some insights that coincide with the findings of our study, concerning (a) the importance of the implementation process of specific agreements for understanding the results of regime complexity vis-à-vis a "fragmentation of international law" (2009); (b) the role of cross-institutional political strategies (such as regime-shifting and forum-shopping); (c) the generation of small group environments and the role of face-to-face interactions in shaping international cooperation (with some affinity to the concept of nodal governance); and (d) the potentially positive impact of competition between multiple actors (increasing available resources, more flexibility to escape deadlocks).

Thus, despite concerns regarding its harmful effects on coordination, there seems to be some recognition that a proliferation of actors in a particular policy field is not necessarily negative. Regime complexity, however, raises one central

---

6 From this perspective, critiques regarding the "over-financing" of HIV/AIDS treatment in relation to other global health priorities (see, for example, England, 2007) ought to take into account that developments in GHG that have originated in the fight against HIV/AIDS have had an impact reaching far beyond this one specific disease ('t Hoen, Berger, Calmy and Moon, 2011).

7 Laurence Helfer has produced a considerable list of publications on regime shifting in IPRs (see Helfer (2004) and as an overview of the problem), Helfer (2009).

problem. In brief: Who is winning? Commenting on regime complexity, Drezner asserts that "we may find that the reality of bounded rationality further advantages the rich and powerful—be they the most resourced states, firms able to hire expensive lawyers, or the most organized activists" (Drezner, 2009). Alter and Meunier are somewhat more optimistic, in line with the findings of our study (see Chapter 9, Section (d)): "... powerful actors will still be interacting with actors who participate in and are shaped by politics in other domains, so that over time powerful actors will have to deal with the reality of parallel institutions that they cannot control" (Alter and Meunier, 2009). Civil society actors (including academic experts) that are not tied to traditional political institutions have the freedom to behave more flexibly even than TNPCs, which have been more focused on lobbying states and exerting their power in international norm-building through governmental institutions.

If the more powerful were always able to protect the status quo, history would reveal no significant social changes. Globalization has resulted in many profound changes, which have allowed for new patterns of political decision-making and significant normative and institutional changes, even if it has not completely overturned hierarchies of power. One important new phenomenon in global politics appears to be the rise of nodal governance and its role in linking fragmented systems of global governance with an increasingly integrated (interdependent and interacting, but not necessarily cooperating) global society. This is closely related to the impact of the emergence of a global society on the cognitive mapping of social belonging and equity. In spite of the continuing dominant role of the nation state in daily politics, transnational identification and solidarity among groups in similar social situations (whether more narrowly defined (e.g. PLHIV) or more general (e.g. the "Occupy" movement)) and advocacy movements yield growing influence. Nodal governance in global affairs is based on the interfaces between CSO, TNCs and hybrid actors with a highly transnational identity on the one hand, and state actors still firmly linked to "national interests" on the other hand.

Informal norms such as the access norm are likely to play a growing role in global governance, even if they might remain informal only for a limited and transitory period of time before becoming codified into more formal rules. The establishment of the International Criminal Court (List and Koenig-Archibugi, 2010, also see Chapter 9) is an example of a political process in which the link between networks of actors supporting informal norms and formal intergovernmental institutions led to an intergovernmental agreement on a new international institution. The broader discourses we are presently observing in various fields of human rights (e.g., regarding the right to water, responsibility to protect), food and agriculture (e.g., food security, land grabbing, bio-piracy, patenting in plant and animal breeding), as well as in environmental issues in general (e.g. equity in responses to climate change, such as who should bear the burden of reducing greenhouse gas emissions), point to the expectation that the dialectics of a densification of global society and changes in norm-building processes are broader phenomena, not only a characteristic of global health governance.

These broader processes offer, perhaps, a reason to hope for the development of more effective responses to global challenges, greater global solidarity, and a progressive realization of human rights.

Annex 1

The 2001 WTO Doha Declaration on TRIPS and Public Health

World Trade Organization	**WT/MIN(01)/DEC/2** 20 November 2001 (01-5860)

MINISTERIAL CONFERENCE

Fourth Session

Doha, 9–14 November 2001

DECLARATION ON THE TRIPS AGREEMENT AND PUBLIC HEALTH

Adopted on 14 November 2001

1. We recognize the gravity of the public health problems afflicting many developing and least-developed countries, especially those resulting from HIV/AIDS, tuberculosis, malaria and other epidemics.
2. We stress the need for the WTO Agreement on Trade-Related Aspects of Intellectual Property Rights (TRIPS Agreement) to be part of the wider national and international action to address these problems.
3. We recognize that intellectual property protection is important for the development of new medicines. We also recognize the concerns about its effects on prices.
4. We agree that the TRIPS Agreement does not and should not prevent Members from taking measures to protect public health. Accordingly, while reiterating our commitment to the TRIPS Agreement, we affirm that the Agreement can and should be interpreted and implemented in a manner supportive of WTO Members' right to protect public health and, in particular, to promote access to medicines for all.

   In this connection, we reaffirm the right of WTO Members to use, to the full, the provisions in the TRIPS Agreement, which provide flexibility for this purpose.

5. Accordingly and in the light of paragraph 4 above, while maintaining our commitments in the TRIPS Agreement, we recognize that these flexibilities include:

    In applying the customary rules of interpretation of public international law, each provision of the TRIPS Agreement shall be read in the light of the object and purpose of the Agreement as expressed, in particular, in its objectives and principles.

    Each Member has the right to grant compulsory licences and the freedom to determine the grounds upon which such licences are granted.

    Each Member has the right to determine what constitutes a national emergency or other circumstances of extreme urgency, it being understood that public health crises, including those relating to HIV/AIDS, tuberculosis, malaria and other epidemics, can represent a national emergency or other circumstances of extreme urgency.

    The effect of the provisions in the TRIPS Agreement that are relevant to the exhaustion of intellectual property rights is to leave each Member free to establish its own regime for such exhaustion without challenge, subject to the MFN and national treatment provisions of Articles 3 and 4.

6. We recognize that WTO Members with insufficient or no manufacturing capacities in the pharmaceutical sector could face difficulties in making effective use of compulsory licensing under the TRIPS Agreement. We instruct the Council for TRIPS to find an expeditious solution to this problem and to report to the General Council before the end of 2002.

7. We reaffirm the commitment of developed-country Members to provide incentives to their enterprises and institutions to promote and encourage technology transfer to least-developed country Members pursuant to Article 66.2. We also agree that the least-developed country Members will not be obliged, with respect to pharmaceutical products, to implement or apply Sections 5 and 7 of Part II of the TRIPS Agreement or to enforce rights provided for under these Sections until January 1, 2016, without prejudice to the right of least-developed country Members to seek other extensions of the transition periods as provided for in Article 66.1 of the TRIPS Agreement. We instruct the Council for TRIPS to take the necessary action to give effect to this pursuant to Article 66.1 of the TRIPS Agreement.

Annex 2
Timeline of Key Events

Reproduced from: 't Hoen, 2009.

1957–1962	The United States Senate Sub-committee on Anti-trust and Monopoly, under the chairmanship of Senator Estes Kefauver, examines the prescription drug industry and recommends legislation to curtail the monopoly powers of the pharmaceutical industry.
	In the late 1950s-early '60s, the US invoked government use powers on a routine basis to order generic medicines from abroad, regardless of the patent status of the products.
1965	Pfizer Corporation unsuccessfully challenges the United Kingdom's routine use of compulsory licenses ("Crown Use") for the provision of generic medicines to the National Health Service.
1969-1992	Canada issues 613 compulsory licenses for importation and/or local production of medicines as part of its cost containment measures.
1986	Launch of the Uruguay Round of the GATT (the predecessor of the WTO).
Early 1990s	Highly Active Antiretroviral Therapy (HAART) becomes available in Europe and North America, changing AIDS from a lethal disease to a chronic illness.
1995	Establishment of the World Trade Organization (WTO) and the adoption of the TRIPS Agreement.
1995	UNAIDS created.
1996	Brazil starts offering universal free ARV treatment to people living with AIDS.
1996	(May) World Health Assembly (WHA) adopts the Revised Drug Strategy and strengthens WHO's mandate in the area of intellectual property; the WHA requests the WHO "to report on the impact of the work of the World Trade Organization (WTO) with respect to national drug policies and essential drugs and make recommendations for collaboration between WTO and WHO, as appropriate."
1997	Brazil starts granting pharmaceutical product patents.
1998	The South African Pharmaceutical Manufacturers Association and 39 mostly multi-national pharmaceutical companies bring suit against the government of South Africa, alleging that the Medicines and Related Substances Control Amendment Act, No. 90 of 1997 violated TRIPS and the South African constitution.
1999	Médecins Sans Frontières (MSF) launches its international Campaign for Access to Essential Medicines.

1999	(March) MSF, Health Action International (HAI) and Consumer Project on Technology (CPTech) organise the first meeting on compulsory licensing of AIDS medicines, held at the UN in Geneva.
1999	MSF, HAI and CPTech organise an international conference on access to medicines in the run-up to the Seattle WTO Ministerial conference.
1999	Seattle WTO Ministerial meeting collapses. For the first time, delegates officially discuss the consequences of the WTO TRIPS Agreement for access to medicines.
2000	(May) US President Clinton issues Executive Order 13155 supporting sub-Saharan African countries in using measures such as compulsory licensing to allow production and import of generic AIDS drugs, without fear of trade retaliation.
2000	(May) Multinational drug companies announce price reductions for AIDS drugs.
2000	(July) The 13th International AIDS conference takes place in Durban, South Africa. This was the first time that this prestigious conference was held in a developing country.
2000	(December) A 3-day G8 summit on infectious diseases takes place in Okinawa, Japan, drawing attention to the need for global action and new financing for health.
2001	(February) The Indian generic medicines manufacturer Cipla announces triple-ARV AIDS treatment for 350 USD per patient/year.
2001	(April) Following a global public outcry against the 39 drug companies' actions in South Africa, the companies are compelled to drop their lawsuit.
2001	(November) The Fourth WTO Ministerial Conference adopts the Doha Declaration on TRIPS and Public Health.
2001	WHO launches the Prequalification Programme to ensure the quality of medicines for HIV/AIDS, TB and malaria.
2002	WHO includes ARV medicines in its Essential Medicines List (EML) for the first time.
2002	The Global Fund to Fight AIDS, Tuberculosis and Malaria is established.
2003	The WHO starts the "3 by 5" initiative to expand access to HIV treatment to 3 million people by 2005.
2003	Thailand offers universal access to ARVs to people living with AIDS.
2003	WTO adopts the "August 30th" decision to allow drugs to be produced under a compulsory license predominantly for export.
2003	In South Africa, the Treatment Action Campaign (TAC) wins its case against GlaxoSmithKline and Boehringer Ingelheim before the Competition Commission, which found the companies guilty of anti-competitive practices.
2003	US President's Emergency Plan for AIDS relief (PEPFAR) is launched.
2003	The Drugs for Neglected Diseases Initiative (DNDi), a not-for-profit drug development organization, is founded.

2003	The UK Commission on Intellectual Property Rights publishes its report, concluding that the new global architecture for intellectual property has serious drawbacks for developing countries, in particular for access to medicines.
2005	(March) India amends its 1970 Patents Act to introduce pharmaceutical product patents, as required by the TRIPS Agreement.
2006	(January) Indian Patent Office rejects the patent application by Novartis for imatinib mesylate (Glivec).
2006	(March) The Indian Network of People Living with HIV/AIDS and the Manipur Network of Positive People file at the Kolkata patent office in India a pre-grant opposition to GSK's patent application for AZT/3TC (Combivir).
2006	(May) Novartis sues the Indian government over its amended Patents Act, attempting to overturn the provision (Section 3d) that establishes higher patentability criteria. The criteria were aimed at only granting patents to highly innovative products, thereby preventing frivolous patenting and "evergreening" of patents.
2006	Establishment of UNITAID, a new mechanism for the purchase of medicines, financed by a tax on airline tickets.
2006	WHO Commission on Intellectual Property Rights, Innovation and Public Health publishes its report, leading the World Health Assembly to establish the Intergovernmental Working Group on Public Health, Innovation and Intellectual Property (IGWG).
2006	(August) GSK withdraws its patents and patent applications on AZT/3TC (Combivir) in India, Thailand and other developing country markets.
2006	Thailand issues a compulsory license for the AIDS drug efavirenz.
2006–2008	IGWG negotiations take place in Geneva.
2007	(January) Thailand issues CL for the AIDS drug lopinavir/ritonavir and the heart disease drug clopidogrel
2007	(May) Brazil issues a compulsory license for efavirenz.
2007	(July) Rwanda notifies the WTO that it intends to use the "August 30" system to import medicines produced under a compulsory license.
2007	(October) In the first use of the "August 30th" system, Canada issues a compulsory license for the production of a triple fixed-dose combination ARV for export to Rwanda.
2008	(January) Thailand issues compulsory licenses for four anti-cancer drugs: docetaxel, letrozole, erlotinib, imatinib.
2008	World Health Assembly adopts the Global Strategy and Plan of Action on Public Health, Innovation and Intellectual Property drawn up by the IGWG.
2008	UNITAID Board decides, in principle, to set up a patent pool for AIDS medicines.

References

Abbott, F. M. (2005). The WTO Medicines Decision: World Pharmaceutical Trade and the Protection of Public Health. *The American Journal of International Law*, *99*(2), 317–358.

Abbott, F. M. (2006). *TRIPS II, Asia and the Mercantile Pharmaceutical War: Implications for Innovation and Access* (Draft paper for the Conference on Economic Challenges in Asia, Stanford Center for International Development). Retrieved from http://www.stanford.edu/group/siepr/cgi-bin/siepr/?q=system/files/shared/pubs/papers/pdf/SCID308.pdf.

Abbott, F. M. (2009). Seizure of Generic Pharmaceuticals in Transit Based on Allegations of Patent Infringement: A Threat to International Trade, Development and Public Welfare. *World Intellectual Property Organization Journal (WIPO)*, Vol. 1, p. 43, 2009. Retrieved from http://ssrn.com/paper=1535521.

Abbott, F. M., Correa, C. M. and Biadgleng, E. T. (2007). *World Trade Organization Accession Agreements: Intellectual Property Issues* (Global Economic Issues Publication. Geneva: Quaker United Nations Office). Retrieved from http://www.quno.org/geneva/pdf/economic/Issues/WTO-IP-English.pdf.

Adelman, C. C. and Norris, J. (2004). *Myths and Realities on Prices of Drugs*. Washington, DC: The Hudson Institute. Retrieved from http://www.hudson.org/files/publications/AdelmanARVWhitePaper.pdf.

Adler, E. and Haas, P. M. (1992). Conclusion: Epistemic Communities, World Order, and the Creation of a Reflective Research Program. *International Organization*, *46*(01), 367. doi: 10.1017/S0020818300001533.

Agence France Press (AFP). (2009, 28 October). Firms Accept Ecuador Plan to Break Pharma Patents. Retrieved from http://www.google.com/hostednews/afp/article/ALeqM5gQ3gR0DaSBmVlSg-luegX4ziFtDQ.

Allen, T., Levin, S., Waxman, H., et al. (2007). *Letter to Susan Schwab*. Retrieved from http://www.cptech.org/ip/health/c/thailand/congressional-schwabletter-thailand-10jan06.pdf.

Alter, K. J. and Meunier, S. (2009). The Politics of International Regime Complexity. *Perspectives on Politics*, *7*(1), 13. doi: 10.1017/S1537592709090033. Retrieved from http://journals.cambridge.org/action/displayAbstract?fromPage=online&aid=3998488&fulltextType=BT&fileId=S1537592709090033RD.

Amendment of the TRIPS Agreement – Second Extension of the Period for the Acceptance by Members of the Protocol Amending the TRIPS Agreement. WT/L/785 U.S.C. (2009).

American University Program on Information Justice and Intellectual Property. (2011). *Trans-Pacific Partnership Agreement.* Retrieved from http://www.wcl. american.edu/pijip/go/tpp.

Anderson, B. (1983). *Imagined Communities: Reflections on the Origin and Spread of Nationalism.* London: Verso.

Anheier, H., Glasius, M. and Kaldor, M. (eds) (2004). *Global Civil Society Yearbook 2004/05.* Oxford: Oxford University Press.

Appelbaum, R. P., Felstiner, W. L. and Gessner, V. (eds) (2001). *Rules and Networks: The Legal Culture of Global Business Transactions.* Oxford: Hart Publishing.

Arts, B., Noortmann, M. and Reinalda, B. (eds) (2001). *Non-State Actors in International Relations.* Aldershot: Ashgate.

AstraZeneca. (2010). *AstraZeneca Corporate Responsibility-Dedicated TB Research.* Retrieved from http://www.astrazeneca.com/about-us/?itemId=7537 532.

Baker, D. (2004). *Financing Drug Research: What are the Issues?* (Submission to the WHO Commission on Intellectual Property, Innovation and Public Health. Issue Brief). Washington, DC: Center for Economic and Policy Research. Retrieved from http://www.who.int/intellectualproperty/news/en/Submission-Baker.pdf.

Baker, G. and Chandler, D. (eds) (2005). *Global Civil Society: Contested Futures.* London: Routledge.

Bale, H. (1999). *IFPMA Position on Compulsory Licensing* Treatment Access Forum Listserve. Retrieved from http://lists.essential.org/pharm-policy/msg 00060.html.

Banerjee, A., Hollis, A. and Pogge, T. (2010). The Health Impact Fund: Incentives for Improving Access to Medicines. *The Lancet, 375*(9709), 166–169. doi: 10.1016/S0140-6736(09)61296-4.

Barbosa-Filho, N. H. (2008). Inflation Targeting in Brazil: 1999–2006. *International Review of Applied Economics, 22*(2), 187. Retrieved from http:// www.informaworld.com/10.1080/02692170701880684.

Barnett, M. and Duvall, R. (2005). Power in Global Governance. In M. Barnett and R. Duvall (eds), *Power in Global Governance* (pp. 1–32). New York: Cambridge University Press.

Bartlett, C., Kickbusch, I. and Coulombier, D. (2006). *Cultural and Governance Influence on Detection, Identification and Monitoring of Human Disease.* (Infectious Diseases: Preparing for the Future) Foresight Project. Retrieved from http://www.foresight.gov.uk/Infectious%20Diseases/d4_3.pdf.

Bartsch, S. and Kohlmorgen, L. (2007a). The Role of Civil Society Organizations in Global Health Governance. In W. Hein, S. Bartsch and L. Kohlmorgen (eds), *Global Health Governance and the Fight Against HIV/AIDS* (pp. 92–118). Basingstoke: Palgrave Macmillan.

Bartsch, S. and Kohlmorgen, L. (2007b). *The Role of Southern Actors in Global Governance* (GIGA Working Paper No. 46). Hamburg: German Institute of Global and Area Studies.

Bartsch, S., Huckel Schneider, C. and Kohlmorgen, L. (2009). Governance Norms in Global Health: Key Concepts. In K. Buse, W. Hein and N. Drager (eds), *Making Sense of Global Governance: A Policy Perspective* (pp. 99–121). Basingstoke: Palgrave Macmillan.

Beck, U. and Lau, C. (2004). *Entgrenzung und Entscheidung*. Frankfurt: Suhrkamp.

Bell, C., Devarajan, S. and Gersbach, H. (2004). Thinking about the Long-Run Economic Costs of AIDS. In M. Haacker (ed.), *The Macroeconomics of HIV/AIDS* (pp. 96–133). Washington, DC: International Monetary Fund.

Berkman, A., Garcia, J., Munoz-Laboy, M., et al. (2005). A Critical Analysis of the Brazilian Response to HIV/AIDS: Lessons Learned for Controlling and Mitigating the Epidemic in Developing Countries. *American Journal of Public Health, 95*(7), 1162–1172. doi: 10.2105/AJPH.2004.054593.

Bermann, G. A. and Mavroidis, P. C. (eds) (2006). *Trade and Human Health and Safety*. New York: Cambridge University Press.

Bermudez, J. and 't Hoen, E. (2010). The UNITAID Patent Pool Initiative: Bringing Patents Together for the Common Good. *The Open AIDS Journal, 4*, 37–40. doi: 10.2174/1874613601004020037. Retrieved from http://www.ncbi.nlm.nih.gov/pmc/articles/PMC2842943/?tool=pmcentrez.

Berndt, E. R., Glennerster, R., Kremer, M. R., et al. (2007). Advance Market Commitments for Vaccines against Neglected Diseases: Estimating Costs and Effectiveness. *Health Economics, 16*(5), 491–511. doi: 10.1002/hec.1176.

Berridge, V., Loughlin, K. and Herring R. (2009). Historical Dimensions of Global Health Governance. In K. Buse, W. Hein and N. Drager (eds), *Making Sense of Global Health Governance: A Policy Perspective* (pp. 28–46). Basingstoke: Palgrave Macmillan.

Betz, J. (2002). Maßnahmen Gegen Kinderarbeit: Nützliches Und Weniger Nützliches. *Peripherie. Zeitschrift für Politik und Ökonomie in der Dritten Welt, 22*(85/86), 144–161.

Bhatiasevi, A. and Maneerungsee, W. (February 2, 2000). HIV/AIDS-Compulsory ddI Licensing Seen Unlikely. *The Bangkok Post*.

Bliss, K. (2010). *Key Players in Global Health. How Brazil, Russia, India, China, and South Africa are Influencing the Game*. Washington, DC: Center for Strategic and International Studies.

Blouin, C., Chopra, M. and van der Hoeven, R. (2009). Trade and Social Determinants of Health. *The Lancet, 373*(9662), 502–507. doi: 10.1016/S0140-6736(08)61777-8.

Blouin, C., Drager, N. and Smith, R. (eds) (2006). *International Trade in Health Services and the GATS: Current Issues and Debates*. Washington, DC: The World Bank.

Bodansky, D. and Crook, J. R. (2002). Symposium: The ILC's State Responsibility Articles. *The American Journal of International Law*, *96*, 773–791. http://www.asil.org/ajil/ilcsymp1.pdf.

Böhringer, C. and Frondel, M. (2002). *Assessing Voluntary Commitments: Monitoring is Not Enough* (Discussion Paper 02–62). Mannheim: Zentrum für Europäische Wirtschaftsforschung.

Boyd, B., Henning, N., Reyna, E., et al. (2009). *Hybrid Organizations. New Business Models for Environmental Leadership*. Sheffield: Greenleaf.

Bradsher, K. (October 12, 2005). Roche Faces Pressure over Birdflu Medicine. *The New York Times*. Retrieved from http://www.nytimes.com/2005/10/11/health/11iht-tamiflu.html.

Braithwaite, J. and Drahos, P. (2000). *Global Business Regulation*. New York: Cambridge University Press.

Braudel, F. (1958). Histoire et Sciences sociales. La longue duree. *Annales. Économies, Sociétés, Civilisations*, *13*, 4, 725–753.

Brown, T. M., Cueto, M. and Fee, E. (2006). The World Health Organization and the Transition from "International" to "Global" Public Health. *American Journal of Public Health*, *96*(1), 62–72. doi: 10.2105/AJPH.2004.050831, http://www.ajph.org/cgi/content/abstract/96/1/62.

Buckley, S. (September 17, 2000). Brazil Becomes Model in Fight Against AIDS; Government, Activists Team to Defy Epidemic through Distribution of Drugs. *The Washington Post*, pp. A22.

Burris, S. (2004). Governance, Microgovernance and Health, in *Temple Law Review*, *77*, 343–362. Retrieved from http://www.ilazarte.com.ar/epss/mt-static/archives/documentos/Microgovernance_Burris.pdf.

Burris, S. C., Drahos, P. and Shearing, C. D. (2005). Nodal Governance. *Australian Journal of Legal Philosophy*, *30*.

Burris, S., Kempa, M. and Shearing, C. (2008). Changes in Governance: A Cross-Disciplinary Review of Current Scholarship. *Akron Law Review*, *41*(1), 1–66.

Busby, J. (2006). *From Benign Neglect to Moral Awakening: Donor Responses to HIV/AIDS* Centre for Globalisation and Governance, Princeton University.

Buse, K. and Walt, G. (2002). Globalisation and Multilateral Public-Private Health Partnerships: Issues for Health Policy. In K. Lee, K. Buse and S. Fustukian (eds), *Health Policy in a Globalising World* (pp. 41–62). Cambridge: Cambridge University Press.

Calcagnotto, G. (2007). Consensus-Building on Brazilian HIV/AIDS Policy: National and Global Interfaces in Health Governance. In Hein, W., Bartsch, S. and Kohlmorgen, L. (eds), *Global Health Governance and the Fight Against HIV/AIDS* (pp. 172–201).

Cancer Patients Aid Association (CPAA), Lawyers Collective HIV/AIDS Unit, Delhi Network for Positive People (DNP+) and Médecins Sans Frontières (August 7, 2000). *Joint Statement by CPAA, MSF, DNP+ and Lawyers Collective on Novartis Judgment*. Retrieved from http://keionline.org/content/view/120/1.

Cardoso, F. H. (1999). In Serra J., Lopes Tápias A. (eds), *Presidential Decree on Compulsory Licensing: Decree 3.201 of October 6, 1999* [Decreto no.3.201 de 06 de Outubro de 1999]. Brasilia. Retrieved from http://www.cptech.org/ip/health/c/brazil/PresDecree.html.

Cawthorne, P., Ford, N., Limpananont, J., et al. (2007). WHO must Defend Patients' Interests, Not Industry. *The Lancet, 369*(9566), 974–975. doi: 10.1016/S0140-6736(07)60473-5,

Cernuschi, T. (2009). Pneumococcal AMC. *Tropical Medicine and International Health, 14*, 103–104.

Champ, P. and Attaran, A. (2002). Patent Rights and Local Working Under the WTO TRIPS Agreement: An Analysis of the U.S.–Brazil Patent Dispute. *The Yale Journal of International Law, 27*, 365.

Chan, M. (February 7, 2007). *Letter to Dr. Mongkol Na Songkhla.* Retrieved from http://lists.essential.org/pipermail/ip-health/2007-February/010538.html.

Chaudhuri, S. (2010). The Indian Pharmaceutical Industry after TRIPS. In Chaudhuri, S., Park, C. and Gopakumar, K.M. (eds), Five Years into the Product Patent Regime: India's Response (pp. 19–72). New York: UNDP.

Chee, Y. L. (2006). Malaysia: 'Government use' Route to Importing Generic Medicines. *Third World Resurgence, 196.*

Chen, L. C., Evans, T. G. and Cash, R. A. (1999). Health as a Global Public Good. In I. Kaul, I. Grunberg and M. A. Stern (eds), *Global Public Goods: International Cooperation in the 21st Century* (pp. 284–304). Oxford and New York: Oxford University Press.

Chequer, P., Cuchí, P., Mazin, R. and García Calleja, J. M. (2000). Access to Antiretroviral Treatment in Latin American Countries and the Caribbean. *AIDS, 16*(Supplement 3), S50–S57.

Chien, C. V. (2007). HIV/AIDS Drugs for Sub-Saharan Africa: How do Brand and Generic Supply Compare? *PLoS ONE, 2*(3), e278. doi: 10.1371/journal.pone.0000278, http://dx.doi.org/10.1371/journal.pone.0000278.

Chow, J. (2010). Is the WHO Becoming Irrelevant? *Foreign Policy*, December 8. Retrieved from http://www.foreignpolicy.com/articles/2010/12/08/is_the_who_becoming_irrelevant.

Clapham, A., Robinson, M., Mahon, C. and Jerbi, S. (2009). *Realizing the Right to Health. Swiss Human Rights Book* (Vol. 3, ed.). Zurich: rüffer&rub.

Clapham, A. (2006). *Human Rights Obligations of Non-State Actors.* Oxford: Oxford University Press.

Clinton, W. J. (1999). Remarks at a World Trade Organization Luncheon in Seattle (December 1, 1999). *Weekly Compilation of Presidential Documents, 35*, 2494–2497.

Clinton, W. J. (2000). *Executive Order no 13155.*

Coleman, M. P., Quaresma, M., Berrino, F., et al. (2008). Cancer survival in five continents: A worldwide population-based study (CONCORD) [Abstract]. *The Lancet Oncology, 9*(8) 730–756.

Commission on Intellectual Property Rights, Innovation and Public Health (CIPIH). (2006). *Public Health, Innovation and Intellectual Property Rights.* Geneva: World Health Organization (WHO). Retrieved from http://www.who. int/intellectualproperty/report/en/index.html.

Commission on Macroeconomics and Health. (2001). *Macroeconomics and Health: Investing in Health for Economic Development.* Geneva: World Health Organization. Retrieved from http://whqlibdoc.who.int/publications /2001/924154550x.pdf.

Commission on Social Determinants of Health. (2008). *Closing the Gap in a Generation: Health Equity through Action on the Social Determinants of Health.* (Final Report of the Commission on Social Determinants of Health). Geneva: World Health Organization. Retrieved from http://whqlibdoc.who.int/ publications/2008/9789241563703_eng.pdf.

Committee on Economic, Social and Cultural Rights. (2000). *General Comment no. 14: The Right to the Highest Attainable Standard of Health* (E/C.12/2000/4, ed.). United Nations Economic and Social Council. Retrieved from http:// www.unhchr.ch/tbs/doc.nsf/%28Symbol%29/40d009901358b0e2c125691500 5090be?Opendocument.

Consumer Project on Technology. (2007). *Thailand: Compulsory Licensing Dispute.* Retrieved from http://www.cptech.org/ip/health/c/thailand/.

Coomans, F. (2005). Progressive Development of International Human Rights Law: Extraterritorial Application of the International Covenant on Economic, Social and Cultural Rights. In M. Windfuhr (ed.), *Beyond the Nation State: Human Rights in Times of Globalization* (pp. 33–50). Uppsala: Global Publications Foundation.

Cooper, H., Zimmerman, R. and McGinley, L. (2001, 2 March). Patents Pending: AIDS Epidemic Traps Drug Firms in a Vise: Treatment Vs. Profits – Suit in South Africa Seeks to Block Generic Copies; U.S. Reverses its Policy – Activists Warn Mr. Papovich. *The Wall Street Journal*, pp. A1.

Cooper, W. H. (2010). *Free Trade Agreements: Impact on US Trade and Implications for US Trade Policy*, No. RL31356 (Updated February 23, 2010). Washington, DC: Congressional Research Service. Retrieved from http:// assets.opencrs.com/rpts/RL31356_20100223.pdf.

Correa, C. M. (2002a). *Implications of the Doha Declaration on the TRIPS Agreement and Public Health* (Health Economics and Drugs EDM Series No. 12). Geneva: World Health Organization. Retrieved from http://apps.who.int/ medicinedocs/en/d/Js2301e/.

Correa, C. M. (2002b). *Protection of Data Submitted for the Registration of Pharmaceuticals: Implementing the Standards of the TRIPS Agreement.* Geneva: The South Centre.

Correa, C. M. (2004). *Bilateral Investment Agreements: Agents of New Global Standards for the Protection of Intellectual Property Rights?* GRAIN. Retrieved from http://www.grain.org/briefings/?id=186.

Correa, C. M. (2006). Implications of Bilateral Free Trade Agreements on Access to Medicines. *Bulletin of the World Health Organization, 84*, 399–404.

Datta, P. T. J. (April 12, 2010). CSIR Open-Source Project for TB Democratises Research. *The Hindu Business Line.* Retrieved from http://www.thehindu businessline.com/2010/04/13/stories/2010041353180200.htm.

David, P. A. (1993). Intellectual Property Institutions and the Panda's Thumb: Patents, Copyrights, and Trade Secrets in Economic Theory and History. In Wallerstein, M. B., Mogee, M. E. and Schoen, R. A. (eds), *Global Dimensions of Intellectual Property Rights in Science and Technology.* The National Academies Press.

de Gucht, K. (DG Trade). (May 5, 2010). *Letter to Mr. Von Schoen-Angerer on the EU-India FTA* European Commission, Directorate-General Trade. Retrieved from http://trade.ec.europa.eu/doclib/docs/2010/may/tradoc_146192.pdf.

Dean, M. (1999). *Governmentality: Power and Rule in Modern Society.* London: Sage.

Deere, C. (2008). *The Implementation Game: The TRIPS Agreement and the Global Politics of Intellectual Property Reform in Developing Countries.* Oxford: Oxford University Press.

Denny, C. and Meek, J. (April 19, 2001). Drug Giants made to Swallow Bitter Pill. *The Guardian.* Retrieved from http://www.guardian.co.uk/world/2001/apr/19/ highereducation.aids.

DFID. (2005). *Increasing People's Access to Essential Medicines in Developing Countries: A Framework for Good Practice in the Pharmaceutical Industry.* London: Department for International Development (DFID). Retrieved from http://www.accesstomedicineindex.org/sites/www.accesstomedicineindex. org/files/publication/dfid_2005.pdf.

DiMasi, J. A., Hansen, R. W. and Grabowski, H. A. (2003). The Price of Innovation: New Estimates of Drug Development Costs. *The Journal of Health Economics, 22*, 151–185.

DiMasi, J. and Grabowski, H. (2004). *Patents and R&D Incentives: Comments on the Hubbard and Love Trade Framework for Financing Pharmaceutical R&D.* Paper submitted to the WHO Commission on Intellectual Property, Innovation and Public Health. Retrieved from http://www.who.int/intellectualproperty/ news/en/Submission3.pdf.

Djelic, M. and Quack, S. (2010). Transnational Communities and Governance. In M. Djelic and S. Quack (eds), *Transnational Communities Shaping Global Economic Governance* (pp. 3–36). Cambridge: Cambridge University Press.

Dodd, R., Schieber, G., Cassels, A., et al. (2007). *Aid Effectiveness and Health.* Working Paper No. 9; WHO/HSS/healthsystems/2007.2. Geneva: World Health Organization.

Drahos, P. (2001). Bits and Bips. *The Journal of World Intellectual Property, 4*(6), 791–808. doi: 10.1111/j.1747-1796.2001.tb00138.x, http://dx.doi.org/10.1111 /j.1747-1796.2001.tb00138.x.

Drahos, P. (2002). *Developing Countries and International Intellectual Property Standard-Setting* (Study Paper 8). Commission on Intellectual Property Rights. http://www.iprcommission.org/graphic/documents/study_papers.htm.

Drahos, P. (2003). *Expanding Intellectual Property's Empire: The Role of FTAs.* Geneva: GRAIN. Retrieved from http://www.grain.org/rights/TRIPSplus.cfm?id=28.

Drahos, P. (2004). Intellectual Property and Pharmaceutical Markets: A Nodal Governance Approach. *Temple Law Review, 77*, 247–289.

Drahos, P. and Braithwaite, J. (2002). *Information Feudalism: Who Owns the Knowledge Economy?* New York: The New Press.

Drezner, D. W. (2006). *The Race to the Bottom Hypothesis: An Empirical and Theoretical Review.* The Fletcher School, Tufts University (unpublished paper). Retrieved from http://www.danieldrezner.com/archives/003076.html.

Drezner, D. W. (2007). *All Politics is Global: Explaining International Regulatory Regimes.* Princeton, NJ: Princeton University Press.

Drezner, D. W. (2009). The Power and Peril of International Regime Complexity. *Perspectives on Politics, 7*(01), 65. doi: 10.1017/S1537592709090100. Retrieved from http://journals.cambridge.org/action/displayAbstract?fromPage=online&aid=3998572&fulltextType=BT&fileId=S1537592709090100RD.

Dugger, C. W. (May 9, 2007). Clinton Foundation Announces a Bargain on Generic AIDS Drugs. *The New York Times*, p. 9.

Dunning, J. H. (1999). A Business Analytic Approach to Governments and Globalization. In Dunning, J. H. (ed.), *Governments, Globalization, and International Business* (pp. 114–131). Oxford: Oxford University Press.

Durkheim, E. (1982 [1895]). *Rules of Sociological Method.* New York: Free Press.

England, R. (2007). Are we Spending Too Much on HIV? *British Medical Journal, 334.*

Enserink, M. (2006). Oseltamivir becomes Plentiful – but Still Not Cheap. *Science, 312*(5772), 382–383. doi: 10.1126/science.312.5772.382. Retrieved from http://www.sciencemag.org.

Epstein, S. (1996). *Impure Science: AIDS, Activism, and the Politics of Knowledge.* Berkeley: University of California Press.

European Commission. (2010). *Trade: Creating Opportunities: Bilateral Relations.* Retrieved from http://ec.europa.eu/trade/creating-opportunities/bilateral-relations/regions/.

European Commission, Directorate General 1. (1998). *Note for the Attention of the 113 Committee (Deputies) Subject: WTO TRIPS/World Health Organisation (WHO) – Revised Drug Strategy; Meeting of the "Ad Hoc Working Group" on 13 to 16 October 1998.* Brussels: European Commission, Directorate General 1: External relations: Commercial Policy and Relations with North America, the Far East, Australia and New Zealand.

European Commission, Directorate Trade. (2009). *The Anti-Counterfeiting Agreement (ACTA): Fact Sheet.* Retrieved from http://trade.ec.europa.eu/doclib/docs/2009/january/tradoc_142039.pdf.

European Commission, Directorate Trade. (2010). *EU-India FTA Negotiations and Access to Medicines: Questions and Answers.* Brussels: European Commission. Retrieved from http://trade.ec.europa.eu/doclib/docs/2010/may/tradoc_146191.pdf.

European Parliament. TRIPS Agreement and Access to Medicines, Resolution P6_TA(2007) 0353. (2007). Retrieved from http://www.europarl.europa.eu/sides/getDoc.do?type=TA&reference=P6-TA-2007-0353&language=EN&ring=B6-2007-0288.

Fairclough, N. (1993). *Discourse and Social Change.* Oxford: Blackwell Publishers.

Falk, R. (1995). Liberalism at the Global Level: The Last of the Independent Commissions? *Millennium – Journal of International Studies, 24,* 563–576.

Farmer, P., Frenk, J., Knaul, F. M., et al. (2010). Expansion of cancer care and control in countries of low and middle income: A call to action [Abstract]. *The Lancet, 376*(9747) 1186–1193.

Ferlay, J., Shin, H., Bray, F., et al. (2010). Estimates of Worldwide Burden of Cancer in 2008: GLOBOCAN 2008. *International Journal of Cancer, 127*(12), 2893–2917.

Fidler, D. (2007). Architecture Amidst Anarchy: Global Health's Quest for Governance. *Global Health Governance, 1*(1). Retrieved from http://www.ghgj.org/Fidler_Architecture.pdf.

Fidler, D. P. (2008a). Influenza Virus Samples, International Law, and Global Health Diplomacy. *Emerging Infectious Diseases, 14*(1), 88–94. doi: 10.3201/eid1401.070700.

Fidler, D. P. (2008b). A Theory of Open-Source Anarchy. *Indiana Journal of Global Legal Studies, 15*(1), Article 11. Retrieved from http://www.repository.law.indiana.edu/ijgls/vol15/iss1/11.

Fink, C. and Maskus, K. E. (2005). *Intellectual Property and Development: Lessons from Recent Economic Research.* Washington, DC: World Bank; New York: Oxford University Press.

Fink, S. and Rabinowitz, R. (2011). The UN's Battle with NCDs: How Politics, Commerce, and Science Complicated the Fight Against an "Invisible Epidemic". *Foreign Affairs* (September), http://www.foreignaffairs.com/print/68197.

Finkelstein, S. N. and Temin, P. (2008). *Reasonable Rx: Solving the Drug Price Crisis.* Upper Saddle River, NJ: FT Press/Pearson Education.

Finnemore, M. (1996). Norms, Culture, and World Politics: Insights from Sociology's Institutionalism, *International Organization, 50*(2), 325–347.

Finnemore, M. and Sikkink, K. (1998). International Norm Dynamics and Political Change. *International Organization, 52*(4), 887–917.

Fischer-Lescano, A. and Liste, P. (2005). Völkerrechtspolitik. Zu Trennung und Verknüpfung von Politik und Recht in der Weltgesellschaft. *Zeitschrift Für Internationale Beziehungen, 12*(2), 209–249. Retrieved from http://www.zib.nomos.de/fileadmin/zib/doc/ZIB_05_02.pdf.

Florini, A. and Sovacool, B. K. (2009). Who Governs Energy? The Challenges Facing Global Energy Governance. *Energy Policy, 37*, 5239–5248.

Flynn, S. (2008). *Using Competition Law to Promote Access to Medicines.* Washington, DC: American University, Washington College of Law: Program on Information Justice and Intellectual Property. Retrieved from http://www.ggp.up.ac.za/human_rights_access_to_medicines/syllabus/2009/day3/3Flynn UsingCompetitionLawtoPromoteAccesstoMedicin.pdf.

Flynn, S. M. (2010). Special 301 of the Trade Act of 1974 and Global Access to Medicines. *Journal of Generic Medicines, 7*, 309–333.

Ford, N., Wilson, D., Bunjumnong, O. and von Schoen Angerer, T. (2004). The Role of Civil Society in Protecting Public Health Over Commercial Interests: Lessons from Thailand. *The Lancet, 363*(9408), 560–563. doi: 10.1016/S0140-6736(04)15545-1,

Furtado, C. (1970). *Economic Development of Latin America.* Cambridge: Cambridge University Press.

Gaventa, J. and Tandon, R. (2010). *Globalizing Citizens: New Dynamics of Inclusion and Exclusion.* London: Zed Books.

GAVI Alliance Secretariat. (2010). *Advance Market Commitment for Pneumococcal Vaccines: Annual Report 12 June 2009–31 March 2010.* Geneva.

Gehl Sampath, P. (2008). *India's Pharmaceutical Sector in 2008: Emerging Strategies and Global and Local Implications for Access to Medicines.* London: DFID. Retrieved from www.dfid.gov.uk/Documents/publications/indiapatentreport.pdf.

George, J., Sheshadri, R. and Grover, A. (2009). India: Intellectual Property and Access to Medicines: Developments and Civil Society Initiatives in India. In R. Reis, V. Terto Jr. and M. C. Pimenta (eds), *Intellectual Property Rights and Access to ARV Medicines: Civil Society Resistance in the Global South* (pp. 110–136). Rio de Janeiro: Brazilian Interdisciplinary AIDS Association (ABIA).

Gereffi, G. (1983). *The Pharmaceutical Industry and Dependency in the Third World.* Princeton, NJ: Princeton University Press.

Gerhardsen, T. I. S. (February 16, 2007). Drug Company Reacts to Thai License; Government Ready to Talk. *Intellectual Property Watch (IP Watch).* Retrieved from http://www.ip-watch.org/weblog/2007/02/16/drug-company-upset-by-newest-thai-license-government-open-to-dialogue/.

Giridharadas, A. (November 30, 2006). Clinton's Foundation Brokers AIDS Deal. *The New York Times.* Retrieved from http://www.nytimes.com/2006/11/30/world/asia/01aidscnd.html.

Glassman, J. (2004). *The Real Obstacle to Treating AIDS, Malaria, and Tuberculosis in Developing Countries. Introductory Remarks.* Washington, DC: American Enterprise Institute for Public Policy Research. Retrieved from http://www.aei.org/speech/health/the-real-obstacles-to-treating-aids-malaria-and-tuberculosis-in-developing-countries-speech/.

GlaxoSmithKline (2007). *GlaxoSmithKline Launches Chinese Research Center with Appointment of Head in Shanghai.* Retrieved from http://www.gsk-china. com/asp/News/client/newconten/5242007105329.htm.

GlaxoSmithKline (2009a). *Big Pharma as a Catalyst for Change.* Speech by GSK CEO Andrew Witty at Harvard Medical School, February 13, 2009. Retrieved from http://www.gsk.com/media/Witty-Harvard-Speech-Summary.pdf.

GlaxoSmithKline (2009b). *GlaxoSmithKline Statement in Response to Paul Hunt's Report on GSK.*

Global Alliance for TB Drug Development (GATB). (November 7, 2008). A Global Effort to Reduce the Costs of a TB Drug Candidate. *TB Alliance Newscenter.*

Glyn, A. and Sutcliffe, B. (1972). *British Capitalism, Workers and the Profit Squeeze.* Harmondswoth: Penguin.

Goldstein, J. L., Kahler, M., Keohane, R. O. and Slaughter, A. (eds) (2001). *Legalization and World Politics.* Cambridge, MA: MIT Press.

Governments of Bangladesh, Barbados, Bolivia and Suriname. (2009). *Chagas Disease Prize Fund for the Development of New Treatments, Diagnostics and Vaccines.* World Health Organization. Retrieved from http://www.who.int/phi/ Bangladesh_Barbados_Bolivia_Suriname_ChagasPrize.pdf.

Governments of Bolivia and Suriname. (April 5, 2010). Submission by the Governments of Bolivia and Suriname (on the WHO EWG Report).

Grace, C. (2004). *Leveraging the Private Sector for Public Health Objectives: A Briefing Paper for DFID on Technology Transfer in the Pharmaceuticals Sector.* DFID Health Systems Resource Centre. Retrieved from http://www. dfidhealthrc.org/publications/atm/India%20China%20ATM.pdf.

Grace, C. (2005). *A Briefing Paper for DFID: Update on China and India and Access to Medicines.*

Grant, A. D. and De Cock, K. M. (2001). HIV Infection and AIDS in the Developing World. *British Medical Journal, 322,* 1475–1478.

Grover, A. (2009). *Report of the Special Rapporteur on the Right of Everyone to the Enjoyment of the Highest Attainable Standard of Physical and Mental Health, Anand Grover* (A/HRC/11/12). United Nations Human Rights Council.

Grover, A. (2011). *Report of the Special Rapporteur on the Right of Everyone to the Enjoyment of the Highest Attainable Standard of Physical and Mental Health: Expert Consultation on Access to Medicines as a Fundamental Component of the Right to Health* (A/HRC/17/43). Geneva: United Nations Human Rights Council. Retrieved from http://daccess-dds-ny.un.org/doc/UNDOC/GEN/ G11/118/42/PDF/G1111842.pdf?OpenElement.

Hanim, L. and Jhamtani, H. (2006). Indonesia: Manufacturing Generic AIDS Medicines Under the 'Government use' Approach. *Third World Resurgence, 196.*

Harris, G. (September 18, 2011). China and India Making Inroads on Biotech Drugs. *The New York Times.* Retrieved from http://www.nytimes.com/2011/09/19/ health/policy/19drug.html.

Hart, H. L. A. (1961 [1997]). *The Concept of Law* (2nd ed.). Oxford University Press: Clarendon.

Hart, H. L. A. (1973). *Essays on Bentham: Jurisprudence and Political Theory.* Oxford: Oxford University Press.

Health GAP et al. (December 16, 2004). *Open Letter to Dr. Manmohan Singh, Prime Minister of India.* Retrieved from http://www.healthgap.org/press_releases/04/121604_HGAP_LTR_India_patent.pdf.

Health Global Access Project (Health GAP). (2010). *Allegation Letter to the United Nations Special Rapporteur on the Right to Health: In the Matter of use of the 'Special 301' Program, Section 182 of the Trade Act of 1974, to Limit Access to Medicines in Violation of the International Right to Health.* Retrieved from http://www.healthgap.org/documents/ComplainttoSpecialRapporteur-1.pdf.

Hecht, R., Bollinger, L., Stover, J., et al. (2009). Critical Choices in Financing the Response to the Global HIV/AIDS Pandemic. *Health Affairs, 28*(6), 1591–1605.

Hein, W. and Kickbusch, I. (2010). *Global Health, Aid Effectiveness and the Changing Role of the WHO* (GIGA Focus International Edition, No. 3). Hamburg: German Institute of Global and Area Studies.

Hein, W. and Kohlmorgen, L. (2008). Global Health Governance: Conflicts on Global Social Rights. *Global Social Policy, 8*(1), 80–108.

Hein, W., Bartsch, S. and Kohlmorgen, L. (eds) (2007). *Global Health Governance and the Fight Against HIV/AIDS.* Basingstoke: Palgrave Macmillan.

Hein, W., Burris, S. and Shearing, C. (2009). Conceptual Models for Global Health Governance. In K. Buse, W. Hein and N. Drager (eds), *Making Sense of Global Health Governance: A Policy Perspective* (pp. 72–98). Basingstoke: Palgrave Macmillan.

Held, D. (1995). *Democracy and the Global Order: From the Modern State to Cosmopolitan Governance.* Oxford: Polity Press.

Held, D., McGrew, A., Goldblatt, D. and Perraton, J. (1999). *Global Transformations: Politics, Economics and Culture.* Cambridge: Polity Press.

Helfer, L. R. (2004). Regime Shifting: The TRIPs Agreement and New Dynamics of International Intellectual Property Lawmaking. *The Yale Journal of International Law, 29*, 1.

Helfer, L. R. (2009). Regime Shifting in the International Intellectual Property System. *Perspectives on Politics, 7*(01), 39. doi: 10.1017/S1537592709090069. Retrieved from http://journals.cambridge.org/action/displayAbstract?fromPage=online&aid=3998524&fulltextType=BT&fileId=S1537592709090069RD.

Henkin, L. (1995). *International Law. Politics and Values.* Doordrecht: Nijhoff Publishers.

Hirschler, B. (November 8, 2010). China seen as no. 2 Drugs Market by 2015. *Reuters,* http://uk.reuters.com/article/2010/11/08/us-summit-china-drugs-idUKTRE6A73SL20101108.

Hoekman, B. and Kostecki, M. (2001). *The Political Economy of the World Trading System – WTO and Beyond.* Oxford: Oxford University Press. doi: http://dx.doi.org/10.1093/019829431X.001.0001.

Hogerzeil, H. V., Samson, M., Casanovas, J. V. and Rahmani-Ocora, L. (2006). Is Access to Essential Medicines as Part of the Fulfilment of the Right to Health Enforceable through the Courts? *The Lancet, 368*(9532), 305–311. doi: 10.1016/S0140-6736(06)69076-4.

Holmes, C. B., Coggin, W., Jamieson, D., et al. (2010). Use of Generic Antiretroviral Agents and Cost Savings in PEPFAR Treatment Programs. *Journal of the American Medical Association, 304*(3), 313–320. doi: 10.1001/jama.2010.993. Retrieved from http://jama.ama-assn.org/cgi/content/full/304/3/313.

Holton, R. J. (2005). *Making Globalization.* Basingstoke: Palgrave.

Hookway, J. (June 18, 2010). Philippines Price Controls Hamper Rise of Generics. *The Wall Street Journal.* Retrieved from http://online.wsj.com/article/SB1000 1424052748703340904575284061202593520.html.

Hubbard, T. and Love, J. (2004a). A New Trade Framework for Global Healthcare R&D. *PLoS Biology, 2*(2), E52. doi: 10.1371/journal.pbio.0020052. Retrieved from http://www.plosbiology.org/article/info%3Adoi%2F10.1371%2Fjournal. pbio.0020052.

Hubbard, T. and Love, J. (2004b). A New Trade Framework for Global Healthcare R&D. *PLoS Biol, 2*(2), e52. Retrieved from http://dx.doi.org.ezp-prod1.hul. harvard.edu/10.1371%2Fjournal.pbio.0020052.

Huckel Schneider, C. (2009a). Global Public Health and Innovation in Governance: The Emergence of Public-Private Partnerships. In S. J. MacLean, P. Fourie and S. A. Brown (eds), *Health for Some* (pp. 105–117). Basingstoke: Palgrave.

Huckel Schneider, C. (2009b). *Legitimacy and Global Governance in Managing Global Public Health.* Unpublished PhD, University of Tübingen. Retrieved from http://tobias-lib.uni-tuebingen.de/volltexte/2010/4526/pdf/ HuckelSchneiderTobiasLib.pdf.

Hunt, P. (2006). *Report of the Special Rapporteur on the Right of Everyone to the Enjoyment of the Highest Attainable Standard of Physical and Mental Health* (A/61/338). United Nations General Assembly. Retrieved from http:// daccess-dds-ny.un.org/doc/UNDOC/GEN/N06/519/97/PDF/N0651997. pdf?OpenElement.

Hunt, P. (2009). *Report of the Special Rapporteur on the Right of Everyone to the Enjoyment of the Highest Attainable Standard of Health, Paul Hunt. Annex: Mission to GlaxoSmithKline* (A/HRC/11/12/Add.2). United Nations Human Rights Council.

Hutter, B. M. (2006). *The Role of Non-State Actors in Regulation.* (CARR Discussion Papers, DP 37). London: Centre for Analysis of Risk and Regulation, London School of Economics and Political Science.

Implementation of Paragraph 6 of the Doha Declaration on the TRIPS Agreement and Public Health, Decision of the General Council of 30 August 2003 U.S.C. (2003).

IMS Health (April 20, 2010). IMS Forecasts Global Pharmaceutical Market Growth of 5–8% Annually through 2014; Maintains Expectations of 4–6% Growth in 2010. *FiercePharma.*

Industria Farmaceutica de Investigacion (IFI) (2009). *Boletin Informativo.*

Inside US Trade (April 15, 2005). Industry Says Indian Drug Law Violates WTO, but no WTO Case seen. *Inside US Trade.* Retrieved from http://www.cptech. org/ip/health/c/india/insideustrade04152005.html.

Intellectual Property Watch (April 21, 2012). Kenya's High Court's Overturning of Anti-Counterfeit Law Hailed. *Intellectual Property Watch.* Retrieved from http://www.ip-watch.org/2012/04/21/kenyan-high-courts-overturning-of-anti-counterfeit-law-hailed/.

International Centre for Trade and Sustainable Development (2011). TRIPS Council: Members Debate Biodiversity, Access to Medicine. *Bridges Weekly Trade News Digest, 15*(8).

International Commission on Intervention and State Sovereignty (2001). *The Responsibility to Protect.* International Development Research Centre.

International Federation of Pharmaceutical Manufacturers and Associations (IFPMA) (March 22, 2005). *Passage of Indian Patent Law: A Step Forward.* Retrieved from www.cptech.org/ip/health/c/india/ifpma03222005.html.

International Federation of Pharmaceutical Manufacturers and Associations (IFPMA) (2007). *Partnerships to Build Healthier Societies in the Developing World.*

International Institute for Sustainable Development (IISD) (2010). *Bilateral Investment Treaties and Regional Agreements.* Retrieved from http://www. iisd.org/investment/bits/.

International Trade Centre (ITC) (2010). *Trade Map: Trade Statistics for International Business Development.* Retrieved from http://www.trademap. org/Index.aspx.

Jenkins, G. W. (2007). Soft Power, Strategic Security, and International Philanthropy. *North Carolina Law Review, 85*(March), 773–846.

Joint United Nations Programme on HIV/AIDS (UNAIDS) (2011). *World AIDS Day Report 2011.* Geneva: UNAIDS. Retrieved from http://www.unaids.org/ en/media/unaids/contentassets/documents/unaidspublication/2011/JC2216_ WorldAIDSday_report_2011_en.pdf.

Joint United Nations Programme on HIV/AIDS (UNAIDS) and World Health Organization (WHO) (2009). *2009 AIDS Epidemic Update* (UNAIDS/09.36E/ JC1700E). Geneva: UNAIDS/WHO. Retrieved from http://data.unaids.org/ pub/Report/2009/JC1700_Epi_Update_2009_en.pdf.

Jones, K. (2009). *The Doha Blues: Institutional Crisis and Reform at the WTO.* Oxford: Oxford University Press.

Kanavos, P., Vandoros, S. and Garcia-Gonzalez, P. (2009). Benefits of Global Partnerships to Facilitate Access to Medicines in Developing Countries: A Multi-Country Analysis of Patients and Patient Outcomes in GIPAP. *Globalization and Health*, *5*(1), 19. Retrieved from http://www.globalizationandhealth.com/content/5/1/19.

Kaul, I. (2003). *Providing Global Public Goods: Managing Globalization*. New York: Published for the United Nations Development Programme by Oxford University Press.

Kazmin, A. and Jack, A. (November 30, 2006). Thailand Breaks Patent for Aids Drug to Cut Costs. *The Financial Times*. Retrieved from http://www.ft.com/cms/s/0/5a5fbfd4-8018-11db-a3be-0000779e2340.html?nclick_check=1.

Keck, M. E. and Sikkink, K. (1998). *Activists Beyond Borders*. Ithaca, NY: Cornell University Press.

Kell, G. and Ruggie, J. G. (1999). Global Markets and Social Legitimacy: The Case for the "Global Compact". *Transnational Corporations*, *8*(3), 101–120.

Kenya Treatment Access Movement (KETAM) and Health Action International Africa (HAI-Africa) (2009). *The Anti-Counterfeit Bill, 2008: Concerns on Access to Medicines for Kenyans* (Briefing Paper). Retrieved from http://www.haiafrica.org/downloads/anti_counterfeit_bill_factsheet.pdf.

Keohane, R. O. and Nye, J. S. (1997). Interdependence in World Politics. In G. T. Crane and A. Amawi (eds), *The Theoretical Evolution of International Political Economy: A Reader*. New York: Oxford University Press.

Khagram, S. (2004). *Dams and Development: Transnational Struggles for Water and Power*. Ithaca, NY: Cornell University Press.

Khagram, S., Riker, J. V. and Sikkink, K. (eds) (2002). *Restructuring World Politics: Transnational Social Movements, Networks, and Norms*. Minneapolis: University of Minnesota Press.

Khor, M. (January 16, 2005). FTA is a 'Matter of Life and Death'. *Global Trends*. Retrieved from http://www.twnside.org.sg/title2/gtrends87.htm.

Khosla, R. and Hunt, P. (2009). *Human Rights Guideline for Pharmaceutical Companies in Relation to Access to Medicines: The Sexual and Reproductive Health Context*. Colchester: University of Essex Human Rights Centre. http://www.essex.ac.uk/human_rights_centre/research/rth/docs/Final_pharma_for_website.pdf.

Kickbusch, I. and Buckett, K. (eds) (2010). *Implementing Health in all Policies: Adelaide 2010*. Government of South Australia.

Kickbusch, I., Hein, W. and Silberschmidt, G. (2010). Addressing Global Health Governance Challenges through a New Mechanism: The Proposal for a Committee C of the World Health Assembly. *Journal of Law, Medicine & Ethics*, *38*, *3*, 550–563, retrieved from http://www.ilonakickbusch.com/global-health-governance/committee-c-2010.pdf.

Kind, R., Smith, A., Tauscher, E., et al. (March 15, 2007). *Letter to Susan C. Schwab*. Retrieved from http://www.cptech.org/ip/health/c/thailand/house03152007.pdf.

Kinderman, D. (2010). Free us so we can do some Corporate Responsibility. *Ökologisches Wirtschaften*, *25*, *1*, 19–20. Retrieved from http://oekologisches-wirtschaften.de/index.php/oew/article/viewFile/680/680.

Kingsbury, K. (November 14, 2007). China's Drug Addiction. *Time.* Retrieved from http://www.time.com/time/business/article/0,8599,1684180,00.html.

Kinney, E. D. and Clark, B. A. (2004). Provisions for Health and Health-Care in the Constitutions of the Countries of the World. *Cornell International Law Journal, 37*, 285–355. Retrieved from http://indylaw.indiana.edu/instructors/ Kinney/Articles/kinney_Constitutions.pdf.

Kirchanski, S. (1993). Protection of US Patent Rights in Developing Countries: US Efforts to Enforce Pharmaceutical Patents in Thailand. *Loyola Los Angeles International and Comparative Law Journal, 16*, 569.

Kohlmorgen, L. (2007). International Governmental Organizations and Global Health Governance: The Role of the World Health Organization, World Bank and UNAIDS. In Hein, W., Bartsch, S. and Kohlmorgen, L. (ed.), *Global Health Governance and the Fight Against HIV/AIDS* (pp. 119–145). Basingstoke: Palgrave Macmillan.

Koivusalo, M. (2003). *The Impact of WTO Agreements on Health and Development Policies* (Policy Brief 3). Helsinki: Globalism and Social Policy Programme. Retrieved from https://gaspp.stakes.fi/NR/rdonlyres/3000F54A-DDCF-48C4-AFFE-056867902724/0/policybrief3.pdf.

Kooiman, J. (2003). *Governing as Governance.* London: Sage.

Koppell, J. G. S. (2001). *The Politics of Quasi-Government: Hybrid Organizations and the Dynamic of Bureaucratic Control.* Cambridge: Cambridge University Press.

Koskenniemi, M. (2007). The Fate of Public International Law: Between Technique and Politics. *The Modern Law Review, 70*(1), 1–30.

Krasner, S. D. (1982). Structural Causes and Regime Consequences: Regimes as Intervening Variables. *International Organization, 36*(2), 185–205.

Laing, R., Waning, B., Gray, A., et al. (2003). 25 Years of the WHO Essential Medicines Lists: Progress and Challenges. *The Lancet, 361*(9370), 1723–1729. doi: 10.1016/S0140-6736(03)13375-2.

Larkin, B. (1999). *US Government Efforts to Negotiate the Repeal, Termination or Withdrawal of Article 15(c) of the South African Medicines and Related Substances Act of 1965.* Washington, DC: US Department of State. Retrieved from http://www.cptech.org/ip/health/sa/stdept-feb51999.html.

Lee, K. (2009). Understandings of Global Health Governance. The Contested Landscape. In A. Kay and O. D. Williams (eds), *Global Health Governance. Crisis, Institutions and Political Economy* (pp. 27–41). Basingstoke: Palgrave Macmillan.

Leonard, D. K. and Straus, S. (2003). *Africa's Stalled Development: International Causes and Cures.* Boulder: Lynne Rienner.

Licht, A. N. (2008). Social Norms and the Law: Why Peoples Obey the Law. *Review of Law & Economics, 4*(3), 23–58.

Liese, B., Rosenberg, M. and Schratz, A. (2010). Neglected Tropical Diseases: Programmes, Partnerships, and Governance for Elimination and Control of Neglected Tropical Diseases. *The Lancet, 375*, 67–76.

Light, D. W. and Warburton, R. (2011). Demythologizing the High Costs of Pharmaceutical Research. *BioSocieties*, 6, 34–50. doi:10.1057/biosoc.2010.40; published online February 7, 2011, 1–17.

Limpananont, J., Eksaengsri, A., Kijtiwatchakul, K. and Metheny, N. (2009). Thailand: Access to AIDS Treatment and Intellectual Property Rights' Protection in Thailand. In R. Reis, V. Terto Jr. and M. C. Pimenta (eds), *Intellectual Property Rights and Access to ARV Medicines: Civil Society Resistance in the Global South* (pp. 137–163). Rio de Janeiro: Brazilian Interdisciplinary AIDS Association (ABIA).

Linklater, A. (1998). *The Transformation of Political Community: Ethical Foundations of the Post-Westphalian Era.* Cambridge: Polity Press.

Linton, K. C. (2008). China's R&D Policy for the 21st Century: Government Direction of Innovation. *SSRN eLibrary.* Retrieved from http://ssrn.com/paper=1126651.

List, C. and Koenig-Archibugi, M. (2010). Can there be a Global Demos? An Agency-Based Approach. *Philosophy & Public Affairs*, 38(1), 76–110.

Long, N. (1989). *Encounters at the Interface.* Wageningen: Wageningen Studies in Sociology.

Love, J. P. (2007). *Recent examples of the use of compulsory licenses on patents* (KEI Research Note 2). Washington, DC: Knowledge Ecology International. Retrieved from http://keionline.org/misc-docs/recent_cls_8mar07.pdf.

Love, J. (September 16, 2011). Will the UN Backtrack on Accessible Medicine? *Al Jazeera.* Retrieved from http://www.aljazeera.com/indepth/opinion/2011/09/201191492714279493.html.

Love, J. and Hubbard, T. (2009). Prizes for Innovation of New Medicines and Vaccines. *Annals of Health Law*, 18, 155–186.

Macan-Markar, M. (February 2, 2007). WHO Chief's Stand on Generic Drugs Slammed. *InterPress Service (IPS).* Retrieved from http://ipsnews.net/news.asp?idnews=36420.

Mackay, B. (2009). *Summary Report of Industry Government Forum on Access to Medicines (IGFAM)* (Meeting Report). London: DFID Health Resources Center.

MacLeod, D. A. (1992). US Trade Pressure and the Developing Intellectual Property Law of Thailand, Malaysia and Indonesia. *University of British Columbia Law Review*, 26(343), 346–348.

Mandelson, P. (July 10, 2007). *Letter to Krirk-Krai Jirapaet.* Retrieved from http://www.actupparis.org/IMG/pdf/Letter_from_Mandelson_to_Thailand.pdf.

Mankad, M. (April 13, 2010). Supreme Court of India to hear Bayer's plea for patent linkage.

Mara, K. (May 21, 2010). World Health Assembly Creates New Initiative for R&D Financing. *Intellectual Property Watch.*

Mara, K. and New, W. (May 18, 2010). Developing Countries Blast WHO Report on IP, Demand "Credible" Approach. *Intellectual Property Watch.*

March, J. G. and Olson, J. P. (1989). *Rediscovering Institutions: The Organisational Basis of Politics.* New York: The Free Press.

March, J. G. and Olsen, J. P. (1998). The Institutional Dynamics of International Political Orders. *International Organization, 52*(4), 943–969.

Marks, S. P. (2009). Access to Essential Medicines as a Component of the Right to Health. In Clapham, A., Robinson, M., Mahon, C. and Scott Jerbi (ed.), *Realizing the Right to Health* (Swiss Human Rights Book Vol. 3, ed., pp. 80–99). Zurich: rüffer&rub.

Marschik, A. (1998). Too Much Order? The Impact of Special Secondary Norms on the Unity and Efficacy of the International Legal System. *European Journal of International Law, 9*(1), http://www.ejil.org/pdfs/9/1/1478.pdf.

Martens, K. (2005). *NGO's and the United Nations: Institutionalization, Professionalization and Adaptation.* Basingstoke: Palgrave.

Martin, J. and Trenado, E. (August 22, 2007). *Letter to Peter Mandelson.* Retrieved from http://www.actupparis.org/IMG/pdf/Letter_from_Aides_Actup-Paris_to_Mandelson.pdf.

Martino, M. (April 9, 2010). Sanofi Opens R&D Center in China. *Fierce Biotech.* Retrieved from http://www.fiercebiotech.com/story/sanofi-opens-r-d-center-china/2010-04-09.

Mathers, C. D. and Loncar, D. (2006). Projections of Global Mortality and Burden of Disease from 2002 to 2030. *PLoS Med, 3*(11), e442. Retrieved from http://dx.doi.org/10.1371%2Fjournal.pmed.0030442.

Mau, S. (2010). *Social Transnationalism. Lifeworlds Beyond the Nation State* (English ed.) Routledge.

May, C. (2008). The World Intellectual Property Organisation and the Development Agenda. *Global Society, 22*(1), 97–113. Retrieved from http://www.informaworld.com/10.1080/13600820701740753.

Mayne, R. (2002). *US Bullying on Drug Patents: One Year After Doha* (Oxfam Briefing Paper No. 33). Washington, DC: Oxfam. http://www.oxfam.org.nz/imgs/pdf/drugs_bullying%20mtf.pdf.

Mayntz, R. (2005). Governance Theory Als Fortentwickelte Steuerungstheorie? In G. F. Schuppert (ed.), *Governance-Forschung. Vergewisserung Über Stand Und Entwicklungslinien.* (pp. 11–20). Baden-Baden: Nomos.

McDorman, T. L. (1992). US-Thailand Trade Disputes: Applying Section 301 to Cigarettes and Intellectual Property. *Michigan Journal of International Law, 14*, 90–119.

Médecins Sans Frontières (MSF) (March 23, 2005). *MSF Statement on the New Indian Patent Bill.* Retrieved from http://www.doctorswithoutborders.org/press/release.cfm?id=1494&cat=press-release.

Médecins Sans Frontières (MSF) (2005). *Untangling the Web of Antiretroviral Price Reductions* (8th ed.). Geneva: Médecins Sans Frontières (MSF). http://www.msfaccess.org/fileadmin/user_upload/diseases/hiv-aids/Untangling_the_Web/untanglingtheweb%208.pdf.

Médecins Sans Frontières (MSF) (June 22, 2011). India Says No to Policy that Would Block Access to Affordable Medicines. Press Release, http://www. msfaccess.org/media-room/press-releases/press-release-detail/?tx_ttnews[tt_ news]=1700&cHash=2f6721d292.

Médecins Sans Frontières (MSF) (2011). *Untangling the Web of Antiretroviral Price Reductions* (Online ed.). Retrieved from http://utw.msfaccess.org/.

Meier, B. M. and Labbok, M. (2010). From the Bottle to the Grave: Realizing a Human Right to Breastfeeding through Global Health Policy. *Case Western Reserve Law Review, 60*(4), 1073–1142. Retrieved from https://docs.google. com/viewer?a=v&pid=explorer&chrome=true&srcid=0Bxj5zdnvGv05NDB mZjM2YjQtODAxOC00OWFiLWJiNjQtNDYxODY4ZjIxNGU2&hl=en_ US&pli=1.

Menou, V., Hornstein, A. and Lipton-McCombie, E. (2008). *Access to Medicine Index: Ranking Access to Medicine Practices.* Innovest Healthcare Team. Retrieved from http://www.atmindex.org/index/2008.

Merletti, F., Galassi, C. and Spadea, T. (2011). The Socioeconomic Determinants of Cancer. *Environmental Health, 10*(Suppl 1), S7. doi: 10.1186/1476-069X-10-S1-S7. Retrieved from http://www.ehjournal.net/content/10/S1/S7.

Ministry of Public Health (Thailand) and National Health Security Office (Thailand). (2007). *Facts and Evidences on the 10 Burning Issues Related to the Government use of Patents on Three Patented Essential Drugs in Thailand: Document to Support Strengthening of Social Wisdom on the Issue of Drug Patent.* Bangkok: Retrieved from http://www.cptech.org/ip/health/c/thailand/ thai-cl-white-paper.pdf.

Modelski, G. (2008). Globalization as Evolutionary Process. In Modelski, G., Devezas, T. and Thompson W. R. (eds), *Globalization as Evolutionary Process. Modeling Global Change* (pp. 11–29). London: Routledge.

Moon, S. (2008). *Research Report on PDPs for Oxfam International.* Unpublished manuscript.

Moon, S. (2009). Medicines as Global Public Goods: The Governance of Technological Innovation in the New Era of Global Health. *Global Health Governance, 2*(2). Retrieved from http://www.ghgj.org/moon2.2medecines publicgood.htm.

Moon, S. (2010). Embedding Neoliberalism: Global Health and the Evolution of the Global Intellectual Property Regime (1994–2009). (PhD, Harvard University).

Moon, S., Szlezák, N. A., Michaud, C., et al. (2010). The Global Health System: Lessons for a Stronger Institutional Framework. *PLoS Medicine, 7*(1). Retrieved from http://www.plosmedicine.org/article/info%3Adoi%2F 10.1371%2Fjournal.pmed.1000193.

Moran, M. (2005). A Breakthrough in R&D for Neglected Diseases: New Ways to Get the Drugs we Need. *PLoS Medicine, 2*(9), e302. Retrieved from http:// dx.doi.org/10.1371%2Fjournal.pmed.0020302.

Moran, M., Guzman, J., Henderson, K., et al. (2009). *Neglected Disease Research and Development: New Times, New Trends*. Sydney, Australia: The George Institute for International Health.

Morin, J. (2008). Dancing with Brazil, South Africa, India and China. *Idées Pour Le Débat, 2008*(02). Retrieved from http://www.iddri.org/Publications/Collections/Idees-pour-le-debat/Id_0802_JF-Morin_Dancing-EN.pdf.

Morin, J. (2009). Multilateralising TRIPs-Plus Agreements: Is the US Strategy a Failure? *The Journal of World Intellectual Property, 12*(3), 175–197. doi: 10.1111/j.1747-1796.2009.00364.x. Retrieved from http://www.allacademic.com/meta/p313466_index.html.

Murray, C., Anderson, B., Burstein, R., et al. (2011). Development Assistance for Health: Trends and Prospects. *The Lancet, 378*, 8–11.

Nankivell, T. (2002). *Living, Labour and Environmental Standards and the WTO* (Staff Working Paper). Melbourne: Productivity Commission.

Nation, Thailand. (October 18, 2005). Ministry Seeks Right to make Tamiflu. *The Nation (Thailand)*.

New, W. (February 10, 2011). Pharma Backs Calls for Extension of TRIPS Deadline for Least-Developed Countries. *IP Watch*. Retrieved from http://www.ip-watch.org/weblog/2011/02/10/pharma-backs-calls-for-extension-of-trips-deadline-for-least-developed-countries/.

Novartis. (2007). *History of Glivec in India*. Retrieved from http://www.novartis.com/downloads/about-novartis/glivec-history-india.pdf.

Novartis. (2009). Novartis Announces USD 1 Billion Investment to Build Largest Pharmaceutical R&D Institute in China. *COMTEX*. Retrieved from http://www.fiercebiotech.com/press-releases/novartis-announces-usd-1-billion-investment-build-largest-pharmaceutical-r-d-institut.

Novartis. (2010). *Pharmaceutical Development*. Retrieved from http://www.novartis.com/research/pharmaceutical.shtml.

Nunn, A. (2009). *The Politics and History of AIDS Treatment in Brazil*. New York: Springer Science+Business Media.

O'Brien, R., Goetz, A., Scholte, J. A. and Williams, M. (2000). *Contesting Global Governance: Multilateral Economic Institutions and Global Social Movements*. Cambridge: Cambridge University Press.

Oakeshott, V. (2009). *The Treatment Timebomb: Report of the Inquiry of the all Party Parliamentary Group on AIDS into Long-Term Access to HIV Medicines in the Developing World*. All Party Parliamentary Group on AIDS. Retrieved from http://www.aidsportal.org/repos/APPGTimebomb091.pdf.

Oberthür, S. and Gehring, T. (eds) (2006). *Institutional Interaction in Global Environmental Governance. Synergy and Conflict among International and EU Policies*. Cambridge, MA: MIT Press.

Office of the High Commissioner for Human Rights (OHCHR). (2010). *EU-India Draft Free Trade Agreement: Generic Medications Under Threat, Says UN Health Expert*. Retrieved from http://www.ohchr.org/EN/NewsEvents/Pages/DisplayNews.aspx?NewsID=10592&LangID=E.

Office of the United Nations High Commissioner for Human Rights. *Special Rapporteur on the Right of Everyone to the Enjoyment of the Highest Attainable Standard of Physical and Mental Health.* Retrieved from http://www2.ohchr. org/english/issues/health/right/.

Office of the United Nations High Commissioner for Human Rights (2011, 16 June). News Release: New Guiding Principles on Business and Human Rights Endorsed by the UN Human Rights Council. http://www.business-humanrights.org/media/documents/ruggie/ruggie-guiding-principles-endorsed -16-jun-2011.pdf.

Office of the United States Global AIDS Coordinator (2008). *The Power of Partnerships: The U.S. President's Emergency Plan for AIDS Relief. 2008 Annual Report to Congress* (Fourth annual report). Retrieved from http://www. pepfar.gov/press/fourth_annual_report/.

Office of the United States Trade Representative (USTR) (2007). *2007 Special 301 Report.* Washington, DC: USTR. Retrieved from http://www.ustr.gov/ about-us/press-office/reports-and-publications/archives/2007/2007-special-301-report.

Office of the United States Trade Representative (USTR). (2010). *2010 Special 301 Report.* Washington, DC: USTR. Retrieved from http://www.ustr.gov/ about-us/press-office/reports-and-publications/2010-3.

Okediji, R. L. (2004). Back to Bilateralism? Pendulum Swings in International Intellectual Property Protection. *University of Ottawa Law & Technology Journal, 1*, 125–146. Retrieved from http://ssrn.com/abstract=764725.

Open Source Drug Discovery. (2012). Retrieved from http://www.osdd.net/.

Our Legal Correspondent (January 20, 2005). MNCs Told to Supply 'Patented' Anti-Cancer Drug. *The Hindu Businessline.* Retrieved from http://www. blonnet.com/2005/01/21/stories/2005012101590400.htm.

Outterson, K. and Smith, R. (2006). Counterfeit Drugs: The Good, the Bad and the Ugly. *Albany Law Journal of Science & Technology, 16*, 525.

Oxfam International. (2007). *All Costs, no Benefits: How TRIPS-Plus Intellectual Property Rules in the US-Jordan FTA Affect Access to Medicines* (Oxfam Briefing Paper No. 102). Oxford: Oxfam International.

Parliament (Kenya). The Anti-Counterfeit Bill, 2008, Paragraph 2 (2008).

Pécoul, B., Chirac, P., Trouiller, P. and Pinel, J. (1999). Access to Essential Drugs in Poor Countries: A Lost Battle? *Journal of the American Medical Association, 281*(4), 361–367. Retrieved from http://jama.ama-assn.org/cgi/ content/abstract/281/4/361.

Penrose, E. T. (1951). *The Economics of the International Patent System.* Westport, Connecticut: Greenwood Press, Publishers.

Perez-Casas, C., Mace, C., Berman, D. and Double, J. (2001). *Untangling the Web of Antiretroviral Price Reductions* (1st ed.). Geneva: Medecins Sans Frontieres/ Campaign for Access to Essential Medicines. http://www.msfaccess.org/ fileadmin/user_upload/diseases/hiv-aids/Untangling_the_Web/UTW%20 1%20Sep%202001.pdf.

Piot, P. (December 26, 2006). *Letter to Mongkol Na Songkhla.*

Pogge, T. (2009). The Health Impact Fund: Boosting Pharmaceutical Innovation without Obstructing Free Access. *Cambridge Quarterly of Healthcare Ethics, 18*(1), 78–86. doi: 10.1017/S0963180108090129.

Porter, M. (1990). *The Competitive Advantage of Nations.* New York: The Free Press.

Porter, M. and Kramer, M. (2006). The Link between Competitive Advantage and Corporate Social Responsibility. *Harvard Business Review, 84*(12), 78–92.

Press Information Bureau, Ministry of Commerce and Industry, Government of India (March 23, 2005). *Important Changes Incorporated in the Patents (Amendment) Bill, 2005 as Compared to the Patents (Amendment) Bill, 2003.* Retrieved from http://pib.nic.in/release/release.asp?relid=8096.

Price, R. M. (1998). Reversing the Gunsights: Transnational Civil Society Targets Landmines. *International Organization, 52*(3), 613–644.

Public Citizen. (2001). *Rx R&D Myths: The Case Against the Drug Industry's R&D "Scare Card".* Washington, DC: Public Citizen. Retrieved from http://www.citizen.org/documents/ACFDC.PDF.

Public Citizen. (2006). *Trans-Pacific FTA.* http://www.citizen.org/more-about-trans-pacific-fta.

Ravishankar, N., Gubbins, P., Cooley, R. J., et al. (2009). Financing of Global Health: Tracking Development Assistance for Health from 1990 to 2007. *The Lancet, 373*(9681), 2113–2124. doi: 10.1016/S0140-6736(09)60881-3.

Reis, R., Vieira, M. F. and Chaves, G. C. (2009). Brazil: Access to Medicines and Intellectual Property in Brazil: A Civil Society Experience. In R. Reis, V. Terto Jr. and M. C. Pimenta (eds), *Intellectual Property Rights and Access to ARV Medicines: Civil Society Resistance in the Global South* (pp. 12–54). Rio de Janeiro: Brazilian Interdisciplinary AIDS Association (ABIA).

Revenga, A., Over, M., Masaki, E., et al. (2006). *The Economics of Effective AIDS Treatment: Evaluating Policy Options for Thailand.* Washington, DC: The World Bank.

Reynolds, J. (July 24, 2007). China's Drive to Promote Invention. *BBC News.* Retrieved from http://news.bbc.co.uk/2/hi/asia-pacific/6912056.stm.

Ridley, D. B., Grabowski, H. G. and Moe, J. L. (2006). Developing Drugs for Developing Countries. *Health Affairs, 25*(2), 313–324. doi: 10.1377/hlthaff.25.2.313.

RiskMetrics Group – ESG Analytics. (2010a). *Access to Medicine Index: Methodology and Stakeholder Review.* Amsterdam: Access to Medicine Foundation. Retrieved from http://www.accesstomedicineindex.org/sites/www.accesstomedicineindex.org/files/general/100621_ATMMethodologyReport_with_correct_back_cover.pdf.

RiskMetrics Group – ESG Analytics. (2010b). *Access to Medicines Index 2010.* Haarlem, The Netherlands: Access to Medicine Foundation. Retrieved from http://www.accesstomedicineindexreport.com/.

Rittberger, V. and Zangl, B. (2006). *International Organization – Polity, Politics and Policies*. Basingstoke: Palgrave Macmillan.

Roche Group, T. (July 1, 2009). *Roche Launches Novel Program to Ease Tamiflu Access to Developing Countries*, Basel, Roche. Retrieved from http://www.roche.com/media/media_releases/med-cor-2009-07-01.htm.

Ronit, K. and Schneider, V. (1999). Global Governance through Private Organizations. *Governance: An International Journal of Policy and Administration, 12*(3), 243–266.

Ronit, K. and Schneider, V. (2000). *Private Organisations in Global Politics*. London: Routledge/ECPR Studies in European Political Science.

Rosenau, J. N. (1995). Governance in the Twenty-First Century. *Global Governance, 1*(1), 13–43.

Rosenau, J. N. (1997). *Along the Domestic-Foreign Frontier: Exploring Governance in a Turbulent World*. Cambridge: Cambridge University Press.

Rosendal, G. K. (2006). The Convention on Biological Diversity: Tensions with the WTO TRIPS Agreement over Access to Genetic Resources and the Sharing of Benefits. In S. Oberthür and T. Gehring (eds), *Institutional Interaction in Global Environmental Governance – Synergy and Conflict among International and EU Policies*. (pp. 79–103). Cambridge, MA: MIT Press.

Ruggie, J. G. (1982). International Regimes, Transactions, and Change: Embedded Liberalism in the Postwar Economic Order. *International Organization, 36*(2), 379–415.

Ruggie, J. G. (1992). Multilateralism: The Anatomy of an Institution. *International Organization, 46*(3), 561–598. Retrieved from http://www.jstor.org/stable/2706989.

Ruggie, J. G. (2004). Reconstituting the Global Public Domain – Issues, Actors, and Practices. *European Journal of International Relations, 10*(4), 499–531.

Ruggie, J. G. (2008). *Protect, Respect and Remedy: A Framework for Business and Human Rights*. (Report of the Special Representative of the Secretary-General on the issue of human rights and transnational corporations and other business enterprises, John Ruggie No. A/HRC/8/5). Geneva: United Nations Human Rights Council.

Rust, S. M. (1992). US-Thai Relations during the 1980s: The Issue of Intellectual Property Rights. *US Air Force Academy Journal of Legal Studies, 3*, 161.

Sakboon, M. (November 13, 1999). Bid to Help Poor Fight AIDS Virus – Drug Agency Seeks to Cut Costs. *The Nation (Thailand)*. Retrieved from http://lists.essential.org/pharm-policy/msg00306.html.

Sanofi-Aventis. (2008). *Sanofi-Aventis Expands its R&D Presence in China*. Beijing: Retrieved from http://www.fiercebiotech.com/press-releases/sanofi-aventis-expands-its-r-d-presence-china.

Schattschneider, E. E. (1960). *The Semisovereign People. A Realist's View of Democracy in America*. Chicago: Holt, Rinehart and Winston.

Schneider, V. and Ronit, K. (1999). Global Economic Governance by Private Actors: The International Chamber of Commerce. In J. Greenwood and H.

Jacek (ed.), *Organised Business and the New Global Order* (pp. 223–240). London: Palgrave Macmillan.

Scholte, J. A. (2011). *Building Global Democracy? Civil Society and Accountable Global Governance*. Cambridge: Cambridge University Press.

Schwab, S. (2007). *Letter to Thomas Allen*. Retrieved from http://www.cptech.org/ip/health/c/thailand/letter.pdf.

Sell, S. K. (1998). *The Power of Ideas. North-South Politics of Intellectual Property and Antitrust*. Albany: State University of New York Press.

Sell, S. K. (2003). *Private Power, Public Law: The Globalization of Intellectual Property Rights*. New York: Cambridge University Press.

Sell, S. K. (2008). *The Global IP Upward Ratchet, Anti-Counterfeiting and Piracy Enforcement Efforts: The State of Play* (IQ Sensato Occasional Paper #1). Geneva: IQ Sensato. Retrieved from http://www.iqsensato.org/wp-content/uploads/Sell_IP_Enforcement_State_of_Play-OPs_1_June_2008.pdf.

Sell, S. K. and Prakash, A. (2004). Using Ideas Strategically: The Contest between Business and NGO Networks in Intellectual Property Rights. *International Studies Quarterly, 48*(1), 143–175. doi: 10.1111/j.0020-8833.2004.00295.x.

Severino, J. and Ray, O. (2010). *The End of ODA (II). The Birth of Hypercollective Action* (Working Paper 218). Center for Global Development. Retrieved from http://kms1.isn.ethz.ch/serviceengine/Files/ISN/118485/ipublicationdocument_singledocument/c4d033da-776c-4cd6-896d-9b121f4bcdc1/en/wp218.pdf.

Sexton, S. (2001). *Trading Health Care Away? GATS, Public Services and Privatization* (The Corner House Briefing 23). Dorset: The Corner House. Retrieved from www.thecornerhouse.org.uk/ pdf/briefing/23gats.pdf.

Shaffer, E. R. and Brenner, J. E. (2009). A Trade Agreement's Impact on Access to Generic Drugs. *Health Affairs, 28*(5), 957–968. doi: 10.1377/hlthaff.28.5.w957. Retrieved from http://www.cpath.org/sitebuildercontent/sitebuilderfiles/cpathhaonline8-25-09.pdf.

Shearing, C. and Wood, J. (2003). Nodal Governance, Democracy, and the New 'Denizens'. *Journal of Law and Society, 30*(3), 400–419.

Sikkink, K. (1986). Codes of Conduct for Transnational Corporations: The Case of the WHO/UNICEF Code. *International Organization, 40*(4), 815–840.

Sklair, L. (2001). *The Transnational Capitalist Class*. Oxford: Blackwell.

Smith, A. (1937 [1776]). *The Wealth of Nations*. New York: The Modern Library.

Smith, R., Beaglehole, R., Woodward, D. and Drager, N. (eds) (2003). *Global Public Goods for Health. Health Economic and Public Health Perspectives*. Oxford: Oxford.

Smith, R. A. and Siplon, P. D. (2006). *Drugs into Bodies: Global AIDS Treatment Activism*. Westport, CT: Praeger.

Songkhla, M. N. (2007). *Letter to Peter Mandelson*. Retrieved from http://www.actupparis.org/IMG/pdf/Answer_Thai.pdf.

Stahl, T., Wismar, M., Ollila, E., et al. (2006). *Health in all Policies. Prospects and Potentials*. Helsinki: Ministry of Social Affairs, Finland. Retrieved from http://ec.europa.eu/health/ph_information/documents/health_in_all_policies.pdf.

Steiner, H. J. and Alston, P. (2000). *International Human Rights in Context: Law, Politics, Morals* (2nd ed.). Oxford: Oxford University Press.

Stokke, O. S. (2001). *The Interplay of International Regimes. Putting Effectiveness Theory to Work.* (FNI Report 14/2001). Lysaker: Fridtjof Nansen Institute.

Strandberg, C. (2008). *The Role of the Board of Directors in Corporate Social Responsibility.* The Conference Board of Canada. Retrieved from http://www.corostrandberg.com/pdfs/08-169The_Role_of_the_Board_of_Directors_in_%20CSR_Report_WEB28.pdf.

Strom, S. and Fleischer-Black, M. (June 5, 2003). Company's Vow to Donate Cancer Drug Falls Short. *The New York Times.* Retrieved from http://www.nytimes.com/2003/06/05/business/05DRUG.html?scp=1&sq=novartis%20strom%20fleischer%20bac&st=cse.

Stuckler, D., Hawkes, C. and Yach, D. (2009). Governance of Chronic Diseases. In K. Buse, W. Hein and N. Drager (eds), *Making Sense of Global Health Governance: A Policy Perspective* (pp. 268–293). Basingstoke: Palgrave Macmillan.

Sturchio, J. L. (February 29, 2008). Response from Merck & Co., Inc. (to Human Rights Guidelines for Pharmaceutical Companies in Relation to Access to Medicines).

Sukkar, E. (April 28, 2010). Kenya's Anticounterfeit Law Halted by Court Over Generic Question. *Scrip World News.*

Sulzbach, S., De, S. and Wang, W. (2011). The Private Sector Role in HIV/AIDS in the Context of an Expanded Global Response: Expenditure Trends in Five Sub-Saharan African Countries. *Health Policy and Planning, 26,* 172–184.

Swenson, J. (2000). *On Jean-Jacques Rousseau.* Palo Alto: Stanford University Press.

Sykes, R. (2002). Commentary: The Reality of Treating HIV and AIDS in Poor Countries. *British Medical Journal, 324*(7331), 214–218. doi: 10.1136/bmj.324.7331.214.

't Hoen, E. (2007). *Intellectual Property, Bilateral Agreements, and Sustainable Development: A Strategy Note* (Intellectual Property, Bilateral Agreements, and Sustainable Development Series: 2). Center for International Economic Law (CIEL). Retrieved from http://www.ciel.org/Publications/IP_StrategyNote_Apr07.pdf.

't Hoen, E. (2009). *The Global Politics of Pharmaceutical Monopoly Power: Drug Patents, Access, Innovation, and the Application of the WTO Doha Declaration on TRIPS and Public Health.* Diemen, The Netherlands: AMB Press.

't Hoen, E., Berger, J., Calmy, A. and Moon, S. (2011). Driving a Decade of Change: HIV/AIDS, Patents, and Access to Medicines. *Journal of the International AIDS Society, 14*(15). Retrieved from http://www.jiasociety.org/content/14/1/15.

Tantivess, S., Kessomboon, N. and Laongbua, C. (2008). *Introducing Government use of Patents on Essential Medicines in Thailand, 2006–2007: Policy Analysis with Key Lessons Learned and Recommendations.* Nonthaburi, Thailand: International Health Policy Program, Ministry of Health.

Tarrow, S. (2005). *The New Transnational Activism.* New York: Cambridge University Press.

Taylor, L. (August 9, 2010). US Senators Seek Incentives for Pharma R&D into Rare Childhood Diseases. *Pharma Times.* Retrieved from http://www.pharmatimes.com/WorldNews/article.aspx?id=18331&src=EWorldNews.

Thakur, R., Cooper, A. and English, J. (eds) (2005). *International Commissions and the Power of Ideas.* New York: United Nations University Press.

Thauer, C. R. (2011). Goodness comes from within. Intra-firm bargaining, asset specificity, and collective good provision. *Presentation at the IPSA-ECPR Joint Conference,* Sao Paulo, February 16–19, 2011.

The Global Fund to Fight AIDS, Tuberculosis and Malaria (2011). *The Global Fund Adopts New Strategy to Save 10 Million Lives by 2016: Reductions in Resource Outlook Limit Funding of New Grants.* Retrieved from http://www.theglobalfund.org/en/mediacenter/pressreleases/2011-11-23_The_Global_Fund_adopts_new_strategy_to_save_10_million_lives_by_2016/.

The Lancet (2010). Drug Development for Neglected Diseases: Pharma's Influence. *The Lancet, 375*(9708), 2. doi: 10.1016/S0140-6736(09)62123-1.

The Office of the President-Elect (2009). *The Obama-Biden Plan to Combat HIV/ AIDS.* Retrieved from http://change.gov/pages/the_obama_biden_plan_to_combat_global_hiv_aids.

The World Trade Organization (WTO). *Whose WTO is it Anyway?* Retrieved from http://www.wto.org/english/thewto_e/whatis_e/tif_e/org1_e.htm.

Thomas, C. (2004). Trade Policy and the Politics of Access to Drugs. In N. K. Poku and A. Whiteside (eds), *Global Health and Governance: HIV/AIDS* (pp. 61–74). Basingstoke: Basingstoke: Palgrave.

Tonelson, A. (2000). *The Race to the Bottom: Why a Worldwide Worker Surplus and Uncontrolled Free Trade are Sinking American Living Standards.* Boulder, CO: Westview Press.

Travis, J. (2008a). Research Funding. Prizes Eyed to Spur Medical Innovation. *Science (New York, NY), 319*(5864), 713. doi: 10.1126/science.319.5864.713.

Travis, J. (2008b). Science and Commerce. Science by the Masses. *Science (New York, NY), 319*(5871), 1750–1752. doi: 10.1126/science.319.5871.1750.

Treerutkuarkul, A. (February 2, 2007). WHO Raps Compulsory Licensing Plan: Govt Urged to Seek Talks with Drug Firms. *The Bangkok Post.* Retrieved from http://lists.essential.org/pipermail/ip-health/2007-February/010493.html.

Treerutkuarkul, A. (February 9, 2007a). Drug Firm Will Cut Cost of Kaletra. *Bangkok Post.*

Treerutkuarkul, A. (March 27, 2007b). Drug-Makers Reject Offer of Royalty Fees. *Bangkok Post.*

Treerutkuarkul, A. (March 16, 2007c). Justice Slams Abbott's Drug Decision. *Bangkok Post.*

Treerutkuarkul, A. (March 15, 2007d). US Drug Giant Hits Back, Says no New Drugs. *Bangkok Post.*

Treerutkuarkul, A. (August 3, 2010). HIV/AIDS Drug Licence Extended. *The Bangkok Post.* Retrieved from http://www.bangkokpost.com/news/health/189154/hiv-aids-drugs-licence-extended.

UN Commission on Human Rights. Access to Medication in the Context of Pandemics such as HIV/AIDS, Resolution 2001/33, 71st Meeting (2001). Retrieved from http://www.unhchr.ch/huridocda/huridoca.nsf/%28Symbol%29/E.CN.4.RES.2001.33.En?Opendocument.

UN Committee on ESC Rights (1999). Statement of the UN Committee on Economic, Social and Cultural Rights to the Third Ministerial Conference of the World Trade Organization (Seattle, November 30 to December 3, 1999), E/C.12/1999/9, November 26, 1999 (47th meeting, 21st session). Retrieved from http://www.unhchr.ch/tbs/doc.nsf/%28Symbol%29/68300503f197ef528025683b004fbbae?Opendocument.

UNAIDS (June 7, 2011). Future of AIDS Response Focus of UN General Assembly High Level Meeting, http://www.unaids.org/en/media/unaids/contentassets/documents/pressrelease/2011/06/20110607_PR_HLM_opener_en.pdf.

UNCTAD-ICTSD (ed.) (2005). *Resource Book on TRIPS and Development: An Authoritative and Practical Guide to the TRIPS Agreement.* Cambridge: Cambridge University Press.

Union of International Associations (ed.) (2004). *Yearbook of International Organizations.* Munich: Saur Verlag.

UNITAID Secretariat (2009). *UNITAID Patent Pool Initiative: Implementation Plan* (UNITAID/EB11/2009). Geneva: UNITAID.

United Kingdom Commission on Intellectual Property Rights (CIPR) (2002). *Integrating Intellectual Property Rights and Development Policy.* London: United Kingdom Department for International Development. Retrieved from http://www.iprcommission.org/graphic/documents/final_report.htm.

United Nations Conference on Trade and Development (UNCTAD) (2005). *World Investment Report 2005: Transnational Corporations and the Internationalization of R&D.* Geneva: United Nations.

United Nations Development Programme (UNDP) (1999). *Human Development Report 1999.* Oxford and New York: Oxford University Press.

United Nations Development Programme (UNDP) (2000). *Human Development Report 2000: Human Rights and Human Development.* Oxford and New York: Oxford University Press. Retrieved from http://hdr.undp.org/en/reports/global/hdr2000/.

United Nations Development Programme (UNDP) (2001). *Human Development Report 2001: Making New Technologies Work for Human Development.* Oxford and New York: Oxford University Press.

United Nations Environmental Program (UNEP) and International Institute for Sustainable Development (IISD) (2005). *Environment and Trade. A Handbook* (2nd ed.). Geneva and Winnipeg: UNEP and IISD.

United Nations General Assembly. 2005 World Summit Outcome, A/60/L.1 (2005). Retrieved from http://www.who.int/hiv/universalaccess2010/worldsummit.pdf.

United Nations General Assembly. 60/262 Political Declaration on HIV/AIDS, A/RES/60/262, 60th Session, 87th plenary meeting (2006). Retrieved from http://data.unaids.org/pub/Report/2006/20060615_HLM_PoliticalDeclaration_ARES60262_en.pdf.

United Nations General Assembly. Political Declaration on HIV/AIDS: Intensifying our Efforts to Eliminate HIV/AIDS. A/65/L.77, 65th (2011). Retrieved from http://www.un.org/ga/search/view_doc.asp?symbol=A/65/L.77.

United Nations Sub-Commission on Human Rights. Intellectual Property Rights and Human Rights, Resolution 2000/7, 25th Meeting. (2000). Retrieved from http://www.unhchr.ch/Huridocda/Huridoca.nsf/TestFrame/c462b62cf8a07b13c12569700046704e?Opendocument.

United States Office of the Trade Representative (USTR) (2011). *Anti-Counterfeiting Trade Agreement.* Retrieved from http://www.ustr.gov/acta.

US Global AIDS Coordinator (2008). *Report to Congress by the US Global AIDS Coordinator on the use of Generic Drugs in the President's Emergency Plan for AIDS Relief.* Washington, DC.

US Food and Drug Administration (2011). *Antiretroviral drugs used in the treatment of HIV infection.* Retrieved from http://www.fda.gov/ForConsumers/ByAudience/ForPatientAdvocates/HIVandAIDSActivities/ucm118915.htm.

Velasquez, G., Aldis, B., Timmermans, K., et al. (2008). *Improving Access to Medicines in Thailand: The use of TRIPS Flexibilities. Report of a WHO Mission (Bangkok, 31 January to 6 February 2008).* Bangkok, Thailand: National Health Security Office.

Vivas-Eugui, D. (2003). *Regional and Bilateral Agreements and a TRIPS-Plus World: The Free Trade Area of the Americas (FTAA).* Geneva: QUNO, QIAP. ICTSD. Retrieved from http://homepages.3-c.coop/tansey/pdfs/ftaa-a4.pdf.

Vogel, D. and Kagan, R. (eds) (2004).*The Dynamics of Regulatory Change: How Globalization Affects National Regulatory Policies.* Berkeley: University of California Press.

Waisbord, S. (2011). Can NGOs Change the News? *International Journal of Communication, 5,* 142–165.

Walt, G., Spicer, N. and Buse, K. (2009). Mapping the Global Health Architecture. In K. Buse, W. Hein and N. Drager (eds), *Making Sense of Global Health Governance: A Policy Perspective* (pp. 72–98). Basingstoke: Palgrave Macmillan.

Waning, B., Diedrichsen, E. and Moon, S. (2010). A Lifeline to Treatment: The Role of Indian Generic Manufacturers in Supplying Antiretroviral Medicines to Developing Countries. *Journal of the International AIDS Society, 13,* 35. doi: 10.1186/1758-2652-13-35. Retrieved from http://www.jiasociety.org/content/13/1/35.

Watal, J. (2001). *Intellectual Property Rights in the WTO and Developing Countries.* The Hague: Kluwer Law International.

Weber, M. (1947). *The Theory of Social and Economic Organization* (A. Henderson, T. Parsons Trans.). New York: Free Press.

Weber, M. (1978). *Economy and Society: An Outline of Interpretive Sociology.* New York: University of California Press.

Wei, M. (2007). Should Prizes Replace Patents? A Critique of the Medical Innovation Prize Act of 2005. *Boston University Journal of Science and Technology Law (Working Paper).* Retrieved from http://www.cptech.org/ip/health/prizefund/files/wei-prizepaper.pdf.

Wellens, K. C. (1995). Diversity in Secondary Rules and the Unity of International Law: Some Reflections on Current Trends. In L. A. Barnhoom and K. C. Wellens (eds), *Diversity in Secondary Rules and the Unity of International Law* (pp. 3–37). The Hague: Nijhoff.

WHO Consultative Expert Working Group on Research and Development (CEWG) (2011). *Report of the Second Meeting of the Consultative Expert Working Group on Research and Development: Financing and Coordination.* Geneva: Retrieved from http://www.who.int/phi/news/cewg_rd_2nd_meeting_report.pdf.

WHO Consultative Expert Working Group on Research and Development (CEWG): Financing and Coordination (2012). *Research and Development to Meet Health Needs in Developing Countries: Strengthening Global Financing and Coordination* (Report of the Consultative Expert Working Group on Research and Development: Financing and Coordination. Geneva: World Health Organization. Retrieved from http://www.who.int/phi/CEWG_Report_5_April_2012.pdf.

Wiener, A. (2008). *The Invisible Constitution of Politics. Contested Norms and International Encounters.* Cambridge: Cambridge University Press.

Wilson, D. (March 6, 2011). Drug Firms Face Billions in Losses in '11 as Patents End. *The New York Times,* http://www.nytimes.com/2011/03/07/business/07drug.html?scp=1&sq=china%20price%20controls%20pharmaceutical&st=cse.

Wilson, D., Cawthorne, P., Ford, N. and Aongsonwang, S. (1999). Global Trade and Access to Medicines: AIDS Treatments in Thailand. *The Lancet, 354*(9193), 1893–1895. doi: 10.1016/S0140-6736(99)06114-0.

Wilson, P. (2010). *Giving Developing Countries the Best Shot: An Overview of Vaccine Access and R&D.* Geneva: Oxfam International and MSF Campaign for Access to Essential Medicines.

Wimmer, A. and Glick Schiller, N. (2002). Methodological Nationalism and Beyond: Nation-State Building, Migration and the Social Sciences. *Global Networks, 2*(4), 301–334. Retrieved from http://www.sscnet.ucla.edu/soc/faculty/wimmer/B52.pdf.

Windfuhr, M. (ed.) (2005). *Beyond the Nation State – Human Rights in Times of Globalization* (Uppsala: Global Publications Foundation).

Wisartsakul, W. (2004). *Civil Society Movement to Revoke the Thai Patent on ddI* (N. Grant Trans.). Bangkok: Medecins Sans Frontieres-Belgium.

Wiseman, G. (1999). *Polylateralism and New Modes of Global Dialogue* (Discussion Paper No. 59). Leicester: Leicester Studies Program.

Wogart, J. P., Calcagnotto, G., Hein, W. and Soest, C. V. (2009). AIDS and Access to Medicines: Brazil, South Africa and Global Health Governance. In K. Buse, W. Hein and N. Drager (eds), *Making Sense of Global Health Governance: A Policy Perspective* (pp. 137–163). Basingstoke: Palgrave Macmillan.

World Health Assembly. Global Strategy and Plan of Action on Public Health, Innovation and Intellectual Property. Resolution 61.21, Sixty-first Assembly. (2008). Retrieved from http://www.who.int/gb/ebwha/pdf_files/A61/A61_R21-en.pdf.

World Health Organization (WHO) (2004). *World Medicines Situation* (WHO/EDM/PAR/2004.5). Geneva: WHO.

World Health Organization (WHO) (2006). *Antiretroviral Therapy for HIV Infection in Adults and Adolescents: Recommendations for a Public Health Approach. 2006 Revision.* Geneva: WHO.

World Health Organization (WHO) (2009). *Rapid Advice: Antiretroviral Therapy for HIV Infection in Adults and Adolescents*. Geneva: World Health Organization.

World Health Organization (WHO) (2011). *Essential Medicines.* Retrieved from http://www.who.int/topics/essential_medicines/en/.

World Health Organization (WHO), UNICEF, UNAIDS (2010). *Towards Universal Access: Scaling Up Priority HIV/AIDS Interventions in the Health Sector: Progress Report 2010.* Geneva: WHO. Retrieved from http://www.who.int/hiv/pub/2010progressreport/en/index.html.

World Health Organization (WHO), UNICEF, UNAIDS (2011). Global HIV/AIDS Response: Epidemic Update and Health Sector Progress Towards Universal Access. Progress Report 2011. Retrieved from http://www.who.int/hiv/pub/progress_report2011/en/index.html

World Health Organization (WHO) and World Trade Organization (WTO) (2002). *WTO Agreements and Public Health. A Joint Study by the WHO and the WTO Secretariat.* Geneva: World Health Organization and World Trade Organization. Retrieved from http://www.who.int/trade/resource/wtoagreements/en/index.html.

World in Brief. (2006, December 1). *The Washington Post.*

World Intellectual Property Organization (WIPO) (2009). *Treaties Statistics: Paris Convention of March 20, 1883.* Retrieved from http://www.wipo.int/treaties/en/statistics/StatsResults.jsp?treaty_id=2.

World Intellectual Property Organization (WIPO) (2010). *A Medium Term Strategic Plan for WIPO, 2010–2015: First Draft Presented to Member States by the Director General on May 27, 2010.* Geneva: WIPO. Retrieved from http://www.wipo.int/export/sites/www/about-wipo/en/pdf/mtsp.pdf.

World Intellectual Property Organization (WIPO) (2012). Statistics on the PCT System; PCT Filings by Country of Origin. Retrieved from http://www.wipo.int/ipstats/en/statistics/pct/.

World Trade Organization (WTO) (2010a). *Dispute Settlement: Dispute DS408: European Union and a Member State – Seizure of Generic Drugs in Transit.* Retrieved from http://www.wto.org/english/tratop_e/dispu_e/cases_e/ds408_e.htm.

World Trade Organization (WTO) (2010b). *Dispute Settlement: Dispute DS409: European Union and a Member State – Seizure of Generic Drugs in Transit.* Retrieved from http://www.wto.org/english/tratop_e/dispu_e/cases_e/ds409_e.htm.

World Trade Organization (WTO) (2010c). *Dispute Settlement: DS224: United States – US Patents Code.* Retrieved from http://www.wto.org/english/tratop_e/dispu_e/cases_e/ds224_e.htm.

World Trade Organization (WTO) (2010d). Members Ask: Is the "Par.6" System on Intellectual Property and Health Working? *2010 News Items.*

World Trade Organization (WTO) (2011). *TRIPS: 'Non-Violation' Complaints (Article 64.2).* Retrieved from http://www.wto.org/english/tratop_e/trips_e/nonviolation_background_e.htm.

Wright, T. (December 12, 2005). Roche Picks Chinese Partner for Tamiflu. *The New York Times.*

Young, O. R. (1996). Institutional Linkages in International Society. *Global Governance, 2,* 1–23.

Ziemba, E. (2005). *Public-Private Partnerships for Product Development: Financial, Scientific, and Managerial Issues as Challenges to Future Success* (Research report for the WHO Commission on Intellectual Property Rights, Innovation, and Public Health).

Index

Abbott Laboratories 31
Accelerating Access Initiative for ARVs
31, 75, 101, 120
access (to medicines) movement/campaign
xi, 2, 5, 10, 28, 73, 78, 101, 140–
41, 160, 163, 164, 168, 176, 195
Access to Medicines Index 112, 169
Accountability 14, 22, 174–8
Activists xi, xiv, 29, 68–9, 96, 118, 170, 190
ACT-UP (AIDS Coalition to Unleash
Power) 73, 92, 166
Advanced Market Commitment 152–3
Advocacy 17, 25–6, 38, 50, 65, 99, 111,
177, 190
Africa (*see also* South Africa) 30, 75, 83,
98, 107, 116, 141, 156
East Africa 140
Sub-Saharan Africa 74, 88, 107, 110, 196
AIDES 92
AIDS Access Foundation 87, 94
AIDS (acquired immune deficiency
syndrome) 5–6, 12, 17, 29–32, 45,
50, 67–71, 74–5, 77, 79, 82, 86, 92,
94–6, 98, 100–101, 103–5, 107–9,
114–18, 120, 122, 132, 142–3,
154, 161, 165–6, 168, 170, 188–9,
193–7
AIDS drugs/medicines (*see also* ARVs)
xi, 31, 52, 67, 71–2, 74, 76, 83,
88–9, 92, 95, 101, 103, 108, 121,
132, 181
HIV/AIDS crisis/pandemics xi, 67, 72,
74, 166
HIV/AIDS treatment 67–71, 83, 85,
95–6, 115, 189
International AIDS Conference 36, 69,
135
Amsterdam Declaration 52, 73
Annan, Kofi 29, 120
Anthrax 76, 104

Anti-Counterfeiting Trade Agreement
(ACTA) 13, 48, 139–41
antiretroviral (ARV) xi, xiii, 5, 6, 8, 11, 13,
31, 49–50, 67–71, 73, 75–6, 82–9,
96–9, 101, 103–4, 109, 113–16,
118, 120, 127, 131–2, 161, 169,
182, 195–7
Argentina 101, 126–8, 134–5, 146–7
AstraZeneca 155
atovaquone/proguanil (Malarone) 30
Australia 81, 133, 139
azidothymidine (Zidovudine) 67, 85–6,
104–5

Bangladesh 127, 156
Barbados 149, 156
Battle of Seattle 73
Bayer 76, 104–5, 119
Bhagwati, Jagdish 63
Bhat, Rawindra 119
bilateral investment treaty (BIT) 13, 139, 183
Bill & Melinda Gates Foundation 100, 152,
156
blaming and shaming 43, 49, 176
Boehringer-Ingelheim 85–6, 104, 109–10
Bolivia 126, 135, 149–50, 156
boomerang effect 171
Brazil xi, 9, 32, 52, 63, 68–73, 75–7, 81,
94, 96–8, 100–101, 103, 105,
110–11, 116, 128, 134–5, 137–9,
147–8, 154, 160–61, 183, 195, 197
Brazilian HIV/AIDS Programme
(BHAP) 68–71, 76, 78, 98
Civil Society (in Brazil) 68, 70
Industrial Property Law 70–71
Trade disputes 71, 101, 127
BRICS 123, 140
Bristol Myers Squibb 31, 85–7, 104
Brundtland Commission 145
Brundtland, Gro Harlem 82

burden of disease 3, 6, 112, 121–2, 126, 128

Cambodia 133, 136, 183
Canada 59, 76, 81, 104–5, 116, 133, 139–40, 195, 197
Cardoso, Fernando Henrique 70
Chagas disease 156
Chan, Margaret 93–4
Chequer, Pedro 70, 101
China 76, 81, 87, 110, 121, 123, 127–8, 136–7, 139–40, 149, 154–5, 157
chronic myeloid leukemia (CML) 117
Cipla 75, 85, 118–19, 196
Ciprofloxacin 76, 104
civil society (CSO) xi, xiii, 5, 10–11, 15–18, 21, 25, 28–30, 32, 37, 41, 49–52, 65, 72–3, 83, 85–7, 91, 93, 95–6, 98, 101, 111, 115–16, 118, 123, 127–8, 135–6, 143, 145–6, 162, 166–7, 169–71, 176–7, 186–7, 190
  advocacy organization (*see also* advocacy) 25
  civil society network 1, 15, 25, 28
  faith-based organization 25, 99
  global civil society 10, 49, 163, 166–7, 170, 175, 179
  philanthropic 6, 25, 41, 43, 168
  social movement 25, 167
Clinton, Bill 74, 92, 196
Clinton Foundation 88, 92, 100
Clopidogrel 89, 105, 107
communicable disease (*see also* infectious disease) 6, 112
compulsory license (CL) 13, 61, 70–71, 73, 76, 78–80, 82–96, 103–5, 108–10, 114–15, 120–21, 123, 127, 139, 141, 181, 195–7
Consumer Project on Technology (CPTech) (*see also* Knowledge Ecology International (KEI)) 72, 196
corporate social responsibility (CSR) 26–28, 110, 169, 185
Correa, Carlos 46, 75, 78, 119, 129
Correa, Rafael 105, 119–20, 132
cosmopolitanism 17
Costa Rica 101, 133, 137

decentration 20–21

democracy 14, 20, 68, 159, 172, 174–5, 177
Democratic Republic of the Congo (DRC) 3
development aid/assistance 1–2, 32–3, 35, 98, 112, 147
didanosine (ddI) 86–7, 104
docetaxel 95, 197
Doha Declaration on TRIPS and Public Health 5–8, 11, 13, 44, 62, 64–5, 71, 75, 77–9, 81, 84–5, 89, 91–2, 96, 101, 103–4, 108, 114–15, 122–3, 129, 134–7, 160–61, 166, 169, 171, 173, 181, 183, 185, 193–4, 196
  (*see also* WTO)
  August 30th decision 80–2, 115–16, 196–7
  Paragraph 6 system (*see also* August 30th decision) 80–81, 101, 105, 169, 181, 183, 194
donation programs 30, 95, 100, 114, 169
Drug Regulatory Authority (DRA) 119
drugs *see* medicines
Drugs for Neglected Diseases initiative (DNDi) 30, 152, 196

Ecuador 13, 105, 109, 115, 119–20, 126, 135, 138–9, 181
Efavirenz 84, 88, 89–93, 95–6, 105, 197
Egypt 126, 128, 137
embedded liberalism 23
emerging market 123, 128–9, 137, 157
epidemiological transition 128
epistemic community 17
Eritrea 3, 104
Erlotinib 95, 197
Ethiopia 3
European Union (EU) 47, 54, 108, 111, 129, 139–40
  Directorate General (DG) Trade 108, 111, 135–6, 140
  European Commission 73, 91–2, 108, 134–5, 139–40
  European Parliament 91–2, 135
European Union-India FTA 111–12, 129, 132, 136
Exclusive Marketing Rights (EMR) 117–18
expert group/expert commission 13, 32, 38, 44, 51, 144–5, 147, 150, 185

Informal Norms in Global Governance

United Nations (UN) 3, 29, 72, 99, 176